Ageing, Corporeality and Embodiment

Key Issues in Modern Sociology

Anthem's **Key Issues in Modern Sociology** series publishes scholarly texts by leading social theorists that give an accessible exposition of the major structural changes in modern societies. These volumes address an academic audience through their relevance and scholarly quality, and they connect sociological thought to public issues. The series covers both substantive and theoretical topics, as well as addressing the works of major modern sociologists. The series emphasis is on modern developments in sociology with relevance to contemporary issues such as globalisation, warfare, citizenship, human rights, environmental crises, demographic change, religion, post-secularism and civil conflict.

Series Editor

Bryan S. Turner – City University of New York, USA
& University of Western Sydney, Australia

Editorial Board

Thomas Cushman – Wellesley College, USA
Rob Stones – University of Western Sydney, Australia
Richard Swedberg – Cornell University, USA
Stephen Turner – University of South Florida, USA
Darin Weinberg – University of Cambridge, UK

Ageing, Corporeality and Embodiment

CHRIS GILLEARD AND PAUL HIGGS

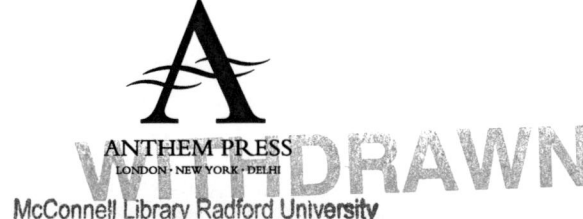

Anthem Press
An imprint of Wimbledon Publishing Company
www.anthempress.com

This edition first published in UK and USA 2013
by ANTHEM PRESS
75–76 Blackfriars Road, London SE1 8HA, UK
or PO Box 9779, London SW19 7ZG, UK
and
244 Madison Ave. #116, New York, NY 10016, USA

Copyright © Chris Gilleard and Paul Higgs 2013

The moral right of the authors has been asserted.

All rights reserved. Without limiting the rights under copyright reserved above,
no part of this publication may be reproduced, stored or introduced into
a retrieval system, or transmitted, in any form or by any means
(electronic, mechanical, photocopying, recording or otherwise),
without the prior written permission of both the copyright
owner and the above publisher of this book.

British Library Cataloguing-in-Publication Data
A catalogue record for this book is available from the British Library.

Library of Congress Cataloging-in-Publication Data
Gilleard, C. J.
Ageing, corporeality and embodiment / Chris Gilleard and Paul Higgs.
  pages cm. – (Key issues in modern sociology)
Includes bibliographical references and index.
ISBN-13: 978-0-85728-329-0 (hardcover : alk. paper)
ISBN-10: 0-85728-329-4 (hardcover : alk. paper)
1. Aging–Psychological aspects. 2. Identity (Philosophical
concept) 3. Aging–Nutritional aspects. 4. Physical fitness for
older people. I. Higgs, Paul. II. Title.
BF724.55.A35G55 2013
155.67–dc23
            2013013870

ISBN-13: 978 0 85728 329 0 (Hbk)
ISBN-10: 0 85728 329 4 (Hbk)

Cover image © Breanna Tallino

This title is also available as an eBook.

CONTENTS

Introduction		vii
Chapter 1	Identity, Embodiment and the Somatic Turn in the Social Sciences	1
Chapter 2	Corporeality, Embodiment and the 'New Ageing'	21
Chapter 3	Gender, Ageing and Embodiment	33
Chapter 4	Age and the Racialised Body	51
Chapter 5	Disability, Ageing and Identity	69
Chapter 6	Sexuality, Ageing and Identity	87
Chapter 7	Sex and Ageing	101
Chapter 8	Cosmetics, Clothing and Fashionable Ageing	115
Chapter 9	Fitness, Exercise and the Ageing Body	131
Chapter 10	Ageing and Aspirational Medicine	145
Conclusions	Ageing, Forever Embodied	159
References		167
Index		199

INTRODUCTION

'In man the changes are familiar: the skin is pale, often yellowish, wrinkled, and inelastic. On the backs of the hands purpura is common and there is patchy pigmentation of brownish hue. The hair is white and often sparse; the back is bowed, the limbs are sometimes tremulous, and the teeth are lost. Movement is slow and often clumsy. There is a tendency to fall, and [...] the fears of accident may be so great that they dominate the life of the old person. Muscular effort entails distress, especially with breathing. Sleep is short and easily disturbed, though drowsiness is frequent. Vision fails and deafness is common. Sexual desire wanes [...]'

—A. P. Thomson, 'Problems of Ageing and Chronic Sickness', *British Medical Journal* 2 (1949): 302

Ageing is not what it once was. That was the premise of our first book, *Cultures of Ageing* (2000) and it continues to guide the present one. From Thomson's time when the above was published to the first decade of the twenty-first century, profound changes have taken place in our understanding and interpretation of ageing and old age. During this period, old age as a distinct social category has collapsed while ageing itself has lost much of its former coherence. Age as 'old age' has been replaced by the feared social imaginary of a 'fourth age' (Gilleard and Higgs 2010) while the ageing 'process' has become caught up in the puzzling, cultural complexity that is the 'third age' (Gilleard and Higgs 2011a). Out of this mix of fear, hope and confusion, some have discerned a new kind of ageing appearing characterised by 'the expansion of more promising possibilities of self-construction' in later life (Gergen and Gergen 2000, 282). Most discussion of this new ageing has concentrated upon issues of the self, citizenship and the changing *social* context of later life. Less attention has been paid to how it is imbricated in the changing relationship between the body and society. This will be the focus of this book.

By 1950, the 'provisional endpoint of modernization' (Kohli 2007, 257), old age, as we and others have argued, had become a status firmly located within the institutionalised life course of white heterosexual able-bodied men. This cultural and economic archetype played an unspoken but important role within the 'modernist' model of social structure where chronological rather than corporeal age provided the principal, legitimised means for men to exit the labour force. Freed from the requirement of continuing to labour, men's old age was supported either by the state alone or by some combination of state, occupational and private pension income. The status of men's 'working age' framed the status of their old age. Women's life course was more loosely marked by chronological age. The nearest comparison to the chronology of working and non-working life for women was defined by 'being of' and 'being beyond' reproductive age. A woman's life course was punctuated by marriage and motherhood, grand-parenting and widowhood, all transitions that reflected personal relationships, health and individual circumstances rather than the institutional arrangements of the economy. The principal marker of women's entry into later life – the menopause – was mostly excluded from public debate. Serving no obvious role within the economy, this particular aspect of women's corporeality was deemed irrelevant for gaining access to the social entitlements and responsibilities of senior citizenship.

In a similar way to the position of women, most disabled people – male or female – were excused (if not denied) from fulfilling the demands of the breadwinner role. Once they had left behind their childhood, the adult life course of disabled people, including their subsequent ageing, was overshadowed by the status given to them by their bodily impairment(s). This status minimised further life course transitions. The choice of whether to become old or remain disabled was not in their hands. Senior citizenship in Europe, North America and Australasia was framed and regulated by the working life of able-bodied white men. The colour of ageing was as implicitly white as were most other institutionalised structures of these societies. In the USA, that most radicalised of Western societies, African Americans were poorly integrated into the national economy, both as workers and as consumers. African Americans benefited little from the corporate welfare structures that provided occupational pensions and healthcare to the majority of the white US workforce (Hacker 2002, 132–33). A similar marginalisation was evident in the benefits dispensed by the state: African Americans were less likely to receive any (Byrd and Clayton 2002, 211–12). Throughout the first half of the twentieth century, the ageing and old age of all so-called 'minorities' were largely irrelevant in framing the institutionalisation of the life course. Its chronology was organised around that of the rational 'disciplined, compliant adult male' by a working life that was embedded within the needs of the productive economy (Sydie 2004, 49).

Those living in the 1960s experienced the culmination of 'first modernity' at the same time as witnessing its dissolution. The cultural ferment of the time saw the status of the white male breadwinner undermined as a new 'normativity of diversity' began to replace the standard life course model. This was achieved less by any deliberate political programme of 'liberation' but more through what Beck has called 'the normalization of diversity' (Beck 2007). Within this normalisation by side effects, the body as a separate cultural entity took on a particular significance. As the body began to orient individuals toward other possible identities, new forms of 'embodiment' emerged whose social distinctions were presaged upon aspects of the corporeal. Social movements based upon gender and race, as well as sexual orientation and the lifestyles associated with them, helped create generalised demands for 'liberation'. As elective communities of association were established that oriented their members toward their own bodies as vehicles of social distinction, bodies other than those of the male white worker asserted their presence in the social polity. In the process, alternative lifestyles were developed, distinct from those that had been standardised within the normativity of first modernity.

These developments were also realised, reflected and promoted by the market and the mass media. The body was exposed in public more than it had been before, not just through the increasing political references to the embodied distinctions of gender, race and sexuality but through the lifestyles and leisure practices that were associated with them. These were widely diffused by the media, the arts and entertainment industries and by the invigorated retail sector. Reflecting upon the somatic turn taken by society in the 1960s, two developments seem particularly salient for this book. One is the importance given by society to the 'embodiment' of identities while the other is the expansion of 'embodied practices' and the ways they served to support and help realise these new identities.

At this juncture it is important to define some of the terms that we have introduced and will use throughout much of this book. The term *corporeality* is used to refer to the relatively unmediated materiality of the body – the body in Donna Haraway's terminology as a social 'actant', standing in contradistinction to the body's role as a social 'agent' (Haraway 1997, 4). Corporeality describes the material actions and reactions of bodies that are realised socially but without recourse to concepts of agency or intent (Haraway 1997). *Embodiment* on the other hand refers to the body as a vehicle or medium of social agency. It encompasses all those actions performed by the body, on the body and through the body which are oriented toward the social and which are both subject to and made salient by the reciprocal actions and expectations of the self and others. In this sense embodiment can be thought of as an 'epigenetic' property of the body arising out of its inextricable engagement with the social, by the processes through which the body is made socially meaningful. The corporeality of ageing – those relatively unmediated bodily changes which occur within individual lifetimes – provides the critical context for age's embodiment and all those practices and narratives that explicitly or implicitly are oriented toward the social expression – or denial – of ageing and agedness.

Embodiment is realised in identity itself, through the various narratives by which an identity is imbricated within society and in the practices by which socially meaningful identities and lifestyles are realised. The term 'embodied identities' refers to identities and lifestyles based around some collectively shared set of bodily distinctions: distinctions of how particular bodies act, look or both. Emerging first in the politics of race and secondly in the Women's Movement, embodied identities subsequently extended beyond the categories of race and gender to include people seeking distinction on the basis of other corporeal differences such as those of disability or sexual preference. If not for the first time then more distinctively, people whose bodies had long been seen to differ from those of able-bodied, white male heterosexuals began to re-position themselves through a common rejection of their cultural, political and economic marginality. Often no longer tolerating the devaluation of their bodies, these groups began to assert the equality of their difference and moreover demand access to the goods and services that were on offer in the newly evolving postwar mass-consumer society.

By 'embodied practices', we are referring to all those practices of self-care and self-expression that are mediated by society in, and through, the autonomous body.

They reflect the culturally mediated body work that writers such as Bauman, Beck and Giddens consider to constitute the modern self and that frame most public and private self-other relationships (Bauman 2000; Beck and Beck-Gersheim 2001; Giddens 1991). Embodied practices serve to realise or repress, completely or selectively, particularly embodied identities and their associated lifestyles. The idea of embodied practices has its roots in anthropology and the work of Marcel Mauss and Maurice Merleau-Ponty, whose relevance to the sociology of the body has already been outlined by Nick Crossley (Crossley 2001, 2007). In the turn towards a more intensely somatic society, many contemporary expressions or practices of embodiment have oriented themselves around the contested identities and alternative lifestyles that were realised in the new social movements and their rapid commoditisation within the market. It is this complex of counter-cultures and consumerism that most distinguishes contemporary embodied practices from those associated with the corporeal ethics of pre-modernity or that were defined by the regimentation and reification of late nineteenth- and early twentieth-century 'first' modernity.

The 'cultural revolution' of the 1960s and the new forms of embodiment associated with it are not simply matters of historical imagination or political rhetoric. They were realised in a distinct set of material conditions emerging after the Second World War, of rising educational opportunities, higher standards of living and the growth of discretionary spending power, particularly among young people. They were diffused across society by a combination of marketing, the new media and the postwar entertainment, leisure and self-care industries, and they consciously and notably privileged youth. Youth sub-cultures and counter-cultures galvanised the market and the market duly responded, rushing to reinforce their claims for autonomy and distinction by promoting the 'democratisation' of fashion complete with a new system of 'age segmentation' (Lipovetsky 2002). The results were not only new clothes, but new hairstyles, new forms of music – in a word, new lifestyles – marketed as signifiers, for those buying into this new culture of consumption, that they had liberated themselves from the oppression of the past and had broken free from all that was old and out-dated (Heath and Potter 2005). Age targeting helped grow sales of non-essential products and services on the back of the consumerist stimulation of young people's desires for self expression, lifestyle choice and enhanced bodily enjoyment. Consumerism, choice and self-expression became linked. Sexuality was similarly distanced from sexual reproduction while 'race' began to acquire a new 'transracial' appeal in the music, the lifestyle and the fashions of those who identified themselves as the young. Political and cultural expressions of identity embodied by a person's gender, race or sexuality were supported by the increasing use of the body as a site for the care of self and the cultivation of lifestyle. Identities were not just about who you were but equally about how you behaved.

During the 1960s, hair salons, beauty parlours, fashion boutiques and dance studios blossomed. In place of the swimming pools and municipal baths that had served as sites of family fun and centres for physical education, fitness and leisure centres increasingly emerged as shop windows for fitness and physicality (Stern 2008). Once limited to the collective callisthenics of future workers and warriors, body work became refashioned and re-individualised through new practices such as aerobics, jogging, and whole body workouts (Bowerman and Harris 1967; Cooper, 1970; Guild, 1971). New and reinvented keep-fit regimes, cosmetic and self-care routines and 'alternative' sexual practices circulated in and through the media influencing the present and the future lives of successive postwar generations of young people.

This embodiment of identity and lifestyle was practiced most intensively by the cohort of young people who were born during or just after the Second World War. Older people, still in the grasp of first modernity, were excluded from participation through a combination of consumer poverty, social exclusion and simple inexperience. The young, defined by their youth, saw little reason to change this age segregation, and in the words of the song, simply 'hoped to die before they grew old'. But, with a few celebrated exceptions, they did not. Instead they recalibrated themselves, abandoning the earlier system of age segregation, not by extending the 'new' cultural practices to the 'old' but by blurring and confounding the boundaries of what or who was 'old'. First evident in the USA but soon extending to Europe and other Western societies, middle age was reinvented. By the 1980s, it had morphed into more pervasively age-resisting, age-denying middle age lifestyles. New cultural narratives and embodied practices emerged that were based upon the reinvention and recalibration of middle age (Featherstone and Hepworth 1983, 1992; Gullette 1997) and by the end of the twentieth century, these mid-life lifestyles had become late-life lifestyles. Sixty was hailed as the new forty and eighty the new sixty (Jagger 2005). The body in late as in early adulthood was open to refashioning as well as rejuvenating. A plethora of self-help books, TV programmes and magazine articles encouraged the no longer young not to let themselves become the old. Adult life was meant to be read neither as 'old' nor 'young' but as a series of passages, each made up of different ways of 'becoming' oneself (Sheehy 1977, 1982; Hepworth and Featherstone 1982).

Earlier versions of modernity had structured age through reified ideas of productivity and the reasonable rewards expected after a life of labour. Ageing bodies were emptied of any other meaning beyond that established by the constricting realms of health and social care. Here, in the infirmaries, hospitals and care homes, the corporeality of the ageing body was exposed; a corporeality defined by illness and infirmity. With the transition to late modernity, ageing became differentiated and the ageing body more distinctly embodied. No longer viewed as a process through which the subject becomes an object to be managed by others, bodily ageing has emerged as (another) arena for self-care, for lifestyle fashioning, even for what Michel Foucault has termed the 'practices of freedom' (Foucault 1994). In a society of busy consumers the body can always be worked on, by the consumer and through the medium of the market, without any agreed end point short of death (Bauman 2005). Much as a fat person is encouraged, through endless dietary and exercise regimes, to realise the slim person within, so agedness has become like fat, something to be sloughed off to reveal the valued 'ageless' self within.

Under the changed conditions of second modernity old age doesn't work, either as a corporeal or as an embodied identity. Unlike gender, race, sexuality or even disability, old age cannot be promoted as a point of somatic distinction or treated as a transgressive 'carnivalesque', alternately threatening or challenging the social and cultural ordering of everyday life. While diversity in and contestation over the expression and understanding of gender, race, sexuality and disability flourish within the destabilising narratives of marketing, market segmentation and the media, few contestations are attempted over alternative embodiments of 'old age'. Diversity exists elsewhere, within other embodied identities, not those of old age. In contemporary society old age exercises its monopoly over the social imagination only in the form of a 'fourth age'. Shrivelled by fear and disgust, old age has become a social imaginary that is realised principally through appeals for charity, alarms over health care and periodic scandals over the nature of welfare provision. There seems to be no scope for other public contestations, only individualised struggles over revealing or concealing the abjection of old age. As desires for self-expression, self-care and self-betterment provide a common rationale behind most forms of body work, old age becomes increasingly invalid, even as an alibi.

The turn toward the body, the transformation from chronology to corporeality and the shifting basis of social distinction from sites of production to sites of consumption have become critical features in today's 'new ageing'. Themes that defined the 'cultural revolution' of the 1960s (self-expression, pleasure and the exercise of choice and personal freedom) have expanded into mid- and now later life (Bennett and Hodkinson 2012). They are fast being integrated into generationally defined life courses. Ageing has changed from a process once described as that of 'structured dependency' to a third age arena, where agency and effort are always expected, not so much through paid employment as by working tirelessly on lifestyle, leisure and consumption. As we have argued elsewhere (Gilleard and Higgs 2011a) much of the cultural fabric making up this third age can be traced to the ferment of the 1960s and its emphasis upon choice, autonomy, self-expression and pleasure. It is from that ferment that the capacity to extend the earlier embodiments of youth into mid and later life derives. The tension that such contradictory forms of embodiment create is what this book explores – the dilemmas of how to age by not becoming old.

The first two chapters provide the main theoretical context for the book. The first chapter outlines the new 'sociology of the body', while the second outlines the emergence of the new ageing paradigm and its 're-orientation' toward the body. The next section explores key aspects of the embodied identities of gender (Chapter 3), race (Chapter 4), disability (Chapter 5) and sexuality (Chapter 6) and their relationship to age and ageing. In each chapter we provide a brief and necessarily selective historical perspective of the emergence of these variously embodied identities before, during and after the cultural ferment of the 1960s, and end with a consideration of their subsequent confrontations with age. In the third section of the book, we turn from embodied identities to embodied practices particularly those which have been imbricated in the identity politics of the post-1960s. We have organised them around those areas of knowledge and practice which the seventeenth century 'philosopher of science', Francis Bacon, described as promoting 'the good of man's body', that is its health, fitness, beauty and its pleasures (Bacon 2002, 208). Beginning with the latter, Chapter 7 explores sexual practices, Chapter 8, cosmetics and clothing, Chapter 9, fitness and exercise and Chapter 10 what we have called 'aspirational' medicine, namely the medicine of health promotion and personal enhancement. The concluding chapter provides an overview and summary of the book's themes of embodiment, corporeality and the ageing body and their utility for exploring and interpreting the cultures of the third age.

It is important to distinguish between the various forms of embodiment that define the cultures of the third age and the corporeality that shapes the social imaginary of the fourth age. We have chosen to avoid discussing issues of illness and physical frailty and those aspects of corporeality whose significance lies in their absence – and exclusion – from the discourses and practices of the third age. Pursuing the themes of the fourth age requires a different perspective and a different book. This book is meant as a specific contribution toward a sociology of the new ageing, exploring its embodiment through the emergence and evolution of later lifestyles. By thinking through the 'ageing' body differently, we hope not only to further an understanding of the new ageing but in the process to use this understanding to re-examine some of the other binary oppositions through which the body is more generally imbricated within society.

Chapter 1

IDENTITY, EMBODIMENT AND THE SOMATIC TURN IN THE SOCIAL SCIENCES

This first chapter is concerned with the contemporary positioning of the body within the social sciences and the implications of the 'somatic turn' for constructing a new, culturally informed approach to ageing (Gergen and Gergen 2000; Gilleard and Higgs 2000). Most conventional accounts of ageing locate it within the body, where it is expressed as a universal, intrinsic, non-reversible and ultimately deleterious process of decline (Strehler 1962). Because bodily ageing is formulated as a more or less unmediated process of corporeal decline, psychosocial attempts to present ageing in a more positive light have focused on its less 'corporeal' aspects, through concepts such as 'seniority', 'integrity', 'wisdom' or 'longevity'. These attempts, which suffuse modern social gerontology, draw upon a much older tradition, dating back at least to Cicero's essay on old age, whereby (mostly men's) ageing and old age are valued because they reflect or 'embody' the accumulation of cultural or symbolic capital in the form of wisdom, maturity or experience. With the coming of Christianity, ageing acquired an additional meaning when it was represented as the gradual 'spiritual' liberation of the individual from the concerns and constraints of his once youthful erring body.

Such positive, 'de-corporealised' views of old age may still be found in modern gerontology, whether in its espousal of a 'good' or 'successful' old age (Havighurst 1961; Schonfield 1967; Rowe and Kahn 1987) or through ideas of gero-transcendence (Tornstam 1996). Where gerontology has engaged with the ageing body, it has either reified the corporeality of ageing, for example by developing indices of functional capacity, transformed it into a chronological marker of individual or collective achievement, in the form of mortality or longevity statistics, dissolved it within a matrix of 'inter-generational relationships' or unproblematically re-inserted it within a bio-medical or social care narrative, where aged outcomes are judged in terms of relative health or disability statuses. It is time for ageing studies to consider other ways of thinking about the body that neither ignore, mask or reify the corporeality of later life but seek to adequately embody it within the social. To do so requires ageing studies to engage more comprehensively with what Bryan Turner has called the 'somatic turn' in the social sciences (Turner 1984). In order to provide a theoretical context for such an engagement, our aim in this chapter is first to outline some of the principal ways that sociological thinking about the body has developed over the last quarter century and then to map its potential significance for a renewed sociology of ageing and its embodiment.

This brings us to the constant theme that will run through this book, namely the impact of the 1960s, both in fostering new developments in the sociology of the body and in creating the conditions for the 'new ageing'. The topics of 'identity' and 'agency', whether at the political or personal level, have acquired a new importance in sociological thinking as the social sciences have oriented themselves toward the concerns of the more differentiated and individualised society that has emerged from this period of cultural ferment. The renewed interest in the representation and oppression of women provided a particularly powerful motivation toward this re-appraisal. Issues of sex and gender rose to prominence as important lines of fracture, as women were identified as suffering from a similar kind of cultural domination, denial of rights and social exclusion that non-white individuals had experienced in the predominantly white societies of the developed Western world.

The civil rights movements in the USA and elsewhere, the anti-Vietnam war protests and other related anti-imperialist movements reshaped left-wing politics around issues of identity and self-determination, creating what Nancy Fraser has described as a new politics of recognition (Fraser 1995). But, while sharing a generalised desire to establish identity as a well-spring for an emancipatory politics, the achievement of a popular front of 'difference' espoused by the new social movements proved as difficult as had been the case for earlier class-based movements. The attempts to create an overarching unity of the different excluded groups based upon their shared *experience* of the oppressions of bodily difference under-played or failed to emphasise the material solidity of the structures by which such diversity was framed. Faced with these difficulties, they opted increasingly for a politics of recognition at the expense of the earlier politics of redistribution (Fraser 1995). For much the same reasons, the theoretical writing developed within these various social movements each produced a particular version or framing of identity – as a woman, as a gay, lesbian or transsexual person, as a black person/person of colour – that has since been viewed as providing a somewhat limited 'sectional' or even 'reductionist' understanding of difference, neglecting considerations of the intersections between class position and the variously oppressed positions of these variously 'embodied' identities. Moreover, while destabilising the hierarchical orderings of the body, they failed adequately to challenge the very dualities through which oppression had been realised.

Several common themes run through the various discourses around the embodiment of identity and agency. As sex has been transformed into gender, race into ethnicity, sexual orientation into sexuality and impairment into disability, each development in thinking about 'difference' has led to what might be called a 'postmodern' problematisation of the relationship between individuals as bounded, corporeal agents and the structures and institutions of society that bind these individual bodies together. Within the academy, feminism and gender studies, black studies and critical race theory, LGBT studies, disability studies and queer theory have all struggled with the contradictions that arise from rejecting the biological essentialism that dominated the categorical thinking of classical modernity, while seeming to replace it with an equally unsustainable cultural essentialism that treats the body's corporeality as a source for unreal yet highly referential signs and signifiers.

Developments in theorising the relationship between people as individually distinct bodies and people as collectively organised members of society form a central theme in this introductory chapter. We concentrate here upon the generic theory that has developed within the sociology of the body and pay rather less attention to the theoretical contributions made by cultural studies. This differential emphasis is not because we feel these latter are less important or less illuminating, but because we shall employ them more extensively in subsequent chapters of the book, particularly those dealing with the embodied identities of gender, race, disability and sexuality and their relevance for the 'new' ageing. Toward the end of this chapter, we consider the potential applications of these general theoretical approaches to understanding the place of the body within the paradigms of the new ageing.

Corporeality and Human Nature: The New Sociology of the Body

Discussions of the relationship between the corporeality of human existence and the society in which this corporeality is embodied have long roots in sociology. Commentators such as Turner (1984) and Shilling (1993), have argued that embryonic ideas about the relationship between the body and society can be found in the works of the 'founding fathers' of sociology long before there was a separate 'sociology of the body'. They have noted, for example, that in nineteenth-century France Auguste Comte was regarded as a key theorist of biology as well as of sociology. Similar concerns with the link between body and society can be found in Émile Durkheim's concept of 'homo duplex' while Max Weber's notion of 'necessary body discipline' has a strong link with his identification of the 'protestant work ethic' as an ideology driving modern industrial capitalism (Weber 1976). Karl Marx's contribution to early classical sociology was not confined to his discussion of the influences on human nature but was also evident in the ways that he saw the exploitation of labour as both a physiological as well as an economic process (Shilling 1993, 27). Despite such recognition, as Shilling points out, 'the overall orientation of the sociological project they (sociology's founding fathers) established mitigated against locating the embodied human as a central area of investigation' (Shilling 1993, 28).

Indeed, upon closer examination, these roots seem neither very deep nor particularly extensive. Issues of gender and the body were mostly reified or ignored. Sydie (2004) has argued that Durkheim, Simmel and Weber saw social structures as essentially 'male', while they considered women a part of a nature that stood in contrast to society. Witz and Marshall (2004) have pointed out that Durkheim's conceptualisation of man is 'both embodied and social [...] while women are denied that liberation from the senses which would truly make them "persons"' (Witz and Marshall 2004, 23–4). While the body's 'absent presence' in sociology is not necessarily a complete reading of the 'classical' sociological canon, what is evident is less the complete absence of the body per se but rather the absence of attention to the role that the bodily distinctions of gender, race and disability had in structuring modern society. It is this masculine, heterosexual and white nature of society and its institutions that is explicitly, or implicitly, conveyed by these writers as is their preoccupation with *man* as the critical social agent. Much of the renewed interest in issues of embodiment has been ignited by sociology's engagement with feminism, and it is this particular engagement that has helped highlight the limited and often reified approach to the body that led to the underplaying of gendered relationships and their role in organising society. As Turner argues, 'greater sensitivity towards gender/sexuality/biology on the part of social theorists' (Turner 1991, 20) has been an important consequence of the encounters between the social sciences and the new social movements in the aftermath of the 1960s.

Yet despite this re-orientation towards the body and growing awareness of the significance of the body as a source of social identity and fracture there has been, with a few notable exceptions, a signal failure to engage seriously with the ageing body. The absence of a viable social movement promoting the interests of older people might be one reason for this failure. However, it more likely stems from the location of the new social movements within postwar youth culture, the impact of the 'campus' cultures of the 1960s, and their rejection of all that was old (Gilleard and Higgs 2009). Whatever the reasons, most key theorists of the sociology of the body have either ignored the issue of age or have subsumed it under issues of 'vulnerability' or 'death' (Higgs and Jones 2009, viii). Given the potential of many of the themes in the new sociology of the body to illuminate ageing as an 'embodied' process, one aim of this book is to address this gap by relating 'embodiment' to age and ageing, and thereby exploring the difficulties that this creates for their developing and sustaining an engagement with ageing itself.

As an inherently dynamic process, ageing threatens to destabilise whatever settlement might be negotiated between the particular embodied identities represented by gender, race and disability and the institutional practices and cultural narratives of operating in society. Just as the classical canon of sociology had difficulties in acknowledging the embodiment of impairment, gender and race, the tendency in the new sociological writing on the body has been to avoid, ignore, or minimise the social and cultural significance of ageing as itself an unsettling influence. In a similar fashion to the earlier 'absence' of the body in sociology, the absence of ageing exposes a critical *lacuna* within these new academic sub-disciplines. Just as the turn to the body has had a galvanising influence on new ways of thinking about society and social identity, an engagement with age and ageing can provide new challenges to the new sociological thinking about the body. Indeed such an engagement offers mutual challenges – to the 'new' ageing studies and to the 'new' sociology of the body. Some of these challenges will be opened out at the end of this chapter before being revisited more fully when we outline issues of embodiment and corporeality associated with the 'new' ageing paradigm in the next chapter.

Foucault and the Cultural Ferment of the 1960s

The cultural ferment that projected issues of identity into sociology in the latter half of the twentieth century was reflected in the work of a number of key writers who were beginning to question the assumptions of classical social science. Prominent among them was Michel Foucault. In a series of books beginning with *Madness and Civilisation* (1970), *The Birth of the Clinic* (1975) and *Discipline and Punish* (1979) Foucault examined how knowledge about the body provided the 'site' of various forms of power relations within society.

In his early work, Foucault undertook what he termed an 'archaeology' of the various 'epistemes' that underpinned developments in the history of human knowledge about the body. A key feature of this approach was his focus upon 'discourse' and the acceptance of its relativist nature, coupled with a rejection of any assumption of progress or teleology that could be ascribed to any particular episteme. In his account of the history of madness, for example, he argued against the view that a more humane 'scientific' understanding superseded earlier 'punitive' understandings of mental illness. Instead he saw the emergence of psychiatry as an example of the growing role of 'reason' in the increasingly rationalised world of modernity. A similar theme is evident in his *The Birth of the Clinic*, where he described the emergence in the late eighteenth century of a new form of 'clinical medicine' which was not simply the development of new, improved technologies for identifying and treating illness but was a result of new forms of power/knowledge by which illness and disease were defined – which Foucault termed the 'clinical gaze' (Foucault 1975, 109). At a time of revolutionary political change, Foucault argued, an equally revolutionary transformation took place in medicine. Medicine began to map the 'body' of a disease onto the 'body' of the sick individual, and using instruments such as the stethoscope and procedures such as auscultation, re-framed discourses about health and disease based upon an 'anatomo-clinical' analysis of pathology. This created new forms of power as it established 'the possibility for the individual of being both subject and object of his own knowledge' (Foucault 1975, 197).

The tendency to relate knowledge of the body to power over it was given more attention in *Discipline and Punish*, Foucault's historical study of punishment (Foucault 1979). In it Foucault outlined the difference between two different modes of power, which he termed 'sovereign' and 'disciplinary' power. Drawing on accounts of public executions in pre-revolutionary France, he posits that *sovereign power* is exercised through the authority of the body of the monarch. Public displays of this power were crucial to its operation. *Disciplinary power*, on the other hand, operates through a 'bio-politics' that over time relies more on public surveillance and the capacity of 'capillary power' to reach down to all individuals, influencing their behaviour and actions. In contrast to the public execution, the most arresting image of disciplinary power was the 'panopticon' a form of prison organisation outlined by the utilitarian philosopher, Jeremy Bentham. A key feature of the panopticon was the way in which prison warders occupied a central location from which they could view all inmates but from which they themselves could not be seen. Because prisoners believed themselves to be always under surveillance, the assumption was that they would follow the desired behaviours of the prison regime whether or not they were in fact being observed at any one time or place, leading each individual prisoner to internalise appropriate prescribed behaviours rather than be made to submit to the regime through the use of force.

Although few prisons were ever built as panopticons, this image was successfully extended to a whole number of social processes and has been influential on how power and governance are viewed in modern society. The metaphor has proved popular with a range of writers interested in moving the focus of politics away from conventional concerns about the role of institutions such as the state or the armed forces and towards a more personalised focus on how power operates in everyday behaviour and relationships. The slogan of the new social movements that 'the personal is political' consequently connected well with Foucault's notions of disciplinary power and its inter-related theorisation of the capillary diffusion of power into the various bodily disciplines enacted in a myriad of individual lives. In this way, issues of bodily difference and identity came to be understood as examples of the micro-politics of such disciplinary 'bio-power' (Sawicki 1988). Writers in the disability movement, for example, found the capacity to produce accounts of the way that power/knowledge constructs and institutionalises disability useful in reframing alternatives to bio-medical discourse (Shildrick 2009; Tremain 1995). Others, especially those from a feminist perspective, were more cautious. Fraser viewed Foucault's early focus on surveillance and the production of 'docile bodies' as creating very little possibility for resistance (Fraser 1989). Here, Foucault's downgrading of the idea of human subjectivity in institutions such as the prison was seen to fundamentally undermine the feminist project by rejecting the idea that liberation was possible outside the framework of bio-power and its insidious systems of surveillance and control.

If Foucault's early writings appeared unrelentingly concerned with the systems of disciplinary power operating within forms of knowledge, a turn towards human subjectivity and personal agency became more evident in his later work marked out by terms such as 'governmentality', 'self-care' and 'technologies of the self' (Foucault 1988, 2008). The three volumes that make up *The History of Sexuality* (Foucault 1990a, 1990b, 1992), represent a perceptible change in approach. Organised around the idea of sexuality as embodied practice, Foucault moved from a concern with the disciplinary discourses of the confessional to a consideration of the uses of pleasure, the cultivation of the self and the practices of freedom (Foucault 1990b, 1988, 1994). While there is considerable debate about whether these later writings represent continuities or discontinuities with his earlier work (Nealon 2008), it is generally accepted that this late or 'final' Foucault allowed for the development of a more expansive, less oppressive and potentially more agentic view of the operation of bio-power and a re-envisioning of power itself.

In his third volume on the history of sexuality, in his later seminars on the technologies of the self and in his lectures on the government of self and others (Foucault 1988, 2005), Foucault addresses the notion of 'self-formation' and the social and political developments that have helped make the modern 'reflexive' individual engage less in face-to-face conflict than in what he describes as a process of 'permanent provocation' (Foucault 1982, 222; Bernauer 1994, 71). Here, Foucault emphasised not only agency but also the productive dimension of power which he saw as constituting freedom. As he put it in one of his last essays before he died in 1984: '[a]t the very heart of the power relationship and constantly provoking it are the recalcitrance of the will and the intransigence of freedom' (Foucault 1982, 221–2). As many critics noted, Foucault had come a long way from his earlier position where he had opined that 'man is an invention of a recent date [...] and would be erased, like a face drawn in sand at the edge of the sea' (Foucault 1973, 387).

Writers such as McNay (1992), Grosz (1994), Bartky (1988) and indeed Fraser (1989), have been much happier to engage with Foucault's 'turn to the personal'. It enabled them to investigate what they identified as the co-construction of the female body, opening up opportunities for examining the practices that were constitutive of both sex and gender. In a similar fashion, critical disability studies have also found the later Foucault more profitable in understanding both the institutionalisation of, and resistance to, the dividing practices that operate in modern society (Thomas 2004). Some writers however have remained concerned that the idea of the body has been effectively removed from Foucauldian discussions of embodiment (Sawicki 1988). Hughes (1995) for example has endorsed Shilling's point that Foucault's bodies do not seem to have much 'prolonged visibility as corporeal entities' (Shilling 1993, 80), while Foucault's perceived failure to engage with the physicality of the body has been seen to hamper the development of truly radical positions about the centrality of the body as 'world forming' (Latimer 2009, 5). This omission has led some sociologists of the body to turn to writers who seem more concerned with actual bodies, their embodied practices and their corporeal agency.

Embodied Experience: Mauss, Merleau-Ponty and Goffman

If the work of Foucault was instrumental in raising awareness of the body in both the social sciences and in the humanities, his somewhat 'cerebral' focus on power/knowledge has made other, non-Foucauldian accounts seem potentially more fruitful in understanding the links between the corporeal and the social. One source has been the work of Maurice Merleau-Ponty. Merleau-Ponty's phenomenological approach to understanding the social and the physical world is based on an acceptance that an inseparable relationship exists between the body and the being of the observer and the world that s/he observes (Merleau-Ponty 1962, 1968). The idea that the actions and perspective of the body render meaningful that which the body perceives while that which is observed in turn influences the experience of embodiment, has proved useful to a number of writers, from Erving Goffman to Judith Butler. Within this phenomenological tradition, social phenomena are seen as 'realised' within the body, just as, through its interactions with the social world, the body forms an inextricable part of that world. Using this approach Nick Crossley (2007, 87) has drawn attention to what he calls 'embodied' knowledge; knowledge that cannot be properly described or discussed but which is only realised in and through bodily performance. Crossley suggests that the study of bodily performances – or 'body techniques' to use a term he borrowed from Mauss (1973) – provides one concrete way for sociology to explore the 'embodiment of the social world' (Crossley 2007, 80). By combining the collective knowledge and performance of body techniques with a mindfulness of the intent and meaning conveyed by such acts, Crossley claims to find a solution to the problem of the 'absent' body in sociology. Researching 'body techniques', in Crossley's view, avoids the problem with the 'cultural studies' approach, identified by Howson and Inglis (2001) where research is focused on meanings and perceptions, and instead provides a more material way of understanding how social actions underpin and are underpinned by bodily practices.

Crossley's exploration of the connections between 'body techniques' and the regulation of social relationships leads him to engage with the work of Erving Goffman. For Crossley, Goffman's importance lies in his *contextualising* of body techniques 'within an interactional order which that activity acknowledges, respects and co-reproduces' (Crossley 1995, 136). This contextualisation of actions and the creation of social meaning in public interactions represent major themes running through many of Goffman's works including *The Presentation of Self in Everyday Life* (1971) and *Stigma: Notes on the Management of a Spoiled Identity* (1970). In these books, Goffman acknowledges the centrality of the body to the 'interaction order' of face-to-face social encounters. In *The Presentation of Self in Everyday Life*, for example, Goffman treats self-presentation as a dramaturgical performance, with the body serving as a 'peg' or a 'back region' which remains hidden from the view of the audience (Goffman 1971, 245). Within this 'dramaturgical' framework, identity and selfhood are realised/performed through scripts, masks and costumes. In *Stigma*, Goffman elaborates on his ideas about the dramaturgical aspects of identity management when he considers how people with impairments selectively present themselves and/or mask aspects of their body in order to prevent 'social discrediting' (Goffman 1970). The extent to which stigma is made salient is less a function of the impairment, Goffman suggests, and more a reflection of the way in which particular social interactions recreate the narrative of stigma – in short how people play their part. What Crossley emphasises in a review of Goffman's work is how 'embodied action drawing from a stock of social techniques or skills is oriented to and articulated within an embodied world (so that) the active body and the social world as a stage of action are completely interdependent' (Crossley 1995, 147).

Some disability activists have criticised aspects of Goffman's work, particularly the unexamined 'personal tragedy' assumptions about disablement that they see inherent in his writings. They view Goffman's approach as being too individualistic, emphasising the individual 'performance' of stigma rather than seeing stigma arising from the social arrangements that separate the conditions of everyday life for the able-bodied from those with impairments (Oliver 1990). This response is similar to other general critiques of the emerging focus on the body; namely that it risks 'individualising' the body and its 'learned' performances rather than placing it and them within a more thoroughly social and historical context. Individual bodies may well learn to perform within and through their social world, but that world is structured by factors that go beyond the history of individual bodies and their individual performances. Bodies are shaped by trajectories embedded in earlier, collective histories whose influence is realised within rather than decided upon by the individual actor. This collective history of the body, or rather the collective histories of bodily practices, were articulated by a sociologist who predates Foucault, Goffman and Merleau-Ponty, but whose work is now seen as an important precursor of the somatic turn, Norbert Elias.

Elias and the Civilised Body

The historical contextualisation of body practices – and by implication forms of embodied knowledge – was pursued by Norbert Elias in his work on the 'civilising process' in fifteenth- and sixteenth-century Europe, in a work first published in 1939 in German as *Über den Prozess der Zivilisation*. It was not translated into English until much later, after Elias had relocated in England, as *The Civilising Process*, (Elias 1978, 1984). Perhaps because of Elias' key role in influencing a number of important sociologists during his time at the University of Leicester in the 1960s and 1970s, *The Civilising Process* became an influential text which has been incorporated into the new sociology of the body (see, for example, Burkitt 1999, 50; Mellor and Shilling 1997, 61–2; Shilling 1993, 150; Turner 1996, 169; and Turner 1991, 15). The two volume work provided a detailed account of the disciplining of the body and bodily habits that emerged during the course of Renaissance humanism (Elias 1978, 1984). Drawing on Renaissance books of manners written for members of the European aristocracy, Elias argued that a civilising process was set in train that sought explicitly to regulate permissible and impermissible bodily habits, establishing standards of civility and virtue that required the exercise of bodily discipline and control within the social settings first of the court and later applied to all public settings. Contrasting the recommendations of these texts with the violent, sexual and toilet behaviour of earlier times, Elias saw in them the explicit development of body-based system 'manners', whereby individuals' bodies were distanced from one another as a growing disdain for unregulated, involuntary bodily functions spread through society. He quotes from a sixteenth-century treatise on good manners to make his point:

> When you come across something distasteful lying in the road, it is improper to turn toward company and show them this filth. Still less is it permissible to present foul smelling things to others, as some are accustomed to doing who lower their nose to it and say 'Do take a sniff; it really stinks'. On the contrary they should say, 'Don't smell it, because it stinks'. (Fontaine, cited by Elias 1978, 247)

Individuals were required to adopt appropriate self-control in relation to their toilet and sexual behaviour as well as become more refined in relation to their eating habits. As these forms of conduct became increasingly standardised into everyday life, Elias argued, this had the effect of 'freeing' individuals from an automatic, unmediated 'corporeality'. This has put him at odds with thinkers like Foucault and Freud who, at least in their earlier writings, saw the civilising process as constraining the bodily passions that animate the self. As Smith writes:

> For Elias, advances in rationality and control make a human existence possible. For Foucault the repression of unreason means losing contact with a major source of human creativity. (Smith 2001, 112)

Elias' work gave greater recognition to both the historical and the contingent in the habits and practices of the body. He argued that bodies are not just oriented to current social relationships, but also act as repositories of past institutions and practices whose history has been so well laid down that it has become 'second nature'. The role of history in shaping current bodily practices and rendering as second nature what was once laboriously learned has had a particular resonance for those theorists of gender, race and sexuality who have emphasised the 'performativity' that is involved in realising these variously embodied identities. It is to this body of knowledge we next turn.

Performing Gender

The historical context of embodied knowledge is echoed most prominently in Judith Butler's work on the 'performativity' of gender (Butler 1986, 1990). Influenced by both Foucault and Simone de Beauvoir, Butler argued that gender is 'not only a cultural construction imposed upon identity, but in some sense […] a process of constructing ourselves' (Butler 1986, 36). While early second wave feminist writers like Shulamith Firestone (1970) and Mary Daly (1978) had tended to view the biological nature of women as a source of their oppression, writers such as Butler followed Simone de Beauvoir's lead in seeing the process of becoming a woman as 'a purposive set of acts, the acquisition of a skill, a "project" […] to assume a certain corporeal style and significance' (Butler 1986, 36). While acknowledging the biological structuring of reproduction as an important part of many women's experiences, for Butler and other feminist theorists the corporeal is refashioned as and through a process of embodiment such that the social meaning of gender is selectively 'read off' or 'performed by' the body.

The lack of any necessary biological foundation to gendered identities in this approach had been stressed by de Beauvoir, who in *The Second Sex*, described gender in Sartrean terms as an 'inapprehensible' entity, having no point of origin, no historical moment of emergence (de Beauvoir 1974). Gender exists always in a state of becoming, a choice made and remade under differing circumstances, through what Butler calls 'an active style of living one's body in the world' (Butler 1986, 40). This mixture of agency and structure, Butler argued, easily goes unnoticed, and individuals perform their gender under conditions of alienation. For Butler, it is because of the 'performative' nature of gender, that the objectification of women's bodies is made possible. As de Beauvoir writes: 'to be a woman means to be the object, the Other' (cited by Butler 1986, 42–3). In this sentence de Beauvoir's 'to be' can be read as Butler's 'to perform as' in order to see the line of continuity between the two authors. This necessary performativity can be contrasted with the 'disembodiment' of men whose project, Butler argues, is to 'dispose' of their bodies, to 'make their bodies other than themselves' (Butler 1986, 44). This binary contrast – between actively becoming versus constantly transcending one's gendered body – is central to the idea that gender and its embodiment can be viewed as both relational and as a mode of re-enactment, with men 'othering' their bodies in order to be men, while women only become themselves in and through their bodies.

While links between Butler's idea of performativity and Goffman's ideas of dramaturgical self-presentation can also be made, Butler has argued that Goffman 'posits a self which assumes and exchanges various "roles" within the complex social expectations of the "game" of modern life' (Butler 1988, 528). Self, for Butler as for the earlier Foucault, is instead 'irretrievably outside' any ascription of interiority or personal essence. Gender as 'a publically regulated and sanctioned form of essence fabrication [...] serves a social policy of gender regulation and control' (Butler 1988, 528). It is through significant institutional impact – through systems of governmentality, in Foucault's terms – that there is an internalisation of the 'right' and wrong' ways of performing gender.

The significance of Butler's work lies in the insistence that there is no particular essence lying underneath gender which 'only takes on a guise of naturalness through repeated, and discursively constructed, performance' (Marshall 1994, 110). Gender appears as second nature. This theme is also evident in the work of Susan Bordo who has acknowledged the particular significance of the 1960s and its 'politics of the personal' in establishing 'culture's grip on the body [...] [as] a constant intimate fact of everyday life' (Bordo [1993] 2003, 17). Bordo notes that whereas in second wave feminism (which she sees as ushered in iconically by the 1968 'No more Miss America' protest) the body was treated as a socially shaped and historically 'colonised' territory, in contemporary feminist discourse this view has been gradually replaced with a more agentic approach that has lauded all body techniques that enable women to shape their anatomy and their destiny (Bordo [1993] 2003, 20). Steering between models of oppression and models of agency, Bordo proposed 'blooming not transcending' the conventional truths about the female body, drawing upon what she calls the 'imaginations of alterity' – i.e. ways of being/becoming 'woman' differently (Bordo [1993] 2003, 41). Significantly, Bordo's proposal that women as women adopt positions of 'alterity' dovetailed with other developments in the sociology of the body that highlighted not just the need for an embodied sociology, but for an embodiment qua embodiment that accentuates and enables agency in the construction of identity. The potential of becoming other, of performing differently, therefore requires consideration of how such socially significant bodily differences are realised and what their implications are. Nowhere has this agenda been more contested than in the new ethnic and racial studies.

Black Studies and the Body

During the 1960s, the Black Power movement in the USA re-energised the quest for civil rights. Blackness was represented as a valued distinction realisable both as a material presence – the black body – and through its embodiment within valued, distinctive lifestyles. The writings of Stokely Carmichael and Malcolm X emphasised the need for blackness to be performed publicly, proudly and distinctively in order to be acknowledged. These attempts to change the relations of representation (West 1990, 103), sought not just to privilege blackness but equally to highlight the particularities of the unacknowledged whiteness that pervaded society generally and the 'academy' in particular. Black power provided a new impetus for the development of Black or African American studies on college campuses across the United States.

These soon 'gained a permanent place in university life, setting the model for the ethnic studies and pan-racial programs that quickly followed' (Rodgers 2011, 115). The discursive infrastructure employed in the construction of the new discipline was, however, fragmentary given that unification around a core theme was difficult when these varied from biological essentialism to socialist class analysis. For some, African studies were intended to provide access to the roots of an 'African' culture that had been lost and suppressed in the tangle of Eurocentric ideology. Race was in essence replaced by ethnicity and blackness revealed through its identification with a suppressed African ancestry, a position made salient in academic circles with the publication of Martin Bernal's *Black Athena* (Bernal 1987). For others, racial studies provided the means for reviving themes that had previously emerged in the 'Negro Renaissance' of the 1920s, serving as an acknowledgement and celebration of black life in America with 'its peculiar brand of irony, oppression, versatility, madness, joy, strength, shame, honor, triumph, grace and stillness' (Morrison 1974, 16). For still others, race was less an embodiment of African or African American culture, but was subordinated to the material reality of class. The roots of oppression and disadvantage associated with race were deemed to lie within the dislocations of a capitalist economy, not Africa, and their resolution required a direct attack on poverty and the conditions that sustained it rather than a retreat into an essentialised culture (Wilson 1980).

Faced with such infrastructural heterodoxy, critical theorists of race began to view the social and ontological status of race as something 'more contingent, fissured, imbued with choice' (Rodgers 2011, 137). Reflecting this cultural landscape of polysemous meanings, writers such as Stuart Hall from across the Atlantic could write of 'the end of the innocent notion of the essential black subject' (Hall 1996, 444). These views were also echoed by a number of other theorists such as Henry Gates, Paul Gilroy, and Cornel West who argued for a more contingent view of 'racial' identity, treating it much the same way that Butler and Bordo had treated gender; as a performance, an identity created and re-created from the embodied practices fashioned within the *hybridity* of cultural diasporisation (Hall 1990). The hybridity of racialised embodiment was held to be separate from its corporeality, and could never be essentialised 'either as a culture or as a breeding group'. It emphasised the importance of 'investigating and interrogating' the otherness of Blackness/Whiteness, demystifying the binary categorisation of racialised bodies in order 'to disclose options and alternatives for transformative praxis' (West 1990, 105). The racialised body and its binaries of white/non-white, black/non-black were seen to be inextricably contingent. Bodies of colour could be freed from the chains of economic disadvantage, social marginality and cultural opprobrium when they became embodied within the plastic rainbow of mass consumer society.

Transgression: The Body as Carnival

Black Power derived much of its influence upon white American society through what has been termed the notion of 'transgression'. One consequence was an interest by the new social movements in the use of the body as a site of boundary transgression. Here the work of the Russian theorist Mikhail Bakhtin began to infiltrate cultural studies associated with the new social movements and came to prominence in the social sciences in the 1980s. Working principally as a literary theorist, Bakhtin is best known for an interest in those acts of bodily resistance which he called 'carnival', defined as impure or abnormal aspects of culture expressed in and through embodiment. In particular, Bakhtin interrogated the 'carnivalesque' activities such as processions and dances that took place in the fairs of medieval and early modern Europe as 'ritual spectacles' (Bakhtin 1981). For Bakhtin, the significance of these rituals lay in how they became sites for the transgression of boundaries, between the mad and the sane, between male and female and between what is seen as sacred and what is defined as profane. In carnival, the world was seen to be 'turned upside down'. Prefiguring Elias, he identified the arenas of food, sex and violence as central arenas of the 'carnivalesque' with rituals celebrating sexuality in forms that if they occurred at other times would be seen as unacceptable. The transgression of social roles was also an aspect of the carnival with a select few being allowed to dress as animals, jesters, clerics or tramps and in doing so inverting the positionalities of social class and status. Carnival in these circumstances represented a temporary inversion of accepted social categories and became forms of resistance where the uncivilised 'lower' body was celebrated over the restraining and restrained 'upper' body. In so doing the carnival provided an opportunity for bodies to perform forms of alterity that literally embodied 'resistance' to the existing social order. While these ideas have been utilised by sociologists investigating the transgressive aspects of contemporary cultural activities, such as tattooing, body art and body-piercing (Pitts 2003), they have also found resonance in ideas of the transgressive performances of age and gender (Woodward 1991), even though, for Bakhtin, a key feature of carnival was its positive emphasis upon youth and youthfulness and its close connections with the 'lower body'.

From a different ontological position but one still focused on the possibilities for embodied transgressive resistance is the work of Gilles Deleuze and Félix Guattari. Introducing the seemingly alarming term 'Body without Organs' (BwO) to the debates surrounding embodiment, they argued that the way bodies are understood and experienced is through processes of inscription that effectively construct a 'Body with Organs' (Deleuze and Guattari [1980] 2004). Bodies can be constructed through a variety of discourses, sometimes these discourses are scientific as in the case of medicine, but equally they may sometimes be political or theological. While drawing on different sources of inspiration such as the work of Freud and Marx, the initial stages of their argument broadly followed Foucault's early structuralist approach. However, in a move towards a more fluid conception of embodiment they signalled the importance of Nietzsche's notion of the 'will-to-power' in what they termed the 'deterritorialising' of knowledge which stressed the active rather than reactive capacity of the human subject (Fox 1999, 125). It is noteworthy that Deleuze and Guattari placed resistance at the centre of their analysis of the relation between the body and society, and it is for this reason they also introduced the concept of 'nomadology' in order to show how knowledge of the body has become a terrain of struggle where knowledge attempts to 'territorialise' the BwO into a more knowable Body *with* Organs. Fox (1999) describes the process as follows:

> For Deleuze and Guattari, there is a constant tension between the forces of the social and the BwO's will-to-power. They describe the construction process as a territorialisation and thus the BwO may be thought of as a territory constantly contested and fought over. (Fox 1999, 127)

This contest has no fixed outcome. It is one of continual flux that reaches a temporary plateau in the course of becoming something else. Unsurprisingly, it is this constant process of conflict that leads them to title one of their works *A Thousand Plateaus* (Deleuze and Guattari [1980] 2004) as a way of representing the unending activity of territorialisation. Consequently, they identify resistance to territorialisation as a progressive action, seeing it as providing a positive note of instability that ensures that different forms of embodied practice can challenge any and all settled identities. For these reasons, Deleuze and Guattari endorse the emergence of the nomadic subject as someone who avoids being tied down by history, who is forever mobile, who is forever becoming 'other'.

The utility of Deleuze and Guattari's ideas lies in their focus on the role of difference in constituting modern social conditions which has mainly become apparent at the boundaries and margins of what is taken to be inscribed as normal. The transgressive, in this account, not only becomes a form of resistance but also tests and remakes the boundaries of what bodies and beings are possible. These ideas have been used in the field of disability studies where Roets and Braidotti (2012) have rejected what they see as the politics of mourning and melancholia that they identify as permeating the field and instead argue for a positive politics that sees the subjectivity of disability and impairment as both embodied and nomadic.

The Body and Consumer Society

If we follow through the arc of thinking about the body that begins with Foucault and which has been picked up by an increasing number of sociologists and cultural theorists we can see there exist tensions between cultural discourses on the body, identities both privileged and marginalised by bodily differences and the various accounts of bodily practices that reflect the incessant and inconsistent dialectic between the social and the corporeal. Most writers from whatever position have generally accepted the idea of embodiment as a space which thrives on instability, however constituted. Thus far we have only marginally discussed the role of consumer culture, but it is in consumer culture and in consumption that the clearest connections can be made with the destabilising of identity and the re-territorialisation of the body. Under the circumstances of a reflexive modernity it is not surprising that the nature of modern subjectivity derives less from an 'unchanging' biology than from the 'disembedding' structures created by commerce and their accompanying ontological instabilities (Giddens 1991, 21).

Restlessness, if not nomadity, characterises modern society. Marshall Berman has made resonant Marx's recognition that under capitalism, 'all that is solid melts into air' (Berman 1982). This incessant instability and contestation is not only a feature of much post-sixties radical thinking, it also has an elective affinity with the mechanisms of consumer culture, the fashionable turnover of goods and services and the endless segmentation and re-segmentation of consumer markets. A fascination with developments in mass consumer society has characterised the work of many sociologists (Sassatelli 2007; Slater and Tonkiss 2001). Part of their fascination has been to do with the way that consumer society has increased the prominence of visual imagery in contemporary culture at the same time as projecting the body as a key point of reference through which consumerism operates and is reproduced.

One of the most influential contemporary social theorists, Zygmunt Bauman places the body and the practices that surround it at the heart of what he identifies as 'liquid modernity' (Bauman 2000). Bauman takes for his point of departure the emergence of a modernity typified by choice and uncertainty, and under the cultural sway of consumerism. Embodiment is an important, if not crucial constituent of these contemporary social relations (Bauman 2000, 76). Drawing a distinction between the way a society of producers understands the body and the way a society based around consumption operates, Bauman sees the body as focused on sensations and on successful distinction. A key component within this is the idea of 'fitness' (Higgs 2012). At an individual level fitness becomes not only an 'unachievable' arena of consumption but also a source of profound dissatisfaction. In Bauman's schema it is not possible to escape this trajectory because to do so is to be placed in the position of the 'failed consumer', a status for which there is no social meaning or purpose other than in its representation as a negation of success. The link that Bauman makes between the body and consumer society echoes the earlier work of Mike Featherstone (1982) which has been influential in directing attention to the enmeshment of the body with consumption. Reflecting on his earlier work, Featherstone pointed out in 2010:

> It has become commonplace that consumer culture is obsessed with the body. There is a preoccupation in the media with images of beautiful bodies, the stars, celebrities and models who exemplify the good life. They are invariably presented as relaxed, smiling and full of youthful energy, surrounded by the latest consumer goods in luxurious settings, enjoying another memorable 'experience'. (Featherstone 2010, 197)

Featherstone makes the connection between these images in the media and individual self-images. Pointing to the role of the photographic image popularised by Hollywood and the film industry in creating desirable self-narratives he argues that these images needed an assemblage of clothing, make-up and adornment to 'realise' the image. From this it is a small leap to the constant need to make perfect outlined by Bauman above. Not only does the image need to be created but it also needs to constantly transform itself to continue to conform to changes in fashion. Transformation does not stop at the viewing of the external body, but equally affects the structure and function of the physiological body. The mass media's fascination with the rise and fall of celebrity lifestyles reflects this. Again as Featherstone writes:

> Stars and celebrities are constantly scrutinised and quizzed on how they maintain their energy, bodily fitness, good looks and appearance, while coping with challenging work schedules and the social whirl. Each fall from grace to deal with weight problems, alcoholism, drugs, or just the ravages of the celebrity lifestyle, is often followed by a period spent in a health farm, clinic or retreat [...] A life which constantly swings between successes and failures, between a beautiful healthy body and an abandoned ill-disciplined body that bears the marks of constant excesses, has a strong media-human interest angle. (Featherstone 2010, 201–2)

Describing this as a 'makeover culture' which is within the reach of all, Featherstone also points to its gendered nature. Even if such concerns about body image are now present among some men, the origins of this makeover culture relied heavily upon the profits that could be made from marketing cosmetics and fashions to women (Jones 2010). It is in these industries that the body as a visual image has been most constantly represented.

The relationship between consumer culture, identity and the body has been, and continues to be, a contested topic. While there are differences in theoretical positions and the positions they seek to represent, what is notable is that they seek to provide a basis for judgements about what is and what is not acceptable as forms of bodily appearance, bodily practice or dressing the body. One element that is distinct about the consumerism of 'liquid modernity' is the democratisation of fashion. As Vinken has observed, the emerging agency of fashion as instigator of cultural change can be dated to the late 1960s and early 1970s, when 'fashion becomes a co-production between the creator and those who wear the clothes' (Vinken 2005, 35). Within this consumerist democracy, the choice of how to look, what to wear and how to conduct oneself has grown and the desirability of making such choices has become an essential feature of 'postmodern' citizenship. Its representation as 'false consciousness' and its consumerist practitioners' 'cultural dupes' seem curiously outdated like the voices from the old 'classical modernity', where the proletarianisation of the masses was seen as corrupting the manly virtues bred in work and war (Livingston 1998, 423). While critics of consumer society's culture of narcissism (Lasch 1979), destructive individualism (Bellah et al. 1996), commodity fetishism (Lefebvre 2002), celebration of the superficial (Wolf 1990) and oppressive dehumanisation (Ritzer 1996) still abound, consumerism and consumption continue to thrive, disembedding selves from older, more stable sources of identity and community into a variety of flexible, for now lifestyles.

Ageing: Corporeal Limits and Embodied Identities

Consumption, as Sassatelli (2007, 106) points out, is a terrain of ambivalence, offering and constraining choice, promising democracy while segmenting difference. Within this incessant ambiguity, the body is no longer the corporeal foundation of what is real, but an embodied platform for what is possible. When the new sociologies of the body confront ageing, such 'postmodern' readings generate considerable theoretical unease. While the various embodiments of gender, race, sexuality and disability have proved controversial, they have mostly been set within the confines of an unstated 'agelessness' of being. The idea that age itself can be ambiguous or indeterminate, that it can be a site of oppression and contestation as well as an arena of choice, has rarely been entertained. For the later Foucault, thinking positively for once, old age was the peak, the culmination of this process of self-care, 'the one who can finally take pleasure in himself, be satisfied with himself is not a limit but a positive goal of existence, an end it itself' (Foucault 2005, 109). But for others it is less a goal in itself and more a status to avoid or resist.

Ageing poses unacknowledged challenges to most other sociological approaches to the body and is consequently omitted more often than engaged with in the majority of social science and cultural studies books on the body. Many of the social distinctions between gay and straight, men and women, black and white require the exercise of personal and social agency in order to avoid becoming locked into the attributions of others. The coming of age threatens the social constructivism of embodied identities rendering everyone equally grey, neutral and invisible. Implicit in most views of embodiment is a position that sees old age in traditional terms as a final limiting condition, a structure beyond the reach of culture and consumption except in opposition. Age is judged differently from other 'embodied identities' in that it is intrinsically a process of 'becoming', but a becoming that is shaped and structured from within the body, unmediated by culture or society.

The negativity involved in confrontations with ageing as a corporeal process differs from the sociological focus upon embodiment when it is related to disability, gender, race, or sexuality. Embodiment privileges ideas about authenticity, autonomy and transgression, making for a 'radical self' that treats the body as both plastic and yet vulnerable. The 'liquidity' of society in second modernity is reflected in the instability of embodied identities and the attention given to lifestyle as 'performance' or 'narrative', embodied forms of knowledge and practice that reflect and reinforce particular ways of being. The problem of viewing ageing as yet another 'embodied' identity lies in the perceived limits of its liquidity, and its consequent restrictions as a site for embodied practice. As such it is an unwelcome guest at the carnival of alterities, passed by in the breathless haste of academics keen to discover yet another distinctive or transgressive mode of embodiment. Ageing seems all too solid for a liquid world.

The Sociology of the Body and the 'New Ageing'

Despite the tendency toward marginalising agedness in the 'new' sociologies of the body, some important beginnings have been made in applying the 'turn to the body' to age and ageing. In their work on the 'mask of ageing', Featherstone and Hepworth (1991) considered how individuals deal with the contradiction between the social discourse of ageing as decline and their own sense of possessing a non-aged identity. The mask of ageing is seen as a surface phenomenon of the body that projects an image at variance with how the person feels 'inside'. This approach – which echoes Goffman's work on stigma – has had considerable influence among gerontologists as they have seen it as a way of locating the oppressiveness of ageism, while at the same time accepting that many older people feel constrained by the images of ageing and its embodiment (Tulle-Winton 1999; Andrews 1999). The theme of the mask of ageing has been taken up by Simon Biggs who has seen the value of examining issues of ageing identity and performativity in ways that recognise the contested nature of the identities that people adopt as they age. Taking an explicitly psycho-dynamic perspective, Biggs (1997) appropriates Woodward's (1991) idea of a 'masquerade' but moves it away from purely feminist concerns about performing gender to a position whereby the older person acts out a 'masque' of youthfulness to avoid the personal consequences of ageing in an ageist society. The idea of the masquerade takes on a contradictory form, one that ultimately confirms the negative evaluation of the ageing body, because in adopting these 'disguising' practices the older person inadvertently draws attention to the very ageing that is being concealed. In his *The Mature Imagination* (1999) Biggs does not see the masquerade simply as a process of conscious deception but as a coping strategy enabling the older person to create a degree of internal psychological stability, thereby controlling social expectations about appropriate behaviours. In Biggs' work, we can see the themes of performativity outlined by Butler (1988, 1990). Not only is identity brought to life through discourse and practice, but through their reiteration such performances regulate and constrain the social norms by which embodied bodies are read.

Ageing narratives also form the central theme in Margaret Gullette's *Aged by Culture* (Gullette 2004). Within the interstices of contemporary consumer culture Gullette seeks to expose the 'central, toxic, unrecognised stories about age and aging', arguing that despite a rhetoric framed by positive ageing, America's obsession with age reveals an underlying fear about the ageing process as a narrative of loss and decline (Gullette 2004, 20). As a result, contemporary culture inevitably draws attention to those parts of the body that are most vulnerable to ageing while 'making other unchanged or improved parts invisible' (Gullette 2004, 33). In a similar fashion to the way that feminist theory has 'denaturalised' male/female differences or that critical theories of race studies have problematised black/white differences, Gullette argues that a new ageing studies is needed that will drag age 'away from nature and toward culture' (Gullette 2004, 102). However, as she seeks to recover a broader canvas from which to study ageing as a series of cultural narratives, Gullette finds herself ceding even more territory to ageing and its totalising effects. To escape this trap she proposes that ageing be studied as 'a set of narratives' fashioned through adult life out of a combination of 'autobiography and mental travelogue' (Gullette 2004, 129). Such individualisation contrasts significantly with her subsequent call for a 'self-conscious movement [...] beating a drum for progressive public policy [...] when the rights of elderly people are threatened' (Gullette 2004, 183). Despite moving toward a more explicitly 'cultural studies approach' to ageing, her position of agency reduces to a social movement agenda, albeit one that is based less upon valuing age as difference than upon establishing equality among age groups.

Turning from narratives to performances, we can address the work of writers who have begun to explore the links between ageing and disability studies. Although the majority of disability theorists have tended to eschew the theme of agedness (book covers of textbooks on disability typically either avoid any depiction of the human body or if they do, invariably choose a young or ageless figure), a few writers have begun to explore connections between the sociology of ageing and the sociology of disability. Michelle Putnam (2002) and Christine Oldman (2000) have both argued that the 'social model' of disability has much that is relevant to understanding ageing particularly its emphasis upon the role of environmental and organisational factors in constraining and disabling people whose bodies are in some way 'different' from the 'mainstream' majority. For Putnam (2002) this means contextualising the study of individual ageing by reference both to the environments in which people grow old and the resources/resourcefulness they possess in 'coping with and adjusting to physical impairment' (805). Minkler and Fadem (2002, 229) also draw attention to the 'environmental accommodations and policy changes' that create the conditions for 'successful ageing'. What these authors emphasise is the role of non-personal, non-corporeal factors in limiting what a body can do and how these can express 'personhood' and 'citizenship'. In the process, they challenge the idea of the body as a corporeal boundary which determines the limits of human agency and performativity, as well as the social spaces that people occupy. At the same time, many barriers to achieving closer political alliances and shared theoretical constructs between those researching ageing and those researching disability remain. For those studying or advocating on behalf of ageing, there can be some discomfort with the assumption that narratives of ageing should be incorporated into a narrative based upon bodily impairments, implying, as it were, the marginality of an impairment free later life. For disability researchers and activists, there is equal unease at confining their ideas about bodily differences, impairments and social barriers to a restricted segment of the human life course. Each fears containment by the other.

Conclusion

The 1960s witnessed a major cultural break in the moral ordering of Western societies, disembedding the relationships that modernity had institutionalised between the body, culture and society. The new sociologies of the body that emerged in response to these changes have continued to deconstruct many of the essentialist assumptions about the body and its role in determining social relationships and social power. Alongside mainstream sociology, gender, race, sexuality and disability studies have all emphasised the multiplicity of ways in which bodies shape and are shaped by culture and society, revealing some of the human contingencies that have shaped historically specific bodies and their freedoms and unfreedoms in society.

Much of this work can be used to help illuminate the changing nature of age and the various interpretations that can be made of ageing in the twenty first century. The rise of the 1960s' counter-cultures, and the identity politics that followed, both privileged and problematised the body – whether as a source or as a signifier both of individuality and of collective identities. The variously embodied identities that emerged from this cultural ferment stimulated new understandings and practices of self-care and self-representation. The transgressive and non-transgressive forms of self-care and the practices of performing as other that these studies have explored are all relevant in making the body a site of negotiation over new forms of power and meaning-making. Their relevance lies as much in what they cannot be as in what they can. Many of these performances, the various masquerades and the stories accompanying them will be unsuccessful. Some already have and many more will never be realised. But all embody the central idea of human beings as 'desiring' subjects, active in creating and sustaining a place for themselves in society and a society in which they can have a place. Acknowledging that human beings can and do influence the conditions under which they live, these new ways of narrating and performing age have emphasised desire, potential and agency over need, vulnerability and limitation.

Without also acknowledging the potential of the various embodying projects and practices to be undermined, such applications however risk building castles out of sand. What is most evident about the new 'ageing' is that it is as much a sociology of 'not becoming' old as it is one of 'becoming' old differently. This struggle over realising new meanings for ageing is most keenly contested around the idea of the body. In second modernity, the body has re-emerged as a once forgotten site of distinction and a continuing source of desire. In this re-emergence it acts as an axis of orientation challenging many of the simple binaries by which twentieth century modernity ordered gender, race, disability, sexual orientation – and age. In place of the old corporeal opposition between youth and age, the new ageing approaches the body differently, as possibility as well as constraint, the site for new practices and new freedoms as much, if not more than, for old vulnerabilities.

Chapter 2

CORPOREALITY, EMBODIMENT AND THE 'NEW AGEING'

For most people, ageing remains a bodily affair. Academic accounts have defined or represented ageing in various ways and from a number of disciplinary perspectives. These have included 'the accelerating risk of mortality' (Strehler 1962), 'the stochastic process of diminishing energy' (Hayflick 2000), the 'process of social redundancy' (Phillipson 1982), 'marginality' (Ward 1984) or the loss of 'role' in society (Burgess 1960). Still, the decline of the body remains ageing's central motif. The personal and social importance of ageing rests upon the changing status of the body and the implications that this has for identity, life chances and lifestyles. It is the body that seems to house selfhood and define individuality. Bodily ageing seems to efface the very site where the self is constructed under conditions of youth, fitness and potential, replacing it with the corporeal marks of decline and defeat. While population ageing, ageing as 'risk' or 'vulnerability' and ageing as status change are important academic preoccupations, it is the ageing of bodies that remains the ineradicable concern of persons, confronting, in their own ageing body, the essential transience of their lives.

Despite engaging with the corporeality of the body as a critical point of reference for social life, social relations and social organisation, the social sciences still seem to find ageing an uncomfortable aspect of corporeality with which to engage. As we have noted earlier, most sociological texts on the body pass quickly over, or ignore entirely, ageing and old age. The new sociology of the body prefers to explore such corporeal topics as anorexia, bodybuilding, sexuality or tattooing. Most sociologists of ageing, in contrast, steer away from the body, choosing instead to reify the ageing body as a social status defined by chronology rather than corporeality. In textbooks on the sociology of ageing, scant reference is made to the body. Social gerontologists have been equally complicit, choosing to engage with the ageing body as a tangential accompaniment of the ageing person who is then defined and understood principally by his or her health and/or functional 'status'. Within the social sciences generally, and in social gerontology particularly, old age is most often treated as a socially constructed identity determined by its relationship to the forces of production and framed within the practices and policies of health and social welfare services. In short, the institutions of the state and the labour market serve as the principal sites where old age has been constructed, to which may be added, possibly, the family. In contrast, much of the social science writing on the body has sought to relocate corporeality and identity elsewhere, in the cultural matrix of power and oppression through which understandings of race, gender, sexuality and able-bodiedness have been filtered.

The new ways of thinking about the body associated with 'post-structuralist' and 'postmodern' writers such as Bauman, Butler, Foucault, Deleuze and Guattari reflect more complex understandings of the way bodies have become a more embodied, fluid presence within contemporary society than the simple reification of the body into a series of essentialised binary oppositions underlying the assumptions of sociology's founding triumvirate. Despite the current neglect of age and ageing in the new sociologies of the body, ageing studies still need to actively engage with these new ways of thinking for a variety of reasons. First these writers can be usefully drawn upon to develop a different understanding of ageing as a site of embodied and contested difference. Secondly they serve to progress a broader dialectic between 'corporeality' and 'embodiment' as a key problematic not just as regards age but in society at large. Third they provide a fruitful source of tension arising from abandoning the old 'corporeal' binaries of age, gender, race and sexuality as well as by embracing the indeterminacies associated with the new forms of embodiment. Lastly, the turn to the body in second modernity provides another prism through which we can review our own ideas about the shift in the social understandings of age in second modernity and the boundaries of a presumed 'third age'.

Before pursuing these very contemporary issues, however, we need to step back and reflect on the history of ageing and especially the changing historical significance of the body in representing ageing and old age. Without such a historically situated understanding, bodily ageing can appear as a relatively unproblematic expression of a life course that pivots naturally around a binary divide between 'age' and 'youth'. Such an unproblematic reading may make it seem 'natural' for sociology and social gerontology to ignore the unchanging nature of the ageing body and focus instead upon the 'non-corporeal' aspects of ageing and the 'status' of the aged. By 'historicising' the ageing body, however, we hope to demonstrate the degree of contingency that is attached to the body as a signifying system for ageing and old age and the different elements of 'corporeality' that have or have not served as signifiers in such systems.

The Transition to Modernity and the Demise of the Ageing Body

Throughout much of recorded history, two responses can be discerned in the attitudes that individuals have held toward ageing and old age. One emphasises its naturalness and inevitability, the other questions both. Whilst accurate records of specific chronological ages are largely, if not exclusively, the phenomena of modernity, dividing the human life course into distinct ages or stages seems universal. Most such distinctions drew upon the contrast between youth and age, whether this is represented as a binary opposition or forms the centre of a more complex system of ages and stages in the life course (Burrow 1986). Central to all such distinctions has been change in the appearance of the body. In most premodern accounts, agedness is represented as much by the loss of youthful features as it is by the emergence of positive signs of ageing. Those who have sought to valorise age in less material terms – by praising the maturity of character, the spirituality of age or the wisdom acquired from a long life – marked the emergence of these qualities by reference to the positive signs of ageing – typically the appearance of grey beards or white hair. Critical views of old age, on the other hand, have treated the unwelcome nature of old age by listing those elements of youth that are lost. Losing one's hair, losing one's teeth, losing one's strength of body and swiftness of movement all serve to mark the loss of youth. In effect, ageing and the decay of the body is the decay of youth.

Accompanying the premodern focus on the changed physical appearance of ageing was the recognition that long lives lead also to illness and disease. In such writing, however, these illnesses and misfortunes are treated more as the accompaniments of ageing than as indices of age's essential nature. The corporeality of ageing that dominated the premodern world was not dependent upon the clinician's gaze, nor was it based on the measuring of the pulse or the colour of the urine. Age emerged as the blush off the rose, a change witnessed first and foremost in the eye of the beholder. Only later would it be marked by the clock and the mirror. Within such a cyclical world, where the passage of time was framed by the changing seasons, the ripening of fruit and the fading of flowers, old age appeared white like winter, drooped like a dying flower, shriven like rotten fruit. The visual culture that dominated the premodern world saw age mostly as the loss of the body of youth which, while commonly bemoaned, was widely but never universally accepted. Premodern philosophers and physicians remained unsure whether ageing should or should not be judged a human inevitability. Faced with such scholastic uncertainty, prolongevity and rejuvenation were always entertained as possibilities; to be achieved through either instant, magical interventions or more commonly through the steady cultivation of health and virtue.

With the coming of modernity from the seventeenth century onwards, the conflict between the preservation of youth and health and the acceptance of age and disease was temporarily suspended, or at least moved from centre stage. As the state sought to judge its health and wealth by the number of its citizens, it began counting and classifying its population. Chronological age emerged as a new source of social stratification and a means of regulating the life course of its citizens (Bois 1988; Gutton 1988). From the eighteenth century, actuarial developments in life insurance and mutual aid societies, taxation registers, national censuses and the compulsory recording of births and deaths established a collective understanding that age was to be determined by time and numbers, not appearance and experience (Gilleard and Higgs 2005). As industrialisation spread, the temporal scheduling of work replaced the cyclical waxing and waning of lifelong labour. As work increasingly defined the life course, working life acquired a beginning and an end, regulated by chronological age not biological function. From the nineteenth century, chronological age determined access to education, to healthcare, to social welfare and to work. Modernity and the machine age effectively institutionalised the life course (Anderson 1985) and chronological definitions of agedness came to regulate the decisions of who was or was not 'old'.

At the outset, of course, there were uncertainties and irregularities, confusions and contestations over the exact chronological parameters of agedness (Roebuck 1979). The majority of the inhabitants of Western societies only acquired an accurate knowledge of their own chronological age during the course of the nineteenth century. Evidence from premodern and early modern censuses – such as the fifteenth-century Tuscan catastas (Herlihy and Klapisch-Zuber 1985), seventeenth-century Russian urban censuses (Kaiser and Engel 1993) and nineteenth- and early–twentieth-centuries colonial censuses (Alborn 1999) demonstrated a phenomenon known as 'age clustering'. In these 'early modern' enumerations of the population, people aged over thirty or forty were typically assigned to an age ending in 0 or 5 – 45, 50, 55, 60 and so forth, and it was typically the enumerator rather than the respondent who aged the individual. By contrast, relatively few people were given the ages 41, 52, 63 or 74 and so forth. As states introduced legislation mandating the official recording of dates of birth, marriage and death, adult ages became more differentiated. Primary school education became universal and knowledge of one's age and date of birth became the norm rather than the exception. Centralised systems for registering these details enabled officials to check people's age. The means for determining an official age for old age became more possible and more necessary as its definition became increasingly important in judging between the deserving and undeserving poor. The transition to an urban industrialised economy had made pauperisation in later life a problem particularly amongst the deracinated urban working class. The determination of individual agedness needed reliable, impersonal methods which had not been necessary in smaller rural communities whose economy had been dominated by the relations of land ownership and systems of household production.

Proposals for state old age pension schemes appeared toward the end of the eighteenth century. Political philosophers such as the Marquis de Condorcet in France and Thomas Paine and Francis Maseres in Britain began making the case for some form of universal pension to support citizens in later life, although the exact ages proposed for these pensions varied from fifty to seventy (Condorcet 1795; Maseres 1792; Paine 1792). As industrialisation progressed local charities and the poor law system struggled to cope with the demands for urban poor relief. Wider political debates emerged about providing for old age through a system of pensions instead of poor relief. While these debates took time to resolve, they succeeded in narrowing considerably the range of ages at which old age was considered to begin (Roebuck 1979).

In premodernity, before chronological age mattered so much, old age had been deemed to start at any point from the late thirties to the early nineties (Zerbi 1988, 29; see also Minois, 1989; Gilbert 1967). The careful counting of one's years was of concern to a literate few. Even after the systematic registration of births and deaths in the nineteenth century, many people remained ignorant of or mistaken about their calculated age. At the beginning of the twentieth century, people would often alter their age to gain entry to jobs, to the military or to help them marry or gain a pension (Budd and Guinnane 1991; Ó Gradá 2002; Woods 2000). Perhaps this had long been the case, but from this point such ignorance and distortions mattered more as the officials of local and national government had the means to check personal accounts of age with 'official' records. By the middle of the twentieth century chronological age and date of birth had become civic identifiers appearing in nearly all forms of private and public documentation.

At this high point of first modernity, agedness was defined and understood almost entirely in chronological terms. The physical appearance of age was gradually pushed from the public sphere, though still residing within the domain of personal concerns.

Exact ages for pension entitlements, for men and women, varied considerably during the first half of the twentieth century, but the debates were not concerned with identifying biological markers and had more to do with identifying acceptable political boundaries and feasible national resources. With one or two exceptions, medicine too showed little concern with the ageing body until the Second World War created a new concern over ageing bodies occupying potential soldiers' beds. Only when modernity underwent its own reflexive transformation, after the 1960s, would the personal concerns of ageing bodies gradually re-emerge as sites of contestation within the newly established somatic society and its cultivation of the desiring, perfectible body. At this point there was a turn to the body but it was to a new ageing body not a return to the body of old age that had dominated premodernity.

Second Modernity and the 'Return' to the Body

The demise of 'classical' modernity has been associated with the rise of a somatic society, where the body re-emerged as an important signifier of social distinction. Beginning in the 1980s a number of sociologists started to draw attention to this phenomenon. Bryan Turner argued that 'the prominence and pervasiveness of images of the body in popular and consumer culture [...] and [...] [t]he emphases on pleasure, desire, difference and playfulness [...] are part of a cultural environment [...] brought about by [...] post industrialism, postfordisnm and postmodernism' (Turner 1984, 2). Another sociologist, Pasi Falk also observed how in modern society [*sic*] 'the signs surrounding the body act [...] as ways of expressing and/or creating the individual identity or self of the subject' (Falk 1985, 124). Similar sentiments were expressed by Mike Featherstone, who wrote that 'within consumer culture, the body is proclaimed as a vehicle for pleasure [...] and the closer the actual body approximates to the idealised images of youth, health, fitness and beauty, the higher its exchange value' (Featherstone 1982, 21). Featherstone was perhaps the first sociologist to see how postwar consumer culture treated the body not as a solid source of meaning but as if it were plastic. He saw it as a form of personal capital capable, with appropriate body work, of increasing in value to the cultural and social credit of its owner. The work of Bauman and Foucault as well as other writers such as Lipovetsky was also equally caught up with the control, exercise and fashioning of the body in the variously termed 'late', 'liquid', 'reflexive', 'post' or 'second' modernity. In this period of transformation what most marked out the changes was the emergence of a mass consumer society, with 'higher standard of living, abundance of goods and services, cult of objects and leisure [...] [and] a hedonistic and materialistic morality' (Lipovetsky 2002, 134). The expansion of the market and the media, alongside the growth in personal affluence, the democratisation of fashion and the increasingly individualised opportunities for recreational leisure, served to establish a 'postmodern' culture in which the body served as a focus, a point of orientation and a canvas for expressing personal identity (Crane 2000). This preoccupation with the body – evident in the various discourses and practices concerning fashion and entertainment, sex and sexuality, leisure and lifestyles – first and foremost affected young people. Significantly, this concern with the body permeated all social classes and crossed the divides of gender, 'race' and sexual identity. It halted, however, at the boundaries of age and generation.

As the 1960s' cultural 'revolution' re-oriented individuals toward the body, various 'repressed' sources of bodily distinction came to occupy the centre ground. Within this ferment of culture and counter-culture, age – or ageing – simply didn't count. Age was either a negative, an absent presence foregrounding youth, or it was simply ignored. 'Youth' and 'youthfulness' defined the outline of the cultural revolution. Youth culture was both process and outcome. Realised in and through 'appearance', the new somatic cultures were oriented away from 'old age' – an orientation exemplified in the iconic lines of The Who's 1964 song, 'My Generation' where they sang 'hope I die before I get old'. Only later, as the members of these bands themselves grew older, would the ageing of youth culture become a more critical element in somatic society.

How should we understand this period of change and how does it help us to understand the changing cultural significance and social importance of bodily ageing? What is perhaps least controversial is that sometime between the mid-1950s and the early 1970s, a cultural shift swept rapidly across much of the Western world setting one generation against another. This was the rebirth of a 'youth culture' that almost before taking flight seemed to have collapsed under the great depression of the 1930s and the subsequent world war; it was a transition from popular to mass culture; from an industrial to a post-industrial society and, for many, a revolution in their personal life and their way of living. Expressed at the time as the 'swinging sixties', it was a time of excitement and rising expectations, when there seemed to be a palpable sense across many groups and classes that things were 'getting better'. What exactly the 1960s heralded is difficult to define with any precision, but for the purposes of this book (as it was for our *Contexts of Ageing*), we shall focus upon this period as primarily a 'cultural' ferment which created a profound, generational schism that set apart the 'old' and the 'new', and by analogy, the young and the aged. This schism set in motion a transformation in the way we think about, understand, represent and even experience all aspects of personal life that eventually included ageing and later life. This latter change was least evident during the 1960s. Why this was so and why it has nevertheless proved so significant in shaping 'the new ageing' is the next topic for this chapter.

Age and the 'Rebel Sell'

During the 'long' 1960s, most of the working age population saw their standards of living rise, their homes become palpably richer and their children's education and health improve. Those exiting the labour market benefited little, if at all, from these changes. The sexual revolution, the democratisation of fashion, the expanding array of self-care cosmetic and beauty products, and the desires for self-expression, authenticity and personal liberation that variously privileged the body depended heavily upon the experience of rising levels of discretionary income amongst young people. While the continuities of kinship and family maintained a moral identity for many older people, this achievement was itself gendered. The links between ageing mothers and their adult daughters survived and even thrived, but men's increasingly regimented retirement left them with little sense of purpose or identity. In the male breadwinner ethos of modernity, men's identities were conferred largely by their work. Their lifestyle was structured by their jobs and their wives. Freedom and self-expression were to be found, if anywhere, in pubs and bars, their consumerism constrained to the consolations of their companions.

Throughout the decades either side of the 1960s, the ageing body was of concern only to the various nationalised health care systems that were being consolidated in Europe and in North America, the latter secured for the old and the poor alone, by the passage of the Medicare and Medicaid legislation that formed part of the 1965 Social Security Act. Unlike young bodies, ageing bodies could only become salient as *objects* of otherness, assessed examined and judged for evidence of disablement and disease, in the case of geriatrics, or of disablement and need in the case of gerontology. There was no other market for the ageing body and without a market no public expression – or recognition – of the ageing body as a desiring body. Outside the hospital and the nursing home, the invisibility of the ageing body was as complete as the economic marginality of the older citizen. Not simply marginalised by their lack of paid labour, older people were equally marginal as consumers throughout the 1950s and 1960s (Goldstein 1968, 1971).

The influence of older people upon the new culture was limited to serving as representatives of everything it was not – not new, but old. Throughout this early stage of second modernity the body that mattered most, mattered principally to the market. The market witnessed its greatest expansion in the entertainment, media, retail and self-care industries that were all oriented toward fashion, beauty, skin colour, hairstyle, sexuality, dance and music, in short to the concerns of a newly affluent youth. Since the late 1950s, makeup had become a universal element in teenage girls' lives; aftershave and hair cream entered the lives of adolescent boys a little later. Throughout the 1950s and early 1960s, makeup and hair cream were unknown amongst most people aged forty and over (Peiss 1998, 170). Likewise for fashion; in the boutiques that flourished in the 1960s and 1970s the principal customers were young people with sufficient discretionary spending power to go shopping regularly. Men and women over fifty were neither seen nor welcome in these age segregated settings of consumption; they were forced to choose their clothes from more traditional outlets such as the large department stores or the cheaper market stalls. People at or approaching retirement age in the 1960s were living and consuming on the wrong side of the generation gap.

Not only were older people on the wrong side of the generation gap, they were also on the wrong side of the material divide separating postwar affluence from the prewar impoverishment that non-working life retained. Most European accounts written in the 1950s and 1960s emphasise the poverty, isolation and unhappiness of old people. Writing of the situation in France, Simone de Beauvoir stated 'It is common knowledge that the condition of old people today is scandalous' (de Beauvoir 1977, 271). She went on to catalogue their near starvation and their dying through hunger (ibid.), their loneliness (ibid., 281) their poor housing (ibid., 279) and the sense of sheer uselessness amongst old people whom she saw condemned to 'a half life that amounts to no more than a waiting for death' (ibid., 308). Similar comments about the hardship faced by French pensioners in the 1950s and 1960s can be found in John Ardagh's book *The New France: A Society in Transition, 1945–1973* when he notes that 'those who live on their pensions alone can rarely afford meat or new clothes or proper heating or any kind of entertainment' (Ardagh 1973, 430). These sentiments were echoed in contemporary English accounts. In his book *The Family Life of Old People*, Peter Townsend wrote how 'so many men talked of retirement as a tragedy. They were forced to recognise that it was not their working life which was over, it was their life [...] their life became a rather desperate search for pastimes or a gloomy contemplation of their own helplessness' (Townsend 1963, 169). For Townsend, writing of life in the 1950s in London's East End, the only real bastion sustaining the well-being of old people, or at least old women's, seemed to be the three generation family 'generally distributed over two or more households near to one another' and the ties of kith and kin (ibid.). Apart from this, ageing and old age had nothing to sell.

From Division to Difference: The Eclipse of the Old Ageing

Even as Peter Townsend was writing his book on old age, the patterns of kinship he was writing about were beginning to disappear. New housing initiatives offered a way up the social hierarchy for more and more families. Many of these old close-knit neighbourhoods were falling apart, a process that a host of British community studies sought to document throughout the 1960s. A decade later and not just the communities but community studies themselves were pronounced dead (Bell and Newby 1971, Macfarlane 1977). Life had moved on, and the position of older people was beginning to shift, though it would take more than a decade before ageing moved from being framed entirely through material neediness and corporeal dysfunction to become a site of contestation over embodiment and identity. For that to happen, further changes were needed.

As first modernity gave way to second modernity, those whose identities and lifestyles had been most inflected by the cultural ferment of the 1960s found themselves growing older. Their youth was fast becoming a view in the rear mirror of their journey through life. The turn to the body and the cult of the new that had once exercised such an energising, liberating effect was beginning to pose new problems through a different kind of 'difference'. Some of the premodern preoccupation with ageing and the appearance of the aged body began to re-emerge, but in a different social, cultural and material form. Looking old and being old were becoming personal problems for those whose sense of identity had been fashioned by the plasticity of 1960s youth subcultures. It was time to give ageing another look.

Thinking through the Body, about Ageing, Differently

From the 1980s, a re-orientation in attitudes toward ageing and the body can be discerned in many Western societies. Fashion and cosmetics and to some extent advertising imagery began to address the prospects not of creating but of sustaining the image of 'youth' longer and later in life. Bodily ageing re-entered popular culture, but in a different way, through the rhetoric of rejuvenation for all. The experiences of those cohorts who were born in the 1940s, of contacts and engagement with bodies both different and similar to their own, of personal discovery and do-it-yourself lifestyles, of enhanced self-care and reflexive self-regard, served to create the conditions under which the old chronological habitus of age could be challenged. Mixed with the old fears about old age were new hopes for ageing differently, for not having to become old on other people's terms.

Age represented a late life return of the adolescent 'identity crisis' first outlined by Erik Erikson (1963) for those growing up in the period after the Second World War. This was a crisis experienced by the members of this particular cohort who were becoming middle-aged in ways quite unlike those of first modernity (Heath 2009). Age, it was increasingly said, 'ain't nothing but a number', just like 'race' was nothing but a colour and gender a matter of how one performed sex. In the neologism of the time sixty was the new thirty (Cravit 2008; Jagger 2005). Earlier promises of remaining 'forever feminine' competed with new promises, of remaining 'forever functional' (Marshall and Katz 2002). Along with smart looks and effective self-care, a healthy sex life was becoming an essential part of 'successful' ageing (Goodson 2010; Vares 2009).

The 'coming of the body' (Juvin 2010), ushered in by the cultural revolution of the 1960s, was reaching later life. While this 'return to the body' contributed positively to the de-institutionalisation/de-standardisation of ageing, it created new uncertainties and stimulated old anxieties about the cultural and social location of age and particularly of old age. The traditional view that linked the social and biological organisation of ageing to old age had been challenged. Alternative embodied identities asserted themselves within the lives of those who were chronologically no longer young. The resilience of these alternatively 'embodied identities', such as those oriented toward ethnicity, gender, fitness and sexuality, rendered more contingent both the nature and the naturalness of ageing. As chronological age ceased to exercise its monopoly over the organisation and control of resources directed toward 'old age', the fears and confusion surrounding its 'identity' rendered age a more unstable and contested system of social categorisation and individual distinction.

It is not just that other competing sources of identity and other forms of bodily distinction intruded into later life. The body itself became subject to a range of 'somatic technologies' whose points of reference outgrew their 'commoditisation' within the 1960s' counter-cultures and sub-cultures. These technologies and practices are no longer so carefully policed and boundaried, as they first were, by age. Variously expressed as 'appearance management' (Cahill 1989; Goffman 1971), 'body maintenance' (Featherstone 1982), 'body work' (Gimlin 2002; Twigg and Atkin 2000) or 'bodysense' (Coleman 1990) the fashioning and refashioning of the body has become a lifelong enterprise and, perhaps, a lifelong chore. The greater their penetration into everyday life, the more they undermine the stability that previously was attached to identities that were embodied as 'foundationalist' social forms. The result is greater individualisation of the body, rendering it subject to the processes of 'lifestyle' rather than 'lifestage' fashioning, as the underlying 'expression of human individuality' (Lipovetsky 2002, 5). Treating one's body as a 'lifestyle' project, always subject to change and betterment, has become an ageless motif in contemporary consumer culture. The possibilities of alternative embodiments once intended only for youth have broken through the boundaries of age. As bodies of difference, whether corporeal or embodied, we are defined, at all times, as forever 'desiring subjects'.

Corporeality, Embodiment and the 'New' Ageing

Bodily ageing – both in terms of its corporeality and its embodiment – has long been contested and the practices of prolongevity and rejuvenation go back centuries (Gruman 2003). There is something distinctive, however, in the way that contemporary contestations over ageing have transformed the way that ageing is interpreted, experienced, represented and understood by a new generation of older people. Chronology and corporeality have become disconnected as the relationship between age's corporeality and its embodiment has become more fluid than before. As sources of social identity, ageing and agedness have become less easily read off the body and chronological age has become less acceptable and less adequate in representing people as 'aged', 'elderly' or simply 'old'. The 'new ageing' that has emerged over the last 20 years or so is more ambivalent about, yet more invested in, age's fleshy corporeality. 'Ageing well' is no longer a matter of transcending the materiality of the body by attributing to age a particular spiritual or civic virtue, such as that attempted by the thinkers of the past, or more recently by those advocating 'gero-transcendence' (Tornstam 1996). Nor is it feasible to return to the issues of first modernity and reify age within the 'moral economy' of the life course (Hendricks 2005; Minkler and Cole 1991). The new ageing seeks a continuing engagement with the body, but under different terms. These include negotiating a wider performative space for ageing and the development of a richer set of narratives through which ageing can be experienced, interpreted, represented or understood.

Within the new ageing, the corporeality of old age, once a central pillar in the construction of a universalised model of ageing, has increasingly been revealed as both less solid and more contingent. Its embodiment – the way people 'act' or 'show' their age – varies more widely than before. As newer cohorts of 'over sixties' replace older cohorts, changes have become embodied in what Bourdieu (1977) might call the 'habitus' of later life, through increased levels of discretionary spending, greater levels of physical activity, more attention to diet and fitness regimes, more frequent recourse to cosmetic and rejuvenative technologies and the rise of what the Gergens have called 'sybaritic lifestyles' in later life (Gergen and Gergen 2000).

Age's 'mattering', to use Cheah's term, (Cheah 1996) is expressed through the social and the contingent while its essentialism as 'old age' has become a more 'imaginary' presence that no longer rests upon unproblematic corporeal foundations. Conceived of as existing within a matrix of corporeality and embodiment, bodily ageing has become increasingly contested as a signifier of identity, position or place. It is negotiated in and through the social– whether this contestation is over the terms of the body's objectification, or over the potential subjectivities that 'desiring' persons still seek, in later life, to express through their bodies.

But even as bodily ageing is re-imagined by the new ageing and in the narratives and performances of its still desiring subjects, agedness itself remains cast within the old discourses and dividing practices of an earlier set of assumptions. Within the responsible social institutions, old age was and still is 'frailed'. Biomedical social and behavioural gerontology persist in representing the ageing body as an object of health needs and social 'oppression'. Only rarely do these disciplines represent it as a site where individuals engage in what Foucault called the 'agonisms', or struggles of modern subjectivity (Foucault 1982, 222). At the heart of the new ageing lies a 'resistance' to these no longer modern gerontological scripts, a declining to decline, as Gullette (1997) has so succinctly put it and a refusal not so much to age, as to become old on other people's terms.

Why the Body?

This then is the aim of our book, to explore the effortful, agonistic processes of identity-work and lifestyling in later life which we see being conducted in and through the body. The body in later life, we will argue, needs to be viewed as a site of 'positive' agency where social 'difference' is performed, contested and renegotiated. The 'new' ageing as practice, narrative and as experience has made it more possible than previously for the body in later life to become a site for the expression of identities and lifestyles that are other than aged, other than old. In making this claim, we do not argue that only the body provides the material base from which to explore the new ageing. As we have argued elsewhere, the body is part of a triumvirate of 'sites' along with 'self-hood' and 'citizenship', where the new cultures of ageing are realised (Gilleard and Higgs 2000). The body is particularly critical to this new agenda, however, because unlike issues of citizenship and self-hood, it has been treated as the 'limiting condition' for developing other forms of citizenship and self-renewal in later life. Major texts of the new ageing, such as Laslett's *New Map of Life* (1989), the Gergens' chapter on 'The New Aging' (Gergen and Gergen 2000) or the edited volume, *Productive Aging: Concepts and Challenges* by Nancy Morrow-Howell, James Hinterlong and Michael Sherraden (2001) have all passed over the question of the body to address more general issues of civic contribution, personal consumption or employment opportunities in later life. We want to focus on the body not as some kind of 'asocial' corporeality out-trumping the capacity of culture, society and the economy to determine human lives, but as itself, an always-emerging site for embodiment from which new ageing lifestyles can be fashioned.

Three developments seem central to us in understanding the changing role of the body and its significance for the new ageing. The first has been the emergence of a politics of identity, concerned with issues of 'embodied difference' as well as the social and personal concerns that have accompanied this; second, has been the somatic turn that postwar mass consumer society has helped shape and support; and third has been the influence of a generational consciousness framed by the 1960s generational schism which has incorporated and retained the cultural turn within its lifestyles and has thereby changed societal expectations about ageing. These developments have created the conditions for a number of alternative embodiments of age. Many of these began by privileging the youthful body as a vehicle through which change comes, actively excluding or marginalising age or treating it as a symbol of all that must be overcome. With time the processes of reconstructing, re-segmenting and revisioning the body have seen 'a return of the repressed' and the issues of ageing have re-emerged within the context of a more personalised politics and a more extensively commodified society.

Much of the emphasis in the texts about the new ageing has been about what people in later life can do, the roles they can perform – their productive 'potential' realised as citizens and selves. Less emphasis has been placed on them as desiring, performing and resisting bodies. Only in the field of cultural gerontology have there been attempts to deal directly with the embodiment of the new ageing and its constant provocation with 'the corporeal inevitability of ageing […] [as] permanent reality' (Blaikie 2002, 107). Refusing to adjudicate in Jones and Higgs' (2010) terms between the natural, the normal and the normative framing of ageing's embodiment, writers working within the cultural gerontological framework have begun to draw upon other intellectual traditions to engage with these new forms of embodiment in later life. Thus ideas from critical race theory, disability theory, radical feminism as well as queer theory have been used to develop alternative understandings of the role of the body in shaping later life narratives and in realising later life performances (Calasanti 1993; Conway-Turner 1995; Oldman 2002; Sandberg 2008). While not uncritical of such post-structuralist theorising, especially its tendency to drift into textual analysis, it is this area of emerging practice with which we too wish to engage in our work on ageing and the body. Consequently, in subsequent chapters we shall explore the relevance that other embodied identities – specifically those of gender, race, disability and sexuality – have for understanding the embodiment of ageing and more generally for helping us think about ageing, through the body, *differently*.

Chapter 3

GENDER, AGEING AND EMBODIMENT

We begin our exploration of corporeality, embodiment and ageing with the issue of gender. We have chosen to start with this topic for two reasons. First, because the transformation of the terms 'sex' and 'sexual difference' into the more socially oriented term 'gender' served as a major vector through which the body emerged as a source and signifier of socially constituted forms of 'difference'; and second, because gender provides one of the most important vehicles through which the embodiment of ageing can be examined. The 1960s' sexual revolution involved a 'rejection of the biological determinism implicit in the use of such terms as "sex" or "sexual difference"' (Scott 1986, 1054). In their place, the growing use of the term 'gender' directed attention away from the individual, isolated body to the relational distinction between men and women, while also reflecting the *social* organisation of both sexuality and gender. The transformation of sex from a biological category into gender as a sociological identity led to a rethinking of the distinction between bodies as corporeal entities and bodies as social identities. In short it allowed for thinking *about* and thinking *through* the body differently. The 'second wave' feminist writers who emerged during the 1960s initiated this shift in approach which has since been incorporated into the new 'sociology of the body' and which is now beginning to impact upon the 'new ageing'.

Writers such as Shulamith Firestone, Betty Frieden, Kate Millett and Juliet Mitchell were instrumental in reconsidering how the position of women in society, the relationships between men and women and the institutions that support these relationships turned the corporeality of sexual difference into the social identity of 'gender'. For them, the term 'gender' became a way of recognising and reading the body as a kind of 'social text' while the signification of sex as gender moved considerations of bodily identity away from the particular shape, size, colour and configuration of bodies to the ways that social institutions framed and organised them in relation to other differently configured bodies. Since the 'deconstruction' of the sexed or gendered body was undertaken within second wave feminism, the emphasis for that deconstruction was placed largely on *women's* identity, *women's* bodies and *women's* roles – initially leaving men's identity as bodies unexplored, until the more recent emergence of 'men's studies'.

Within second wave feminism, Caddick has argued that two distinct, if related, approaches toward gendered identity can be discerned, which she has described as following a structuralist or a cultural reading of 'difference' (Caddick 1986). While both approaches shared the view that women's bodies are oppressed by the constraints placed on their identity as women and that women needed to be 'liberated' from this oppression, the way that gender and sex are 'embodied' by these approaches differed considerably. The first re-positioned the body by moving its 'nature' or 'corporeality' into the background, foregrounding a more 'structural' account of men and women's position and role within modern society and specifically its relations of production. This deconstruction of sex and gender was influenced by Engels' idea that gender relations constituted the source of class relations. While critically aware of the long history of Marxist approaches to the problem of gender, or what was often called 'the woman question', these writers sought not so much to replace them but rather to expand and enlarge their materialist foundations (Millett 1972; Mitchell 1971). To understand how men and women are positioned in relation to each other, they argued, it was first necessary to understand the economic and social relationships of men and women to each other, as well as their physical and sexual relationships. Just as the proletariat cannot be defined in Marxist theory without reference to the bourgeoisie or disabled people defined without reference to able-bodiedness, so men and women in these revisions could not be defined without reference to their social relationship to each other. This formulation led to the identification of a distinct power differential that advantaged men and oppressed women. This binary relationship, whose corporeal distinction as 'sex' had been essentialised in historically particular social and economic circumstances, was seen to be imbricated in the power relationships of a theory of 'patriarchy'.

The term 'patriarchy' has been used in different ways by different writers (Cliff 1984; Vogel 1995) but it has generally been used to describe women's social and economic oppression in a society that privileges men. The corporealities of sexual difference – the material, biological distinctions between men and women – were seen to be particularly problematic in that they constituted a key dimension of women's oppression. To overthrow such oppression it was necessary to re-embody gender in ways that enabled men and women to occupy more equal positions within the relations of production, while minimising the significance and consequences of corporeal difference – for example through state supported infant and childcare, and flexible working arrangements. As Mitchell wrote in terms very redolent of the early 1970s: 'feminism is the terrain on which a socialist analysis works [...] the oppressed consciousness of all groups contributes to the nature of this socialist ideology [...] [and] if any oppressed awareness is missing from its formation that is its loss' (Mitchell 1971, 96).

In contrast to this structuralist approach to gender relationships, a number of other feminist writers sought to deconstruct the nature of 'difference' itself, focusing upon the oppression suffered by and through women's *bodies* rather than by the inequalities they faced in the labour market. Calling for women to develop a new consciousness, to think about their sense of self and identity 'through the body', writers like Betty Friedan, Germaine Greer and Gloria Steinem sought to connect the oppression of women with the oppression of their bodies, and particularly, with their sexuality. Beginning with Friedan's feminist classic *The Feminine Mystique* (1963), this approach was developed in the book *Our Bodies, Ourselves* which was collectively written by the Boston Women's Health Book Collective ([1973] 1984). Written as a guide for women to take control over their own bodies and to maintain and manage their own health and sexuality themselves, self-care was promoted as a route to liberation. Attention to one's body served as evidence of one's self-esteem, while such 'thinking through the body' (Gallop 1988) reflected the way that the political awareness of women's position as an 'oppressed other' was necessarily mediated by and through personal experience. A more reflexive understanding of gender was realised by 'consciousness raising', a technique linked to the Chinese Cultural Revolution's practice of 'speaking bitterness', whose aim was to explore the collective political dimensions of personal experience. 'Consciousness raising' within the women's movement helped women discover a shared identity in their gendering and the commonality of an oppression that had been hidden by the isolating privacy of women's experience of sex and their bodies (Mitchell 1971, 62).

While many of the radical elements of women's liberation and its advocacy of difference have survived, the structuralist approach espoused by Firestone, Millett and the early Mitchell has receded, perhaps because, as Marshall has suggested, they still equated 'the masculine with the human' and advocated a model of society 'in which the female body disappears – transcended in the name of individualist and implicitly "malestream" culture' (Marshall 1994, 254). The search for a unity of the oppressed, one to which all marginalised groups could connect (in the 1960s, this included black people, the young, women and the poor) was short lived. The market for such revolutionary radicalism rapidly fragmented and by the early 1970s, individual bodies were aligning themselves with distinct 'communities' of difference, each claiming its own identity and pursuing its own struggles to create and sustain 'authentic' lifestyles.

Out of this feminist tradition of difference, however, a more culturalist approach to understanding bodily difference emerged. It was influenced particularly by the work of Michel Foucault, as we have previously asserted. As McNay noted, Foucault's 'theory of power and the body indicate[d] to feminists a way of placing a notion of the body at the centre of women's oppression' (McNay 1992, 11). In place of earlier concerns over the nature of 'patriarchy' and its role in exerting oppression, these 'post-structuralist' approaches sought to problematise the body as the key site of oppression. To counter oppression, they argued, demanded a fundamental questioning of the stability of the corporeal boundaries and the material and social 'constituents' that framed the embodied identities of 'men' and 'women'. The fluidity and 'relationality' embodied by the identity of gender was a theme subsequently pursued by writers such as Judith Butler (1990, 1993) Elizabeth Grosz (1994) and Luce Irigaray (1985).

As stated in Chapter 1, for some feminist writers theorising bodily identity as a social process has become something of a balancing act. As Cheah has noted there is a danger either of repeating modernity's binary 'essentialisms' of sex and gender but stripped of their modern corporeal referents or of losing sight entirely of the body's substantive corporeality by an 'ideology of the body' that is only understandable as and through disembodied text (Cheah 1996). This difficulty is illustrated when Butler states 'it must be possible to concede and affirm an array of "materialities" that pertain to the body, that which is signified by the domains of biology, anatomy, physiology, hormonal and chemical composition, illness, age, weight, metabolism, life and death' (Butler 1993, 66).

Here Bulter lists age as one of an array of 'materialities' that include anatomy, biology and physiology but which exclude gender (and race and other 'embodied' identities). Yet if one is not born but becomes 'a woman' or a 'man', how much less is one born 'old'? The problem is not whether sex or age matters to men and women (or to those who feel no allegiance to either genders) but the ways in which they matter. To quote Elizabeth Grosz: 'the specificity of bodies must be understood in its historical rather than simply in its biological concreteness' (Grosz 1994, 19). To make sense of the contingent relationship between gender and ageing, then, that relationship itself needs to be viewed in its historical perspective. It is to the history of this relationship we now turn.

Ageing and the Traditions of Gender

Expectations of how older people look and behave and the status attributed to ageing have long been understood through a gendered lens (Shahar 1994). In pre-modern European society, older men were traditionally invested with the *'patria potestas'* of seniority; older women benefited little if at all from their longevity. Differentials in age at marriage – men typically marrying women younger than themselves – made widowhood a common experience at all points in women's married life. As a result, along with orphans and the chronic sick, widows formed one of the principal groups amongst the deserving poor. Morally deserving, they were seen as weak, frail vessels, lacking in intrinsic authority. While older men were unconstrained in their freedom to remarry and to father children when and as they wished, older women were not. Marginalised within civic society, individual widows did on occasion exercise considerable economic and social influence, managing large estates and controlling significant resources of both capital and labour. But despite these anomalies, most men managed to maintain or improve their status with age while women experienced a diminution in theirs. Even in early nineteenth century France, de Beauvoir claimed that 'the patriarchal family continued to exist in the country and the authority of the old man who ruled it might be tyrannical' (de Beauvoir 1977, 218). Such seems to have been the case throughout the pre-modern era.

Just as seniority tended to confer status through maleness, so the male appearance dominated portrayals of age. In the illustrations, paintings, sculpture and writings of the pre-modern period, the old people who appear are principally old men, highlighted by their white hair, sallow faces, jowled cheeks and high, domed foreheads. In so far as the appearance of ageing serves to represent its status, until the dawn of modernity ageing and agedness retained a distinctly masculine appearance (Minois 1989). If present, old women were portrayed as hags or paupers, with their agedness typically clothed in rags (Sohm 2007). The nude ageing body was rarely painted or sculpted and when it was it was typically modelled on the sculpture of Ancient Greece, placing an old man's head on a young man's body. Most pre-modern representations of aged men were of their heads and faces or as fully clothed figures given stature by their long cloaks of wisdom and authority. Narratives of ageing and the bodily changes accompanying ageing were equally men's accounts of men's ageing. Until the modern period, little interest was shown in describing women's ageing, beyond the occasional expressions of scorn and distaste activated by thoughts of older women as sexually active, predatory beings, or in Leonardo da Vinci's words, as 'infernal furies' (Sohm 2007, 21).

With the emergence of industrial society, age came to be understood through the different, if equally limiting, discourses of productive labour. From the eighteenth century, ageing was typified for both men and women as a time of declining powers and increasing impoverishment. At the same time, men and women were represented in a less unequal manner and by the nineteenth century old men and women were both painted more accurately and more sympathetically, 'usually framed in order to demonstrate the physiognomic evidence of a virtuous character' or to demonstrate that 'old age does have a part to play' (Blaikie and Hepworth 1997, 107–8). Modernity began to roll back the pre-modern stereotyping of ageing as embodied by an exclusive masculinity as the earlier focus on the bodily appearance of age and ageing was replaced by concerns over age's economic and social significance, and particularly its significance as an indicator of poverty, lack and want. But even as a non-corporeal, chronologically framed age began to replace the earlier gendered versions of ageing it was still men's ageing that dominated its representation. Nevertheless, having moved the focus from the visible corporeality of age to its reified chronology, the old gendered dominance of age by men would become less complete as modernity advanced.

The modern nation state located men's ageing within an 'institutionalised life course'. Education, employment and retirement from work provided the social template governing the various transitions from childhood to old age (Anderson 1985; Kohli 1986). While these socialised transitions became the defining features of men's life course, 'nature' and the somatic still framed those of women. For women, education and employment were squeezed together into childhood and youth, while marriage, child rearing and household management provided the domestic anchors of an adulthood that continued more or less uninterrupted, unless, and until, illness or widowhood intervened. Old age, tragic old age was, for most women, confined to the experience of an impoverished widowhood. As men's age at death increased, widowhood increasingly marked women's transition to later life. The menopause remained a matter of relative indifference; a silent marker of women's ageing that only began attracting medical attention in the nineteenth century. More than before, the bodily experience of women's – and men's – ageing was rendered subservient to their functional role in the production and reproduction of labour.

Industrialisation and the transformation of social and to some extent economic relations saw the first wave of the women's movement emerge at the end of the nineteenth and beginning of the twentieth century (Rowbotham 2011). Unlike second wave feminism, this first phase was not confined to youth nor was it pre-occupied by youth's fears and desires. As Kate Millett pointed out, it began with the women's emancipation movement, a movement that was consciously linked to the movement for the emancipation of slavery initiated earlier in the nineteenth century (Millett 1971, 80). It was framed within a distinctly Victorian ideology that assumed women's right to the vote was based upon the civic equality of men and women, an equality that existed as an ideal within the conjugal family. It assumed a differential in the development of maturity, since women's initial political enfranchisement occurred at an older age (30 years) than men's (21 years). Few, if any, presumptions were made concerning biological or economic equality. Even Engels, who supported the idea of women having universal access to education and employment, wrote within the framework of a Victorian understanding of sexuality – as witness his view that the emergence of patriarchy and women's consent to the 'rule' of monogamous marriage was because women felt this arrangement 'protected' them, by its very exclusivity, from their being exposed to the sexual and social predations of 'the ancient community of men' (Engels cited in Millett 1971, 116).

Throwing off the shackles of the domestic sphere led suffragettes to be labelled 'unsexed' by their opponents. Their public claim to be heard was seen as proof of their lack of 'femininity' (Carstens 2011, 64). Despite the impact of the First World War, women's improved access to education and employment, much 'scientific' thinking about sexual differences was still dominated by the late Victorian belief that an inner biological destiny determined women's lives (Jordanova 1989). Nature, expressed in terms of the 'inner secretions' that ruled women's lives, was seen as governing women's life course, from the onset of menstruation to the menopause and beyond. In contrast, men's lifecycle was framed not by the workings of their bodies but by the work their bodies performed.

The late nineteenth and early twentieth century pre-occupation with the impoverishment consequent upon old age and the need for some form of old age pensions reflected the pre-occupation with men's ageing and their associated loss of earning power (Rowntree 1902). Their ageing appearance and declining sexuality remained private concerns that only 'leaked' into the public sphere in the 'roaring twenties', 'an era that celebrated youth and the [...] cult of outdoor vitality, strength and beauty' (Haycock 2008, 182). Since women's social and economic status throughout adult life was seen to depend upon the stability and longevity of her marriage, her husband's earning powers and the support available from her family, the somatic course taken by women's ageing remained of less concern to all but members of the elite.

The Western representation of women and their life course that had been built up during the late nineteenth and early twentieth centuries began to unravel in the 'roaring' 1920s, at the same time as older men were beginning to express more publicly their concerns over maintaining intellectual vigour and physical and sexual prowess (Hirshbein 2000). The First World War had required women to 'man' large sectors of the productive economy. The impetus this gave to demands for civic equality did not end with the gaining of the vote. A growing number of young women stayed on in the work force, acquiring 'white collar' positions and exercising a degree of financial independence, buying into the new fashions, hairstyles and cosmetics that the new media – the cinema and magazines particularly – advertised. Many women cut their hair short, flattened their chests and some began wearing suits in what was seen at the time as an excessively 'mannish' fashion. The emergence of this 'new' woman, though demographically exaggerated, nevertheless brought new anxieties. As one US survey put it: 'modern women have awakened to the knowledge that they are sexual beings. And with this new insight, the sex side of marriage has assumed sudden importance' (Blanchard and Monasses 1930, cited in Dumenil 1995, 131).

This 'first wave' fragmentation of the divide between the sexes was soon overshadowed first by the Depression and then by the Second World War. Politically enfranchised, but economically constrained, women's equality was still largely confined to the domestic sphere. Even in the USA, the leading economic power of the period, less than one woman in three was in paid employment before the country entered Second World War (Dumenil 1995). Since the early decades of the twentieth century, women's sexuality had been acknowledged – and celebrated – but strictly within marriage. Outside it was still condemned and despite the momentary stimulus of the 'roaring twenties', women's civic status remained located in their role in reproduction, child rearing, domestic management and the exercise of moral influence over family (Rowbotham 2011). Subject to a nature now represented by her recently discovered 'fluctuating hormones' (Oudshoorn 1994; Roberts 2000), yet charged with the stabilising responsibilities of being both mother and wife, women's position at the mid-point of the twentieth century was presaged upon a dubious domestic equality that never really challenged the dominant model of the male breadwinner household. Men still controlled and over-determined the public sphere while understandings and representations of ageing were still shaped by men's presence – and by their anxieties (de Beauvoir 1977). Ageing, as a woman's issue, would only emerge after the generational schism of the 1960s and its *soi-disant* sexual revolution.

Gender and the Generational Schism of the 1960s

Second wave feminism began as part of the 'youth oriented' new social movements of the 1960s. Developing and expanding the work that had been started earlier in the twentieth century, second wave feminism was linked to the civil rights movement of the 1950s and the demand in the USA for a materially and culturally realisable racial equality. This desire for 'liberation' reflected the postwar decolonisation movements in Africa and Asia and the globalised desire of the young everywhere to be free of the old (Mitchell 1971). The 'sexual politics' that emerged from this ferment went beyond questions of suffrage and civic representation that were so central to 'first modernity'. Feminist activists and writers were not just challenging women's social and economic inequality; they were challenging women's invisibility and exclusion, and the taken for granted assumptions of maleness that pervaded all aspects of the public sphere. Denying the once privileged but now questioned biological determinants of male power, the new women's movement argued that gender differences stemmed first and foremost from the social arrangements of a patriarchal society which placed women as men's property rather than their partners, and not from any assumed inferiority in their corporeal constitution.

Relationships of 'real' equality were represented through the enactment of alternative sexualities. Lesbian (and gay) relationships were viewed as particularly challenging to patriarchy. The new birth control technologies gave young women direct access to the means of controlling sexual reproduction in a way that previously had not been possible, freeing them from the constraints of marriage and monogamy. Second wave feminism centred as much on freedom from oppression and equality within all social relationships as it did on political representation or arguably economic position. Like the other new social movements of the time, it was fuelled by the energy and desires of youth and youthful aspirations for autonomy and identity. Like these other movements, it sought to draw a line between those who were 'oppressed' – youth, women, blacks and 'the poor' – and those who were the 'oppressors' – i.e. old, rich, white men. Like them, it sought unity in youth against the barriers of race, sex and class; and like them it failed to achieve such unity with the result that the bodies of 'difference' remained. For women, as for other embodied and politically engaged identities, however, the generational schism between 'old' and 'young' grew more salient altering the balance of power between the generations. As Betty Friedan remarked of the women's movement of the 1960s: 'we all felt young' (Friedan 1993, xv). While the unity of oppression could not contain the embodied differences of sex, race, sexuality and disability, youth – or at least not being identified as 'old' – provided an unquestioned boundary uniting nearly all the counter cultures and sub-cultures of the 1960s.

While changes in sexual attitudes and behaviour led to the 1960s being characterised as a time of 'sexual revolution', change in the performance of gender was not confined to personal relationships. From the 1960s onwards, women began entering the work force in greater numbers and across a wider range of jobs. Increasingly they stayed at work after marriage and after childbirth, and by the late 1970s the model of the male breadwinner was being more or less replaced by the dual earner household. In Britain, the USA and elsewhere, legislation for equal pay enacted during the period of the 'long' 1960s began to reduce the economic inequalities of gendered labour, while the more liberal divorce laws enabled women to break out of unhappy marriages without their facing the consequences of personal ruin. Sexuality was liberated from marriage, gender from sexual relations and sexual relations were liberated from economic dependency. Whatever caveats are placed around these claims, there was a widespread recognition that throughout the 1960s and early 1970s a sexual revolution was taking place, from which, this time, there would be no going back.

Like the other counter-cultural social movements, the women's movement was soon interpellated in the market's 'radical sell' (Heath and Potter 2005). Women's magazines, women's hairstyles and women's fashions were quickly positioned to capture the aspirations of the newly liberated woman. Higher education saw a rise in the number of women students, equal pay became formally established and sexual discrimination in the workforce was made illegal. Young women's earning power, and hence their economic independence, increased. Yet despite these gains, and their potential for reducing the oppression directed towards women's bodies, women were becoming even more incorporated into the consumer society against which they had earlier railed (Mitchell 1971). Writers such as Naomi Wolf argued that the new consumer capitalism used women's growing economic independence to market an ethos of 'self-presentation' and 'self-fashioning' which acted as a counterweight against women's growing independence (Wolf 1990). One key element in the process of stimulating this corporeal consumerism was the use made by the beauty industry of women's fears of ageing, 'hooking' them into a cycle of compulsive consumption and self-dissatisfaction.

As much as it stimulated it, consumer capitalism responded to the new cultural understandings of sex, gender and the body. Agedness and being old had been the antithesis of the 1960s counter-cultures. Older people, women as well as men, seemed to embody the inauthenticities and oppressions of the past. Youth, not age, expressed the authenticity of difference, a desirable difference that seemed to demand youthfulness in image, identity and lifestyle in order for it to be maintained. For a generation to whom the body had become a highly visible, polysemous signifier of self and identity, the cultivation of the body as the embodiment of identity was important in sustaining a sense of personal worth and esteem. Ageing challenged both the embodied sense of identity that this generation had acquired and the embodied technologies of self-care that sustained it. Faced with this dilemma, the question was whether gender could prove the undoing of age, or whether age would undo the achievements of gender (Silver 2003). If the performativity of gender became more closely allied with the performativity of age, could an explicitly feminist gerontology lead the way to rethinking bodily ageing?

Gendering Gerontology and Ageing Women's Studies

Within academia, the realignment of age and gender in late modernity has seen women and their bodies become the dominant source for representing and understanding ageing. In the 1950s and 1960s, a notionally un-gendered but implicitly male orientation was evident in much of the academic literature on ageing (Beeson 1975; Russell 1987). *The Gerontologist,* which began publication in 1961 as the official organ of the Gerontological Society of America, had until the late 1970s, devoted only a small number of papers on issues concerning women and ageing (e.g. Heyman 1970; Kline 1975). By 1985 it had instituted a regular section on the topic of 'Women's Issues'. A journal devoted specifically to that topic, the *Journal of Women and Ageing* began publication four years later, in 1989. While journals such as *Women and Health* and *The Psychology of Women Quarterly* had also been publishing research into women and ageing since the late 1970s, the balance of research interest in implicitly 'men's issues' that had once filled the pages of academic journals like *The Gerontologist* and the *Journal of Gerontology* had shifted overwhelmingly to 'women's issues' by the 1980s.

Few signs of the former 'gender-blind' but inherently masculinist perspective now survive in the gerontological literature, and the gendered nature of age and ageing is widely acknowledged (McMullin 1995). A large body of evidence has been accumulated that indicates that both inside and outside their bodies, men and women age differently. Much of this research has focused upon 'objective' differences in life expectancy, in the appearance of agedness, in functional capacity, in the relative risk of developing age associated illnesses and in the prevalence of functional impairment (cf. Arber and Ginn 1993; Deutsch, Zalenski and Clark 1986; Henss 1991; Levy 1988; Manton 1988; Verbrugge 1986; White 1988), and some of these corporeal differences appear to be conserved across species (Clutton-Brock and Isvaran 2007). One consequence of these emerging findings – that women's bodies seem to 'age' more visibly and become ill more often while surviving longer – may help explain why bodily ageing is more often and more overtly expressed, experienced and represented as women's business, and why ageing men's bodies have become less central to the ageing enterprise.

Objective findings of differential rates of illness, impairment and mortality in later life, however, do not tell us how these 'objective' differences mediate the performance and representation of gender in later life, nor do they reveal how men and women orientate themselves as subjects in their own and others' bodily ageing. The focus in gerontology on gender differences is still dominated by a structural approach based on recording 'objective' markers of age, illness, health and disability (Morley 2004). Such findings, though important, can easily mask or misrepresent the 'subjectivity' of the body that is ageing and its role in expressing the agency of individuals as men and women. In short, they tell us little about the practices of embodiment that imbricate gender with age.

Age Gender and the Cultural Turn

If elements within the women's movement initially 'exploited, patronized and stereotyped' older women, the ageing observed since around the edges of feminism has become 'a major issue for graying feminists' (Silver 2003, 385). In both ageing studies and in women's studies, a growing number of qualitative and quantitative accounts have begun to examine women's orientation toward their body's ageing, as well as their access to and the use they make of various resources, services and narratives to mask, minimise or otherwise moderate the more adverse experiences of ageing (Calasanti 2004; Calasanti and Slevin 2001; Cruikshank 2003; Hurd-Clarke 2011; Krekula 2007; Morrell 2003). Since 1987, the *Journal of Aging Studies* has provided one of the main outlets for the publication of academic papers on ageing that reflect what might be called the 'cultural turn'. Research on gender published by this journal provides a useful, but still limited, empirical perspective on gendered forms of ageing and the everyday practices, lifestyles and narratives by which gender and ageing are embodied (e.g. Hurd-Clarke and Griffin 2007a; Twigg 2004).

This more culturally oriented research on the ageing body reveals as many gendered differences in later life as have more 'positivist' approaches to gender. Differences have been described in the use of hair dyes, anti-ageing cosmetic procedures, self-examinations and physical health check-ups, hair removal, consumption of nutreceutical, dieting regimes, and sport and outdoor exercise activities (Bennett 1998; Harris 1994; Hennessy 1989; Holly, Lele and Bracchi 1998; Leontowitsch et al 2010; Oliveria et al. 1999; Tiggemann and Kenyon 1998). While older women display and report a greater focus on their physical appearance and link their sense of self more closely to their bodies (Pliner, Chaiken and Flett 1990), they also appear more flexible in the deployment of such technologies as well as being more open and sharing in their practices and experiences of embodiment (Basting 1998; Furman 1997, 21–9; Hurd-Clarke 2011). The earlier experience of a generation of women 'performing gender' through the body differently has helped provide new prototypes for similarly 'performing age'. Other divisions in the embodied practices of gender reflect the relative balance in performing age or gender. This is evident in the split between procedures aimed at producing anti-ageing effects, such as fillers and concealers, and procedures designed more generally to make women look attractive as women, such as makeup, lipstick, eyeliners, body lotions, and new outfits. Although the balance – toward ageing or toward gender – may vary, 'appearance management' amongst older women seems to contribute, directly and indirectly, to positive self-esteem (Kligman and Graham 1989). Research conducted by Hyun-Mee Joung and Nancy Miller found older women who looked after their appearance raised or reinforced their sense of personal well-being while, by implication, those not styling and/or dyeing one's hair, not using anti-ageing skin products, not wearing makeup, and not applying body lotions and fragrances felt less good about themselves (Joung and Miller 2006). Interestingly, the 'therapeutic' impact of cosmetics upon older women's sense of well-being had been demonstrated two decades earlier by Kligman and his colleagues (Graham and Kligman 1984).

If 'the body as an object of display is significant throughout their [women's] lives' (Halliwell and Dittmar 2003, 682), it is not so surprising that women express more concerns over age associated changes in appearance than they do over functional decline (Halliwell and Dittmar 2003; Pliner, Chaiken and Flett 1990). By continuing to engage in practices of self-care, by continuing to dress smartly and wear fashionable clothes, women of all ages, it is claimed, still seek to 'look their best' (Gosselink et al. 2008, 318). Looking one's best is not necessarily looking young. It can also mean constructing viable lifestyles for growing older gracefully, for maintaining one's 'style' across the years. The embodied practices that support a 'forever feminine' narrative may serve to escape the neutering of old age even when they are not consciously oriented toward that aim. They may also make failing to do so more difficult. As Laura Hurd-Clarke points out in her studies of older women's embodied appearance, for many 'throwing off of the burden of beauty ideology was ultimately a call for individuals to resign themselves to exclusion, invisibility and social devaluation' (Hurd-Clarke 2011, 67). Retaining the embodied practices of 'becoming' gendered individuals risk turning the virtues of self-care into the vices of endless vanity, while abandoning vanity risks abandoning one's self.

No such risks seem to be attached to men, who continue to be men as they age. While appearance management is not the only way that women 'embody' the new ageing it is often commented upon and agonised over. In contrast to the appeal of being 'forever feminine', men's desires not to become old have been framed around being 'forever functional' (Marshall and Katz 2002). Once an unexamined point of reference for the human sciences, masculinity too has begun to be understood as a 'performance', one that emphasises 'doing' rather than 'being' (Spector-Mersel 2000, 69). A 'hegemonic script of masculinity' (Spector-Mersel 2006, 67) is said to orient men toward treating their body as a machine, an instrument or tool directed toward personally and socially valued accomplishments and the competitive accumulation of power and status. Men's bodily ageing, when and if acknowledged, is represented as a decline or loss of powers, of reduced instrumentality and goal directedness and less as declining erotic capital or corporeal smartness (Higgs and McGowan 2012).

All gendered perspectives toward ageing are, as we have tried to show, contingent. With the rise of consumerism and the postindustrial economy, the individualised pursuit of a better body has started to engage men as well as women in the practices of 'appearance management' (Haiken 2000; Luciano 2001). Masculinity as a consumerist project has begun extending its influence over a range of male body practices. Stimulated in part by the rise of gay liberation and the 'gender-bending' of popular culture during the 1960s and 1970s, increasing numbers of straight and gay men seek not just to maintain their inner fitness and health but to display these virtues through the appearance of their bodies. Alongside the benefits arising from this new performativity have come the risks once confined to the gay community of 'premature ageing', when men's bodies and their masculinity are seen as becoming 'old' and 'invisible' before reaching 'mid-life' (Gagnon and Simon 1973).

Pre-modern attempts to embody alternative ways of ageing involved diet and a little light exercise, combined with the studied maintenance of civic virtù and the retention of economic power (Gilleard 2013). For most men in classical modernity, however, their main concern was less with their bodily appearance and more with carrying on working and maintaining their breadwinner role. Fitness was a concern of a small number of enthusiasts and eccentrics who took to regimes of weights and gymnastics in order to strengthen their sense of masculinity without any evident concern for preserving a sense of youthfulness. Most men neither dieted nor exercised and male conscripts in both First and Second World Wars were generally viewed as anything but 'fighting fit'.

The collective practices of masculine exercise associated with school and military service were sloughed off during the postwar period. In their place emerged the newly individualised practice of fitness, publicly displayed but privately provided (Stern 2008). From the 1970s, jogging grew in popularity and the rise of gym culture fostered the display of the exercising body. A new 'cross-gender' sports-fashion took off for sweat pants, tracksuits, trainers, lycra and jogging pants, as both men and women routinised their visits to the gym and the 'fitness centre' (O'Connor 2008). Fitness 'switched gears' from the 'group callisthenics and national goals' of the 1950s to the quest for individual perfection in the 1980s (Luciano 2001, 121). The new technologies of the self saw 'men's health' measured by the muscular definition of their bodies rather than by the work they performed. The cosmetic attention and concern over physical appearance that had seemed such a gendered part of the early 1960s crossed to the male side. Men were becoming embodied actors too, ready to modify their 'never-aging stories of hegemonic masculinity' (Spector-Mersel 2006).

Fewer accounts of men's embodied experience of and engagement with self-care and physical ageing no doubt reflect their historically more limited engagement with the market for 'appearance management' and health related 'self-care'. Taking responsibility for managing one's own ageing – for ageing with agency – remains less common and operates within a more restricted arena for older men. Although this seems particularly to be the case for 'appearance management' practices and engagement with the new 'rejuvenative' technologies, practices framed around health, fitness and functioning that are also implicitly oriented toward not becoming old seem to comply more readily with hegemonic narratives of masculinity. This is exemplified on the one hand by the take up and continuance of jogging – an activity explicitly designed for the no longer young athlete (Bowerman and Harris 1967; Wiersma and

Chesser 2011) – and on the other by the increasingly common use of performance enhancing pharmaceuticals such as Viagra (Marshall and Katz 2002).

Ideas held by younger adults about older men retain a strong sense of 'gender' – of 'masculinity' (Thompson 2000) – even if men's ageing appearance is less often used in judging their attractiveness (Vares 2009). Investment in rejuvenating their appearance might be less of a priority for older men to take up, but there are signs of a cross-gendered appeal in several 'anti-ageing' practices. Thus, while some studies have reported that older men purchase fewer 'anti-ageing' nutreceuticals (Gray et al. 1996) others have found no marked differences between men and women (Marinac et al. 2007). Indeed it could also be argued that notions of 'hegemonic masculinity' which underpinned a focus on the younger man as the ideal have been challenged by the introduction and availability of drugs such as Viagra and Cialis, which 'return' older men to a state of sexual capacity previously seen as the domain of much younger men and, in so doing, provide a different template for the performance of masculinity at older ages (Higgs and McGowan 2012).

Ageing in Culture as Gendered Performance

The cultural scripts defining gender, what it means to be 'a man' or 'a woman', privilege younger adulthood and the reproductive years. The ageing of those men and women whose experience of youth and early adulthood occurred within the context of the cultural ferment of the 1960s has given a new edge to performing gender in later life and, equally, performing age through gender. This has involved negotiations between the older agonisms of gender and the newer ones of age. The de-gendering, negating, neutralising or transforming effects of age challenges men and women's ability to assert a gendered identity in later life (Cruikshank 2008). At the same time, the new ageing has become a point of reference in the contemporary performance of gender, stimulating new embodied practices designed specifically to sustain positive and more differentiated views of masculinity or femininity in the face of ageing. The embodiment of gender provides the base for the embodiment, not so much of 'pure' ageing but of ageing 'in culture', an ageing that is not 'old', 'de-gendered', 'neutralised', 'unproductive' or 'sexless'.

In reviewing the variously gendered performances of 'ageing in culture', four distinct fields of practice can be identified. First and most publicly evident is the use made of and engagement with 'anti-ageing' consumerism and the 'pursuit of somatic enhancement'. Rejuvenative surgery (face lifts, fillers and skin peels) has grown in popularity over the last three decades as has the marketing and sales of anti-ageing products such as creams, serums, injections and so called nutreceuticals (Kennedy 2005). Women have been the leading consumers of these products and services, perhaps because of their greater reported anxieties over physical ageing and the salience that the body has had in fostering women's rethinking of gender (Delinsky 2005; Hurd-Clarke and Griffin 2007a; Muise and Desmarais 2010). Yet even here there are signs of a growing market for men, albeit for a differently nuanced form of anti-ageing, that still includes the pursuit of youthful looks and youthful performances (Haiken 2000).

The second dimension is the turn toward exercise and fitness – part of what Ekerdt has called 'the busy ethic' of the third age (Ekerdt 1986; see also Katz 2000). Whether it is line dancing, swim aerobics or pilates, women outnumber men in such communal 'embodied' activities, but active participation in 'senior' sports remains more popular among older men, perhaps, as much an assertion of youthful competitiveness as age resistance (Dionigi 2006). One important difference in men and women's orientation toward exercise, for example, is whether their focus is upon form or fitness, appearance or performance with men tending to seek to sustain their masculinity through solo performances while women more often seek socialised routes in keeping their bodies 'in shape'. If women are more concerned over the impact on their appearance (maintaining youth, health and good looks) and men more concerned about their performance (becoming faster, stronger, or simply lasting longer), the different meanings attached to male and female identity make approaches toward fitness different – in ways that the self-care and cosmetic industries have already started taking account of in their 'representations' of anti-ageing products and practices to potential later life consumers. Even so, such gendered differentiation in the orientation toward physical activity and exercise may itself be unstable, as new cohorts of ageing women master athletes take to the track (Tischer, Hartmann-Tews and Combrink 2011) and new cohorts of ageing men turn to the mirror (Haiken 2000).

The third dimension of embodying practices oriented toward gender and not becoming old involves dress, fashion and personal self-care or 'appearance management'. This term covers a wide variety of activities in which bodily ageing, or the ageing of some part of the body, becomes the focus for consuming various goods and services. This may involve masking or covering over observable signs of 'agedness' or serving to distract attention away from such signs, such as depilation techniques and practices, the selection and use of hair dyes, the choice of particular clothes and shoes or more generally 'managing' a wardrobe mindful of age. In each of these arenas of practice, the gendered nature of what Foucault termed 'technologies of the self' is significant (Foucault 1988). If women have realised – or performed – their gender in part through activities that make salient their physical appearance as women rather than, say, as workers, any perceived neglect of self-care implies a loss of interpersonal power, whether in relation to their own or the opposite sex. Since men have made less use of, or found less useful, this kind of gendered appearance management at most points in their adult life course it is not surprising that the decline in reported attractiveness associated with ageing has proved less critical in expanding men's embodied practices oriented toward their own ageing.

The fourth arena is that of sexual practice. If sexual practice in first modernity was dominated by marital and extra-marital coitus with limited exposure of the body and limited variation in positions and performance, the 1960s sexual revolution introduced changes and variations in sexual practice and increased corporeal intimacy as sex and reproduction became effectively separated. These changes in sexual practice were facilitated by the various youth counter-cultures and their valorisation of choice, autonomy self-expression and pleasure and, more specifically, by the market for self-help materials and the expansion of what was deemed acceptable in books magazines and film. Books provided more explicit accounts of sex, films and magazines gradually increased their nudity and sexual activity quotients, while 'good sex' manuals from sexed up summaries of the *Kama Sutra* to Alex Comfort's *The Joy of Sex* became bestsellers. After the 1960s, forms of non-penetrative and non-heterosexual sex were opened out to the wider world. A general belief grew that more and better sex equated to a better life and better relationships. Cohorts reaching sexual maturity during the 'long' 1960s lead the way in pioneering sex as a route to liberation. This cohort's own ageing, as we have already pointed out, has changed the landscape, first of middle age and now of later life. The rise of sex manuals designed for older consumers and practitioners, developments in sex technologies to maintain desire and performance and the reframing of age associated sexual inactivity as age related sexual disorders have contributed to maintaining sex as an important element in gendered later lifestyles (Hayes et al. 2007; Leiblum et al. 2006; Marshall and Katz 2003).

Gender, Generation and the New Ageing

The recent historical fashioning of gender and its various embodied lifestyles have enhanced the salience of generational differences. Research conducted by Gosselink and colleagues found that later born 'late life' cohorts, whom they term boomer women, 'have experienced lifelong beauty culture media imaging [and the] constant exposure to idealized beauty standards [...] which has shaped boomer women's fear of looking and becoming old' (Gosselink et al. 2008, 322). The sexual revolution of the 1960s, these authors suggest, has only increased the pressure for women to maintain an attractive appearance for longer, in effect of signing them up for lifelong 'body work'. Ageing is now an additional point of reference, another parameter of performativity in becoming 'gendered'. As the 'agentic' responsibility for looking good and acting smart expands for both men and women, there is less excuse for not caring about one's body and its ageing, without seeming also to give up on oneself or to fail to respond to the appropriate forms of 'governmentality'. As Jones and Higgs (2010) have pointed out, while the new normativity of ageing may accept diversity, there is also an expectation of adherence to appropriate modes of self-care which in a more overtly somatic society now include activity, appearance and attitude.

Alongside the pressure to look after one's body and perform at all times, ambivalence exists about the acceptability of these variously embodied practices of being and becoming gendered, an ambivalence which grows more acute as it is oriented towards ageing (Higgs and Jones 2009). While more women than men may want to look younger than they are and to 'conceal' evidence of agedness – through the use of clothing choices, anti-ageing creams, concealers, hair dye, etc. – even as these choices are exercised, there is resistance and rejection of such behaviour (Harris 1994). The more 'clinical' the interventions the more problematic they are considered. Even within the clinical realm those practices that seem 'less intrusive' such as the use of injections, fillers or various forms of dermabrasion are deemed more acceptable than invasive anti-ageing surgery, such as face and forehead lifts, where the risks are greater and the exposed desire for age reversal more unambiguously revealed (Hurd-Clarke, Repta and Griffin 2007).

Practices of 'appearance management' in later life can be distinguished between those that emphasise continuities in 'performing gender' and those practices that are taken up in response to the perceived ageing of one's gendered identity. Changes in the former highlight changing generational practices associated with the postwar democratisation of fashion and the mass consumption of cosmetics. Lipstick, hair dye, face creams or tights may have been first used in youth, during the 1950s and 1960s, but their continued use into later life conveys the message of being 'forever feminine'. Changes in gendered practices oriented toward ageing such as removing facial hair (bristles) from the chin or upper lip, undergoing non-surgical cosmetic procedures like Botox, fillers or anti-ageing creams, convey a similar message but they require more agency. Part of what distinguishes these two types of practice is that they require different degrees of agency and choice. The latter require a deliberate decision to start; the former the lack of any decision to stop. Whilst most adult women in contemporary society have engaged with fashion and makeup since their youth, only in the last quarter century have distinctive 'anti-ageing' practices, products and procedures become popular methods of reducing the physical signs of ageing.

Cultural changes in the acceptability of these latter procedures has perhaps been slower to spread to all sectors of the middle aged and older population since youth is traditionally more open to change and does not need to shed so many existing habits of embodiment as those whose adult lives are longer. Nevertheless, increasing numbers of men and women now aged fifty and over are turning toward the use of products and services aimed at their not becoming old (and/or de-gendered) while current cohorts of younger women are more prepared than earlier cohorts to consider using such anti-ageing procedures, in future, particularly the so-called minimally invasive methods of rejuvenation (Wollina and Payne 2010). Reflecting the growing acceptability of somatic interventions to combat looking old, the psychological profile of those undergoing rejuvenative plastic surgery has become increasingly 'normal' (Delinsky 2006). Whether measured by prescriptions for Viagra and Cialis, sales of anti-ageing creams, lotions and serums, participation in physical activity and master sports, or engagement with fashion and 'beauty culture', the embodiment of gender is delivering more market power in later life than corporeal ageing is depressing it.

Conclusions

The changing role of gender in representing age and ageing provides a key theme in the embodiment of ageing. From the classical period in Western history through to the Renaissance, the male body had dominated representations of age. Public concerns over ageing from Cicero and Plutarch to Cornaro and Paleotti were men's concerns. The coming of 'modernity' was in some historians' eyes the point when ageing was 'born', or at least transformed from a civic or aesthetic issue to a matter of societal significance (Gilleard 2002; Gutton 1988). Modernity reconceptualised men's age as chronology, where the appearance of men's age became less important than their longevity and productivity. These disembodied concerns over chronological age became matters of growing importance in both state formation and social policy during the late nineteenth and early twentieth century. Throughout this period and beyond, however, the dominant concerns over ageing remained those of men. But while men's ageing remained the modern state's key concern, issues concerning women's position in society and the difference between the sexes rose to prominence in the first wave of the women's movement. Despite the setback of the Depression and the Second World War, the gender of ageing became more salient as a result of the radical rethinking of gender that took place in the wake of the 1960s' sexual 'revolution'. As feminists began to rethink the position of women in society, their economic and cultural marginality, and the cultural constraints that surrounded their lives, the gendered body became a site of increasing cultural contestation. Difference and particularly the difference that could be attributed to the body became the site for a new politics of identity.

These new ways of thinking about and understanding the body were incorporated into a mass consumerist culture that was thriving in part through market growth and segmentation. Consumerism helped redirect the generational schism between the old and the new, between age and youth, into a 'radical sell' that privileged youthful lifestyles and youthful difference (Heath and Potter 2005). Gender was at the centre of this transformation. The male breadwinner model was undermined by the habitus of a mass consumerist society that dominated the second half of the twentieth century. Well-being was marked less by income than by consumption and particularly consumption displayed through embodied lifestyles and embodied practices. The 'performativity' of gender and the realisation of self-identity through the body formed the basis for new identities and flexible lifestyles. As the confrontational era of the 1960s faded away, members of the cohort at the heart of its counter-cultures found themselves facing, in mid-life and beyond, new challenges to maintain and develop their newly achieved embodiments of gender.

Within this changing landscape, ageing became an increasingly important point of reference against which these new lifestyles were positioned. The embodied practices of gender shaped the habitus of a generation that is now no longer young. As a result, the narratives of bodily ageing constructed around decline and loss are being challenged across a much broader front than was the case for the small mostly male elite who dabbled in rejuvenation during the inter-war period. While the embodiment of gender and the practices supporting it have been central to this process, other bodily identities, intersecting with and confounding already existing gendered identities, have provided further sites around which the embodiment of ageing could be reconstructed. As Öberg and Tornstam have noted, 'youthfulness and fitness' have become identity ideals for all – across gender, cohort, class and other cleavages (Öberg and Tornstam 2001). But whilst engagement with a less chronologically bound form of ageing may have universal appeal, it can only be realised within distinct embodied practices whose histories are inflected by differences other than those of age, generation or gender. Practices shaped by and inflected with other embodied identities such as race, sexuality and disability also helped define the cultural ferment of the 1960s and its turn toward the body. In the next chapters we explore how these 'other' embodiments of identity are impacting upon the 'new' ageing.

Chapter 4

AGE AND THE RACIALISED BODY

In the previous chapter we argued that men and women's ageing made salient different aspects of an aged identity. Furthermore we argued that this could give rise to different ways of 'performing' age while maintaining a still gendered identity in later life. Part of performing gender in later life we suggested meant not acceding to the 'neutralising' corporeality of old age. This then opens up the possibility that if it is possible to retain in later life the distinctions of gender without necessarily embodying its past oppressions, might a similar situation apply to racialised identities? Putting it slightly differently, might retaining a racialised identity through later life be another way of not becoming old? Or does ageing 'in culture' serve merely as a revisiting of past oppressions with present ones – leading only to a different and potentially more debilitating way of becoming old? In this chapter we address the historical forms by which race has been embodied in people's lives and its contemporary significance for understanding and interpreting ageing without becoming old.

At this juncture it is important for us to be clear how the term 'race' is being used before we consider how race has been used in studying ageing. Without bodies race has no social signification, and without social institutions and practices race has no bodily identity. In this chapter we will concentrate primarily upon skin colour as the site for the embodied distinction between 'black' and 'white' and use the term racialisation to indicate the imbrication of social relations by this 'black/white' skin colour divide. 'Ethnicity' in contrast to race exists primarily within the realm of institutions and embodied practices – without the need of particular corporeal distinctions. So long as corporeal signifiers are used in the mediation of social relationships, 'race' and 'ethnicity' remain separate and 'race', not ethnicity, functions as an embodied identity.

Granting this terminology, two distinct approaches to the relationship between 'race' and bodily ageing can be identified. The first associated with the notion of 'intersectionality' studies the relationships among multiple dimensions and modalities of social relationships and subject formations (McCall 2005). This approach emphasises 'racialised identity' as a structuring institution, whereby blackness becomes the point of reference in defining an embodied hierarchy within society, making 'bodies of colour' marginal to the organisation of an implicitly 'white' life course. From this perspective, 'race' defines a position of advantage or disadvantage based upon a socially registered corporeal distinction while ageing represents the accumulation of advantages and disadvantages realised within these given 'racialised' identities. The merging or intersecting of 'age' with 'race' results, as one writer has put it, in 'different shades of grey' (Newman 2003).

The second approach focuses upon the 'meaning-making' associated with racialised identities, the narratives and performativities that express sites of struggle over the meanings of 'race'. Historically, within the United States such meaning-making has been more evident among younger adults, leaving 'a less than ideal situation for the aged black' whose life and 'meaning-making' has been dismissed on account of its inevitable out-datedness (Kent 1971, 49). It could therefore be argued that ageing and old age risk neutering the body's desire and power to challenge and transgress the old oppressive structuring of 'race'. Even were this to be the case, however, it is unclear whether such 'neutering' is something that must be mourned or whether it could also be celebrated as a liberation from the bonds of a racialised identity – to no longer be forever 'coloured' much as Germaine Greer has argued that the menopause could set women free from being forever 'feminine' (Greer 1991). Such cultural approaches to 'race' reject the unproblematic structuring of a racialised identity into a social binary by arguing instead for a more agonistic relationship within and between those ascribed an identity that is 'black' or 'white'.

Within the social sciences and in social gerontology, particularly, the structuralist approach to race has been dominant. Within cultural studies, while the narratives and practices of racialised identities have been explored through the complex negotiations between a desire for and a fear of such corporeally externalised identities, such as being 'black' in a 'white' society, little has been written about the destabilising impact of age upon such 'meaning-making'. While historically situated in inequalities of power and voice, the cultural studies approach recognises that such identities retain the potential to be viewed as 'other' than through the 'permanent prism of race' (Marable 1995, 191).

Within the disciplines of gerontology, it could be argued that a de-gendered and de-racialised corporeal ageing has occupied the foreground of research. The embodied identities of gender and 'race' have been treated primarily as supplemental categories of structural disadvantage. Arguably this has been more the case with 'race' than it has been with gender, as a number of feminist gerontologists have foregrounded gender as a lens for examining age (Arber and Ginn 1993; Calasanti and Slevin 2001). Equally, more slowly and more cautiously, ageing has begun to be used to inform understandings of gender (Marshall 2011).

Within cultural studies of ageing and 'race', racialised identities have rarely been used to extend or reframe our understanding of ageing and later life, nor has age been used to do similar work for 'race'. African American, Black and Critical Race Studies have examined racialised identity through a distinctively cultural lens, emphasising the unacknowledged contingencies of whiteness and the double consciousness of 'race' fostered by classical modernity's attempt to 'naturalise', and thereby 'order', human variety and variability (Malik 1996; Smaje 2000). But cultural studies of 'race' and racialised identity have rarely explored the dominant 'whiteness' of ageing, let alone concerned themselves with black or African American narratives and performances of 'age'. Although cultural studies have explored how racialised identities are enacted through the body, they have never been contextualised by considering the changes associated with the bodily ageing. It is as if race is still used as an ageless, ahistorical prism through which to understand the non-corporeal social world. As a result, the challenge that ageing brings to the identity of 'race' and its embodied lifestyles goes mostly unremarked.

In gerontology, one of the earliest structural framings of 'race' and age was expressed by the concept of 'double jeopardy'. This was the title of one of the first reports on the health and financial well-being of ageing African Americans published by the National Urban League (NUL) in 1964. The term was used to reflect a view that older African Americans laboured under the dual disadvantage that age and blackness created in postwar American society. Actions to remove the disadvantages of age therefore required differential responses, informed by the different positions that black and white Americans occupied in society. Two decades later this position was elaborated by the term 'triple jeopardy' as 'race' (blackness), gender (femaleness) and age (agedness) were seen to 'triple' the marginalisation of non-white, non-male, non-young people in contemporary Western societies (Norman 1985). These narratives, however, risked limiting the potential agency attached to the identities of 'race', gender and age by emphasising their structural characteristics and becoming in Foucault's terminology 'docile bodies'. Narratives of embodied identity and the cultural practices through which they are realised were subsequently ignored in favour of framing racialised (or gendered or disabled) identities as positions of structured social (dis)advantage.

Many of the themes raised in Chapter 3 recur when exploring the nature of racialised identity. These include the historical contingencies that have shaped the way 'race' has been embodied as 'whiteness' in ageing much in the same way gender was once embodied in ageing as 'maleness'. In exploring 'race', in this fashion, we are strongly influenced by the dividing colour line of 'black' and 'white' that has particularly marked the history of the United States. It is this distinctively American 'blackness' that has been the modern test bed where 'race' has been configured, embodied and identified, in the political discourses of power, in the cultural assertions of privilege, and in the market segmentation of consumers. If 'race', in a similar fashion to 'sex', can be seen as an example of a difference mystified into a corporeal signifier of hierarchy and status, the renegotiation of the terms of its embodiment could potentially offer a model also for renegotiating the structural embodiment of ageing. Engaging in such renegotiations, however, is not just a matter of creating alternative narratives to those currently dominating society. Renegotiation requires bodies to act differently, to perform other forms of embodiment, and to practice new technologies of self-care in order to be able realise such changes. Being racialised differently, like ageing differently, requires *doing* things differently, whether as individualised consumers or as collectivised communities.

Racialisation in Modern America

The inter-continental trade in slavery between Africa, America and Europe provides the inescapable historical context for discussions on racialised identity in modern America. The history of slavery, and the processes of European colonisation in which it was embedded, have given the distinctions between black and white bodies their peculiar and pernicious social and cultural significance (Smaje 2000). This history has established the terms of knowledge and power by which people with lighter skin understood and were understood by people with darker skin. It has pervaded the modern era, creating the 'widespread assumption among intelligent people that there are [...] ineradicable and for all practicable purposes unchangeable racial differences' between peoples (Du Bois 1928, 6). These assumptions became reified in the formulation of 'the Negro problem' that dominated the early work of American social scientists such as Dow, Ellwood and Ross (Dow 1922; Ellwood 1918; Ross 1921).

Within this 'modern' perspective, the 'problem of the Negro' was predicated upon the 'social' fact 'that the Negro is an inferior race because of either biological or social heredity or both; that the Negro because of his [*sic*] physical character cannot be assimilated; and that physical amalgamation is bad and undesirable' (Frazier 1947, 271). These assumptions were widely held within the African and European American populations of the USA and made prospects for healing the divide after the abolition of slavery particularly difficult. Though criticised by 'white' and 'black' radicals they remained one strand in the dominant ideology of twentieth-century American society, radically shaping the life chances of white and black individuals, to the advantage of the former and the detriment of the latter. This profound racialisation of American society continued up to and beyond the Second World War, when its power to diminish and demoralise those deemed 'non-white' began slowly to subside (Fairclough 2001).

In the 1960s an irreversible change took place in US society, a change which has lead, if not to the realisation at least to the emergence of, a viable, 'post-black' American society, where racialised identities expand more than they confine individual experiences and expectations (Neal 2002; Taylor 2007). Despite undermining the solidity of the social and cultural hierarchies of modernity, the break of the 1960s should not blind us to the pervasive influence that the processes of modernisation have had and still have in affecting black and white America throughout the entirety of the twentieth century. The many economic and cultural changes that influenced the development of modern American society, from the growth of the media, the rise of mass consumerism, the expansion of higher education and the postindustrialisation of the economy, permeated both black and white communities. The 1960s represented the period when the pace of this common twentieth-century modernisation accelerated and in accelerating brought them closer together.

Blackness before 'Black Power'

While 'Black Power' can be viewed from the vantage point of the radical politics of the 1960s, it can also be seen as a constituent part of the broader cultural changes that led from a 'first' to a 'second' modernity (Beck, Bonz and Lau 2003). The embodiment of blackness celebrated by the Black Power movement and the 'self-presentational' style of the Black Panther Party can be connected to developments in the 'body work' and 'self-presentation' that emerged earlier in twentieth-century African American society. The inter-twining of commercial enterprise, body culture and ideas of racial uplift formed a constant background for debates over ancestry and identity throughout much of the twentieth century. Indeed, the history of American consumer society and its privileging of the body cannot be considered complete without reference to its active incorporation within the African American community (Chambers 2006). Blackness, as both identity and lifestyle, was built in America and, like Coca-Cola, exported across the world.

Claude Barnett, Madame C. J. Walker, Anthony Overton and Annie Turbo Pope Malone, near contemporaries of Helena Rubenstein and Dorothy Arden, were fellow advocates and engineers of twentieth century beauty culture. These early twentieth-century African American entrepreneurs played a significant role in shaping a mass market for 'black' beauty products. In the process their commercial activity was linked to issues of racialised identity within the African American community. While the rejection of 'artificial practices' such as hair straightening, skin colouring and skin lightening in favour of more 'natural' and more 'authentic' fashions and hairstyles became part of the Black Power ethos, their message reiterated themes that had already been played out in the African American communities of an earlier 'first modernity'.

One of the central concerns in the process of becoming a modern (black) American was – and remains – the rights and wrongs of 'dressing up'. Debates about the rights and wrongs of African American women 'straightening' their hair, 'lightening' their skin and pursuing the 'worship of fashion' were evident in post–Civil War nineteenth-century America (Rooks 2004, 77), reflecting the longstanding policing of gender and racialised identities within the African American community. Almost as soon as commercial hair straightening and skin lightening products were marketed, debates about such practices appeared in the African American press. Rooks cites an article written in 1859 by one Martin Freeman decrying the mentality of those African American women who chose to emulate 'white' ideals of beauty by 'pinching up their noses and oiling, pulling, twisting up, tying down and sleeking over their "kinky hair"'(Rooks 1996, 35). But though some senior male figures within the African American community were castigating women's use of 'unnatural' cosmetics and hairstyling, and chastising the 'Negro' for emulating 'European' fashions, others were adopting a different approach, aimed at 'reconstruct[ing] the very idea of who and what a Negro was or could be' (Gates 1988, 148). These advocates of a 'black renaissance' focused less upon issues of economic and political equality, and more upon establishing a cultural status for black people that was both equivalent to European Americans and yet distinctive of African Americans.

As Gates has put it, the 'Negro' renaissance of the 1920s was an attempt 'not only [...] to rewrite the black term [...] [but] also to rewrite the [white] texts of themselves' (Gates 1988, 148). African American writers of the period consciously sought to undermine essentialist attempts to pin down the 'Negro' as a social mass, instead playing with change and transformation in ideas about 'blackness and whiteness' (Favor 1999, 10). Others within the African American community criticised what they perceived as the 'white' 'elitist' assumptions lying behind the 'New Negro' movement, and viewed its aims as evidence of racial self-hatred. Advocates of 'Negro separatism', such as Marcus Garvey or Elijah Muhammed, were critical not only of the penchant for 'prettification', but of all expressions of popular culture within the African American community that might serve as indicators of their seduction by a morally corrupt, 'white' consumerist culture. As Kathy Peiss notes, 'the contradictory rejection and embrace of Euro-American aesthetic standards surfaced repeatedly as black writers, reformers and educators responded to the new beauty culture that spread throughout black communities in the early twentieth century' (Peiss 1998, 206). Despite criticisms from both 'black nationalist' and black conservative leaders, ideas of racial uplift were woven into African American discourses of beauty, fashion and consumer culture throughout the twentieth century. Just as the early advocates of 'white' beauty regimes were criticised for turning 'respectable' young women into 'scarlet women', Madame C. J. Walker and other African American entrepreneurs in the beauty and culture industries were criticised for betraying the purity of their 'race' by artificial means.

In the same fashion as Elisabeth Arden and Helena Rubinstein, these entrepreneurs of the modern beauty industry recognised and helped validate the desire for personal enhancement that was part of the newly emerging African American middle class. Unlike the radical movements of the time, they operated within an explicitly petit-bourgeois framework, providing goods and services to the African American community. Whether through art, culture, fashion or leisure, they offered modern new lifestyles as alternatives to the culturally and symbolically subaltern position that black bodies had possessed within a slave-owning society. While by no means unaware of the racism that was endemic within American society, (Madam C. J. Walker contributed actively to organisations such as the National Association of American Colored People (NAACP)), these pedlars of art and beauty aligned themselves with the ethos of consumer capitalism and its spirit of exhortatory self-improvement.

During the period 1900–1950, a number of middle class African American women had begun to shift their relationship to body work, not just as producers but as consumers of its products and services. Through the intermediaries of small but influential entrepreneurs, opportunities arose to set up African American beauty parlours and hairdressing salons, which became important sites for the performance of 'race' and gender. Other service sectors also contributed to this re-positioning of blackness, including the cinema, the photographic studio and mass circulation magazines. Noliwe Rooks has described how 'successful photography studios owned by and catering to African Americans were a ubiquitous feature of the urban landscape' where 'the resulting photographs offered African Americans proof that they could fashion an image and, by extension, portray a life markedly different from that represented in mainstream popular culture and in the white imagination' (Rooks 2004, 16–17). Similar developments were evident in the press and publishing industries, as mass circulation African American women's magazines appeared, advertising and advising on personal lifestyles oriented toward fashion and 'home management' (Rooks 2004). Some of the first movies of the period were also directed toward an African American audience and formed a key part of the 'Negro Renaissance'. One of the most famous African American directors was Oscar Michieux, inventor of the cross-shot whereby scenes showing one set of events were juxtaposed with other events taking place elsewhere in time or place. Michieux was a leading exponent of racial uplift who sought, through his films, to show that 'the colored man [*sic*] can be anything' (cited in Weiss 2000, 11).

In short, the twentieth century's 'turn toward the body' and the rise of its 'glamour industry', exemplified by beauty parlours and hair salons, movie houses and photographic studios, fashion and home improvement magazines and numerous cosmetic companies, were part of a new 'modern' society that cultivated consumerist aspirations across both classes and 'races'. Both African and European Americans were (albeit unequally) involved in these developments. The resulting debates over the virtues of nature, the value of artifice, the critique and the celebration of what was 'new' and 'modern' (and youthful) were shared by both communities. What was added to these debates within the African American community was a contestation over the identity and meaning of 'blackness' and more generally of 'race'. As with the broader transition toward 'modernity', these issues concerned a relatively privileged minority within the black community and were overshadowed by the depression and the Second World War. But they served as precursors for changes to come, the rehearsal for a more profoundly somatic society that would be ushered in during the decades after the Second World War when it would become possible to celebrate being 'young, gifted and black'.

Reconstructing Blackness after the 1960s

The somatic turn that formed such an important element in the cultural ferment of the 'long' 1960's was evident in the celebration of 'blackness' as a source of identity and distinction that was promoted by the Black Power movement. The radicalisation of the US Civil Rights Movement and 'the rise of radicalized black nationalist discourse, symbolism and activity in the 1960s' (Ogbar 2004, vii) created new narratives of black nationalism, black power and black liberation. These narratives, framed within the more general cultural, demographic, economic and political changes taking place in the wake of the Second World War, were realised in the context of the progressive urbanisation of African Americans, the expansion of a significant black middle class, the flourishing of the counter cultures of youth and the increasing democratisation and individualisation of affordable, fashionable lifestyles. Youth culture was critical in the struggle to develop new meanings of 'race', particularly those sections of the young who were most distant from the productive processes of the economy. Within the college campuses' counter-cultures, old people were the 'other', parents and professors marked by their pasts. The times were changing, and those identified as old were actively rejected as sources of moral authority and social influence. A generational schism in attitudes and expectations took place, including attitudes about 'race' which separated those African Americans who had grown up and grown old in the largely rural Jim Crow society of the South from those whose adult lives were fashioned in the urban black world of the North (Ogbar 2004, viii).

As the personal became political, the political was increasingly aligned with issues of difference and distinction, with authenticity and liberation. But as these political positions were presented increasingly in personal, individualised terms they came closer to 'the market' and open to the iconography of branding. As Heath and Potter have pointed out, 'consumerism manages to engage our central political ideas – freedom, democracy, self-expression – in ways that are accessible, personable and immediately gratifying' (Heath and Potter 2005, 188). As market segmentation replaced legal segregation, images of the 'revolution' were sold as t-shirts, berets, sunglasses and hairstyles. While the material conditions facing people in the African American community were slow to improve, a profound change was taking place in the face that American society presented to itself. Black pride, Black Power and black fashion became iconic sources for product placement and market segmentation. Black culture, once limited to mirroring mainstream America, now merged with it and helped shape its mainstream elements through the postindustrial industries associated with music, media, entertainment and fashion.

Reflecting this confluence between racial identity and consumer culture, the 1960s saw the first major US TV series with black heroes (Bill Cosby in *I Spy*, first broadcast in 1966 and followed two years later by Diahann Carroll in *Julia*). Films were produced with an explicit cross-racial appeal – leading to the so-called 'blaxploitation' movies, such as *Shaft* and *They call me MISTER Tibbs!*. The first black models appeared in the mainstream Anglo-American fashion industry, Beverley Valdes in 1962, Donyale Luna in 1964 and Naomi Sims in 1968 (Cheddie 2002). Magazines such as *Ebony* developed into 'mass circulation black-owned entertainment oriented' fashion journals, offering similar styles and content to that of white-oriented magazines such as *Cosmopolitan* and *Vogue* (Cheddie 2002, 67). In the words of Jeffrey Ogbar, Black Power 'sanitized and repackaged by various forces [...] liberal to conservative [...] as well as corporate America [...] had marketing power' (Ogbar 2004, 199). Such marketing power formed part of a more general trend that saw the rapid take up and refashioning of 'youth oriented' counter cultures by a market increasingly attuned to the radical sell (Heath and Potter 2005). Youth was at the heart of this yearning for the new and the market was listening increasingly to its beat.

In short, the growing affluence of the young was not confined to white society: young African Americans were no longer peripheral to the economy, nor were they so excluded from higher education. A new 'black' culture was emerging more closely attuned to the mass consumer society that America had signed up to at the start of the twentieth century. Ongiri quotes the ex-Black Panther and Soledad Sister, Angela Davis, who, when looking back on the 1960s said: 'it is both humiliating and humbling to discover that a single generation after the events that constructed me as a public personality, I am remembered as a hairdo' (cited in Ongiri 2010, 51). Afro hairstyles, which Davis sported with iconic success during this period, were created to celebrate the 'authenticity' and 'naturalness' of people of African descent, but they spread as fashion statements. By the 1970s the Afro had become a hairstyle choice for people of diverse origins, just as dreadlocks and cornrows would be for subsequent generations of 'urban' youth.

Old Black or Post-black?

Civil rights, black pride and Black Power movements overturned the traditional prewar racial dividing line in American society. They marked 'a decisive turn' in the history of blackness and 'race' (Taylor 2007, 639) replacing the old 'Negro versus White' divisions of first modernity with more complex and more contingent forms of racialised identity. These revised identities were no longer confined within a homogenous black community. They supported a more diverse set of lifestyle and bodily practices, loosely and more flexibly attached to the corporeal distinctions that had been used to mark racialised identities. While racialised disadvantage and inequality existed at all ages, race thinking had, to quote Taylor again, 'entered a post-historical phase [...] at which the future of the practice is not assured or clear' (Taylor 2007, 638).

There are now more ways for African Americans to grow older than existed in the enclosed diversity that characterised those cohorts of African Americans born before the Second World War. For them, retirement meant little more than an end to a life of unrewarding labour; a release without a role or the resources to refashion one (Hearn 1971, 23). Within the new diversity of difference that is African American society, is it more possible to retain the distinction of racialised identities – of being black – in later life, without losing contact with the richer narrativity and performativity through which racialised identities came to be expressed 'after the revolution'? In *Soul Babies*, Neil uses the term 'post-soul' 'to describe the political, social and cultural experiences of the African American community since the end of the civil rights and Black Power movements' (Neal 2002, 3). He sees this transformation as the culmination of a black nationalism whose roots lie in the black politics of the early twentieth century, but which has been reconstructed in the context of mass consumer society. The result, he suggests, is a more fragmentary set of positions that challenge the normativity of any particular black identity within American society.

Growing older in the context of a greater variety of 'black' lifestyles created new opportunities as well as presenting new challenges. Being 'post-youth', in a 'post-soul' cultural context seemed particularly difficult for those African Americans who were born in the 1940s and early 1950s. From their childhood the hardships of race had formed a continuing social reality, in systems of structured disadvantage; from their youth the hope, anger and pride associated with being 'black' burned as a memory. As these cohorts face negotiating a later life in an America that is more 'post-black', 'multi-ethnic' and yet perhaps more unequal than it was at the start of their adult lives, there seems to be more of a disconnect between the old ways of growing old and the new than that facing white America.

This is compounded by a 'second' generational gap, which has emerged within the African American community, one that appears as significant as that which emerged in the 1960s (Ogbar 2004, viii). African Americans born in the decades after the 1960s have been called a 'post-soul' generation, 'collectively different from previous generations of blacks – a hybrid of past struggles, the need for self determination and a desire simply to succeed on America's terms' (Neal 2010, 193). While the existence of such a 'post-soul' or 'post-black' generation is contested by writers who argue that the cultural changes that followed the 1960s have 'in reality' made little or no impact on the 1960s' aspiration for America to become a 'post-racial' society (Teasley and Ikard 2010), there seems at least some sense in which the practices of 'racialisation' and its embodiment have become more reflexively performed by later generations (Taylor 2007, 638).

Age and the Legacy of 'Race'

Those who grew up during the 1960s, whose experiences were shaped directly or indirectly by the Civil Rights Movement and the Black Freedom struggle, have witnessed the incorporation of many elements of 'black culture' into mainstream America – and vice versa. Many African Americans from the 'baby boom' cohorts occupy different material positions from those of African Americans from earlier generations. They also occupy different positions from those of young adult African Americans in the twenty-first century. For both generations, significant changes have taken place. In 1950, one third (36 per cent) of adult white Americans had graduated from high school; only 14 per cent of black Americans did so. By 2010, over 80 per cent of Americans, black and white, were high school graduates while the proportion of white American college graduates has risen fourfold – from 7 to 30 per cent – over the last half century, and tenfold – from 2 to 20 per cent – for black Americans. Improved education has been accompanied by higher incomes. In 1949, the median income of black Americans was half that of their white counterparts – a disparity that did not change during the 1960s (Batchelder 1964) but which did by the 1980s, even if not as much as might have been anticipated from the growing equality in educational attainment between black and white America (Sakamoto, Wu and Tzeng 2000; Wilson 1980).

Over the same period – from the 1950s to the 2000s – later life seemed to prove something of a leveller. Measures introduced since the mid-1960s reduced persistent poverty in later life for all racialised groups, through the redistributive impact of Social Security and Medicare. These policy initiatives have incrementally benefited successive cohorts of African Americans of retirement age. In 1968, older African American families (i.e. those headed by someone aged 65 and over) had a median income less than two thirds that of whites (64 per cent); by 2008, their median income had risen to three quarters of that of whites (77 per cent). The percentage of non-white American men aged 60–69 experiencing poverty fell from 39 per cent in the period 1968–84 to 22 per cent between 1985 and 2000. The percentage of white American men of similar ages experiencing poverty actually rose from 14 to 19 per cent. Although the gap was greater, change for women has been in the same direction – with poverty rates *falling* from 66 to 48 per cent for non-white American women aged 60–69, but *rising* from 21 to 24 per cent for white American older women (Sandoval, Rank and Hirschl 2009, 732; see table 5). Home ownership also suggests a narrowing of the black-white divide in later life. Using data from the *US Panel Study of Income Dynamics*, Hirschl and Rank found that 61 per cent of white people were home owners by age 30, but only 34 per cent of non-white people were (Hirschl and Rank, 2010), but by age 55, the figures had risen to 92 per cent for whites and 77 per cent for non-whites (an inequality ratio decline from 0.55 to 0.66). Although much of this change predated the civil rights legislation of the 1960s (Collins and Margo 2011, 22), what is noticeable is that from 1940 to 2000, the greatest increase in home ownership was amongst black householders aged over 50.

The divide in life expectancy between black and white Americans has also lessened over this period. Figure 4.1 illustrates the changing life expectancy of African American men and women at ages 55–64 and 65–74 over the period from 1968 to 2008.

Figure 4.1. Standardised mortality rates at ages 55–64 and 65–74 for US black and white populations, 1968–2008.

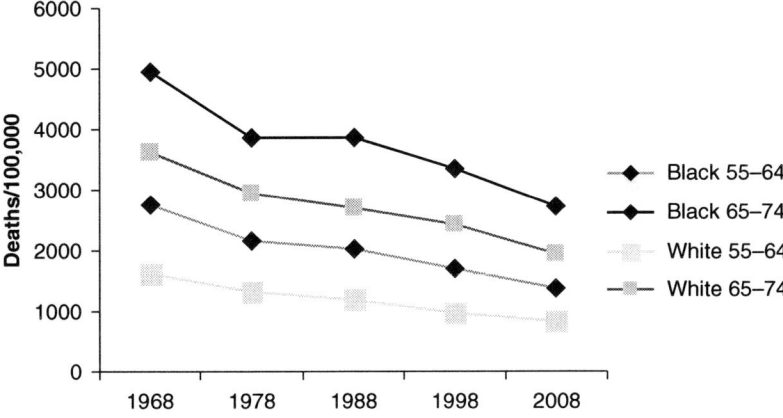

Not only have racialised divisions in the educational, income and health status of older Americans changed over the last half century, personal relationships have also begun to change. After the 1960s, inter-racial marriage became more common with rates of 'intermarriage' doubling between 1980 and 2008 (Taylor et al. 2012). Studies of internet dating suggest that amongst recent cohorts of 'older' people, those born after 1945 show more willingness to date people who are racially different from themselves compared with those from prewar cohorts (Tsunokai and McGrath 2011). Though limited, such statistical evidence suggests a diminution in the racial divide between black and white older Americans in terms of their economic, physical and social well-being – as well as in their levels of racial prejudice (Kleg and Yamamoto 1998; Wilson 1996).

In some ways this decline in difference is surprising, since there is a general belief that the impact of childhood poverty, more limited educational opportunities and greater disease burden should weigh particularly heavily upon African Americans in later life, through the processes of double jeopardy or 'cumulative disadvantage' (Mutchler and Burr 2011, 87–9). Despite evidence of an overall reduced life expectancy for those individuals identified as 'black' compared with those designated 'white', evidence of a racially structured process of cumulative disadvantage has been difficult to establish. As one researcher put it, findings have been 'fragmented and inconsistent, with some studies finding a persistent gap at the oldest ages [...] others one that increases across time or age [...] and still others, convergence at the latest ages [...] or no significant differences' (Taylor 2008, 230). Attempts to control such factors as selective attrition, differential health and disability status in younger adult life are now being made to better test the hypothesis of cumulative disadvantage, and recent research suggests that African Americans are still more likely to experience an earlier onset of ill health and a faster rate of deterioration in their health in later life (Taylor 2008).

Such findings have been viewed as a form of 'premature' ageing that derives from social rather than bio-medical or genetic factors (Geronimus 2001).

Central to this process is the over-exposure of African Americans to chronic stress arising from their position of material disadvantage and prolonged and persistent racialised oppression (Geronimus et al. 2010). Such socially mediated 'weathering' implies that 'US blacks may be biologically older than whites of the same chronological age due to the cumulative impact of repeated exposure to and high effort coping with stressors' (Geronimus et al. 2010, 2). Granted that such weathering can be demonstrated, is there any sign that it has become less severe over time, rendering the current cohort of African Americans approaching later life less aged than their predecessors?

If education, health care and affluence are major determinants of bodily health and well-being in later life, improvements in these areas over the last half century should have altered the extent to which ageing selectively disadvantages and depletes the still racialised bodies of American society. Black and white adult mortality rates have declined over this period. Death rates in later life among the older black population, for example, are lower in the twenty-first century than was the case for their parents' generation in their midlife. Even so the relative mortality differential between blacks and whites has shown little sign of lessening, reinforcing observations made earlier that despite overall improvements in health and well-being amongst the baby boom generation, 'the relative magnitude of the black-white differential has remained remarkably constant over time' (Cooper 1993, 139). Mortality among African Americans born between 1944 and 1953 remains higher than their white American peers, and the mortality differential between the two differs little from that of cohorts born before the First World War. At the same time the probability of African Americans dying before they reach old age (i.e. between ages 16–60) has declined dramatically over the last half century (Elo 2001) as has the prevalence of disability and the number of years spent with a chronic disability (Crimmins 2001; Manton and Gu 2001; Yang and Lee 2009). Whether or not the relative difference in rates of improved health and life has changed, the improvements for both black and white Americans have been substantive (Kramarow et al. 2007).

Analysing and understanding the structural disadvantages associated with being 'black' is rendered more contingent by the increasing disparities within American society; disparities that are replicated within both black and white communities. The cumulative benefits of better education, higher pay, greater home ownership and richer opportunities has favourably impacted on bodily ageing, irrespective of racialised identity. This leaves those without such benefits at risk of 'premature' ageing and with fewer of the bonds of race that once reached across the divisions of class. As improved standards of living have combined with greater diversification in the life course, expectations of a healthy later life have become more widespread at the same time as becoming more contingent. For those, whether they are black or white, favoured by good health in childhood, extensive education, well paid work and access to healthcare, the costs of longevity are considerably less and the capacity to age well considerably better whether measured by lower rates of disease, less functional impairment or the subjective experience of feeling healthy – compared with those not so favoured. As the number of African and European Americans in the middle classes has risen, so have the benefits attending that position and – it should be added – the disadvantages from not reaping these benefits.

Studies on the returns to health of educational advantage illustrate this point. Educational advantages strongly influence health and well-being for black and white populations alike, while the returns on poor education are much poorer health in mid-life (Walsemann, Geronimus and Gee 2008). Poorer health in mid-life, in turn, increases the risk of subsequent disability setting the conditions for a more limited and restricted later life (Taylor 2008). Nor is it just the experiences of childhood and youth that are embodied in later life. Policies and practices operating across working life and after play equally important roles. Estimates suggest that 'medical care amenable' morbidity may contribute up to one third of the black-white differential in mortality *before* age 65 (Macinko and Elo 2009). Changes in access to quality healthcare are evident across the population, but these changes have left a disproportionate number of African Americans without adequate health insurance during their working lives. How much a universal healthcare system after age 65 compensates for those earlier differences remains to be seen, although there is some suggestion that it may go some way to doing so (Banks et al. 2006; Sherkat et al. 2007).

In short, African Americans as a category seem to be ageing 'on the inside' at a faster rate than their white counterparts, even if the deleterious effects of the 'ageing process' are declining for both. A large part of such differential ageing must be located in the past and present social structuring of racialised identity within US society. Black and white differences in health and disability are much less evident in Canada, for example, implying that 'health inequalities are a reflection of much deeper and systematic racial inequalities in the US' (Prus, Tfaily and Lin 2010, 391). Secular changes in health and disability are, however, evident in both African American and European American populations, showing that 'more recent cohorts fare increasingly better in mean levels of physical functioning and self assessments of health […] because of large overall cohort improvements in health capital' (Yang and Lee 2009, 2117–18). Time and place impact equally upon age's corporeality.

Later life however may not be the principal site where the structural disadvantages of 'race' are realised. People defined as 'black' or 'white' reach later life in America through differing trajectories of ageing. To (mis)use Taylor's phrase, the old black are not yet the post-black (Taylor 2007) though they are becoming more diverse as a category of persons than those earlier generations of old 'black folk' born, raised and 'weathered' in Jim Crow America (Trotman 2002). Whatever the virtues born out of ageing during and after Jim Crow, for good or ill, contemporary and future cohorts of ageing African Americans will continue to share less of the common legacy of 'black' America as the black demographic continues to diversify and fragment (Berlin 2010).

Race, Ageing and the New Somatic Technologies

For most of the twentieth century, ageing and the anti-ageing enterprise were white endeavours. Ageing white faces dominated the displays 'describing' the ageing process and these same white faces appeared in the commercial, professional and academic literature to illustrate 'rejuvenation' or 'age reduction' interventions. Most indices of facial or skin ageing were based upon analyses of white skin. European models of facial youth and facial beauty provided the template against which rejuvenative interventions were measured. All this is beginning to change. Rising affluence, the changing demographics of 'race' and an increasingly common cultural concern for resisting the oppression of age have contributed to these market trends. The twenty-first century has seen a significant increase in the number of Asian Americans, Hispanic Americans and African Americans requesting cosmetic procedures, including blepharoplasty, fillers, Botox and chemical peels (Sturm-Obrien, Brissett and Brissett 2010, 70). Where cosmetic interventions amongst non-white, non-European populations once focused upon the reduction or minimisation of non-European features, such as minimising eyelid folds amongst people of Asian ancestry or narrowing the lips or nose amongst people of African ancestry, the analysis of attractiveness and the signs of ageing is increasingly set inside a matrix of distinct racial phenotypes. If aesthetic surgery acts as 'the canary in the coalmine' (Wong et al. 2010), reflecting the state of the economy in developed nations, its expansion and segmentation within multi-ethnic, multi-racial societies can be seen as indicative of the mass consumer market's developing emphasis on what some writers have described as 'masstige' or mass luxury for the multi-cultural middle classes (Silverstein and Fiske 2003).

Dermatologists have conventionally classified skin types and their vulnerability to sunburn and photo-aging using a classification developed to categorise white skin. As Taylor notes, set against this white template 'all skin of color was initially classified as type V' (Taylor 2002, S43). Studies of ageing skin classified the various depth and extensiveness of wrinkling according to measures developed on and for white aging faces. Until 1989, Herzberg and Dinehart claimed, '[skin] changes that occur with aging in blacks [were] almost un-documented' (Herzberg and Dinehart 1989, 319). Although there was an assumption within both black and white communities that black skin ages less quickly and less extensively than white skin, evidence to document and explain racial differences in skin aging did not started to appear until the end of the twentieth century. Research demonstrates areas of similarity and difference. On the basis of histological analyses of skin punches taken from 8 black individuals with ages from 6 weeks to 75 years, Herzberg and Dinehart argued that 'chronologic aging in white and black skin is similar' (Herzberg and Dinehart 1989, 319). However a subsequent comparative study noted that 'most of the older white women […] had wrinkles beside the lateral canthi of the eyes (crow's feet) and on the corners of the mouth, none of the […] black women had obvious wrinkles' (Montagna and Carlisle 1991, 934–5) – a result, the authors suggested, that arose from the emergence of large collagenous fibre bundles that 'result in an overall shrinking or withering of the dermal volume' (Montagna and Carlisle 1991, 936).

The demand for anti-ageing products from older people of African American and Asian American backgrounds has stimulated applied research into ethnic skin ageing. In 2003, L'Oréal USA opened its Institute for Ethnic Hair and Skin Research in Chicago; in Washington DC, Howard University's Ethnic Skin Research Institute was established in 2004 with substantial support from L'Oréal USA and Johnson & Johnson. In 2005, the Ethnic Skin Care unit was set up at the University of Miami Cosmetic Center, while in 2007 Rush University Medical Center opened a new Ethnic Skin and Hair Clinic. These developments have created new technologies for the measurement of the colour, appearance and structure of hair and skin which in turn have altered the significance of these features from matters of collective to matters of individual concern.

Research into ethnicity and skin ageing is beginning to extend understanding of ageing's corporeality beyond gerontology's dominant 'white' template. Various forms of alopecia that particularly affect African American women from early middle-age have become significant research themes in contemporary dermatology (Taylor 2002, S57). Hairstyles widely adopted within the African American population such as braids, microbraids, twists and cornrows can also result in alopecia and premature aging through receding hair (Taylor 2002). Some have suggested that links between promoting hair care and promoting health care may be profitably pursued particularly within the African American community (Browne 2006).

As demographic projections indicate that populations with skins 'of colour' will become a majority in the United States, 'the cosmetic and dermatological industries are [...] confronted not only with the issue of treating a population of increasing age but also one of increasing ethnic diversity' (Rigal et al. 2010, 168). The growth of civil rights, consumerism, market segmentation and migration that was set in motion during the 1960s is now impacting on the embodied diversification of ageing. Basic and applied researchers are examining issues of skin colour and hair texture not in the context of a racialised science of hierarchy that pervaded classic modernity, but as part of a market driven interrogation of previously taken for granted aspects of the body – whether in terms of age, gender or 'race'. New technologies are being deployed to measure the structure, smoothness, colour and degree of skin wrinkling. The 'subjects' of this research are no longer young and white – even if they remain overwhelmingly female. Blackness as a 'foundational' source of identity – like agedness – is becoming subject to interrogation, not by state sponsored scientists driven to discover a justification for evident social inequalities, but by a global consumer capitalism, keen to develop effective anti-ageing cosmeceuticals that will work for and be consumed by 'people of colour'. In seeking to resist the common oppression of bodily ageing, people of colour have become engaged not only with the beauty industry and its more conventional 'technologies of the self' but with the new somatic technologies of self-improvement that have flourished in second modernity (Reel et al. 2008).

The new ageing resists any simple identification of what is 'old'; it also undermines some of the previous certainties of 'race'. It is in these 'postmodern' approaches to bodily ageing rather than in traditionally welfare oriented social gerontology where racialised and aged identities are being 'deconstructed'. As one group of cosmetic dermatology researchers have noted: 'the human brain cannot memorise color and weak color variations precisely. Correct measurements and knowledge of slight color variations or changes in color evenness associated with aging [are] of great interest in improving the adaptation of cosmetic products to these variations [...] [and] protecting against [...] these age-induced phenomena' (Rigal et al. 2010, 169). Skin colour in young adults is primarily the consequence of the distribution of melanin granules and blood microcirculation; it varies less than it does in later life. Ageing is associated with increasing skin colour heterogeneity within and between populations. The skin of older people is less regular and less constant in both its shading and colouring. As youthfulness gains in value, it, more than racial authenticity, reflects individual desire. The desire to retain youth and delay, prevent or mask ageing is shared by growing numbers of people from white and non-white racial groups (Sturm-Obrien, Brissett and Brisset 2010, 72; see fig. 4). Attitudes toward rejuvenative procedures are changing. According to Odunze et al. (2006), 'a generation ago [...] African Americans hesitated [...] to entertain the idea of cosmetic plastic surgery fearing that a change in their appearance would efface their ethnic identity or heritage [...] The view of ethnic plastic surgery has changed dramatically [and] the awareness of the benefits of cosmetic plastic surgery is becoming ever present to patients [...] transcending cultural and racial boundaries' (Odunze et al. 2006, 1011). Once concepts of youth and beauty were 'universally influenced by European standards [...] [and] during the 1960s through the 1980s, these features were considered the goal for many surgeons' now, the goal for each rejuvenating procedure is 'maintaining the patient's racial characteristics while addressing the patient's specific desires' (Sturm-Obrien, Brissett and Brisset 2010, 73). Statistics released by the American Society of Plastic Surgeons (ASPS), showed 'ethnic' cosmetic procedures increasing by 11 per cent in 2008, with more than 3 million performed, while procedures among 'Caucasians' dropped by 2 per cent. For African Americans the increase was 8 per cent, for Hispanics 18 per cent and for Asians 3 per cent. Figures from the American Academy of Facial Plastic and Reconstructive Surgery (AAFPRS) indicate that African Americans now make up to 7 per cent of all plastic surgery patients (Brissett and Naylor 2010).

Although rejuvenative interventions are more commonly used by white rather than non-white populations in the USA, and presumably in other affluent societies, trends show that these disparities are lessening. The results of research undermine much previous 'scientific' work that organised bodily differences into a hierarchy based on 'race', replacing it with studies presaged upon the acceptance of a normativity of difference. While such developments might be restricted to the elites within consumer society and while racial difference may have a less benign import for the majority of older African Americans, the new somatic technologies are bringing a new colour into ageing and with it a broader acknowledgement of the diversity of the ageing body. The lens by which classical modernity saw black and white is being replaced by one that refracts colour. Part of this comes from a desire, shared by many African Americans from the baby boom cohorts, to not become old, to not become part of a colourless community homogenised by the attributions of whiteness.

Conclusions

The study of bodily ageing has mainly been the study of white bodies. In so far as they have figured in gerontology, racialised identities have been framed as sources of structural inequality where black is equated with 'lack'. Older people who 'pass' their bodily identity as 'not old' have, in the past, been treated as behaving in ways similar to people who have sought to 'pass' their bodily appearance as 'not black' – behaving inauthentically and even 'unnaturally' (Schonfield 1967, 270). The contemporary experience of ageing by people of African and other non-white ancestries has expanded beyond the structural stereotypes of 'race' and 'age'. Throughout the twentieth century and into the twenty-first century African Americans have bought into the same ideas of personal betterment and individualised distinction that pre-occupied modern white America (Chambers 2006). The development of self-care and the accompanying 'technologies of the self' did not take place exclusively in white society. The struggle of African Americans to escape the policing of the essentialised identities of 'sex' and 'race' through a more diverse set of embodied practices of self-care has resonance for the contemporary agonistic representations of ageing (Bailey 2008).

The turn to the body associated with identity politics has destabilised all forms of embodied identity even as it has sought to privilege them. Unlike the needs of the modern state to count and classify its citizens, the market thrives upon creating, fashioning and dissolving identities into lifestyles; within contemporary consumerism, authenticity and ethnicity have become lifestyle themes, not positions of permanence. The marketisation of self-care practices products and procedures has shifted ageing from a position framed within the expectations of a stable white male life course to one that sees ageing as shifting and changing through its relation to gender, ethnicity and other competing forms of embodiment. Second modernity situates the body through the performativity of diverse and often transient distinctions, some oriented towards and others orientated against ageing. These performances are supported and sustained by the multi-cultural consumerism of the third age, even as these distinctions are now incorporated within the structures of the state.

The racialised structure of American society has subjected black bodies to what has been called 'premature' ageing, leading to lower expectations of later life than those of the white majority of Americans. The distinctiveness of race in structuring that disadvantage is slowly dissipating. Poverty, educational disadvantage, interpersonal and institutional discrimination have weighed heavily upon the health and well-being of previous generations of African Americans in mid- and later life. Lack of access to good quality health care has compounded the problem. However, many African Americans are now reaching later life with increased human capital in the form of better education, better paid work, better housing and safer neighbourhoods. Many are participating in and helping to shape America's distinctive third age cultural habitus. In the process the ageing of people of colour is adding to age's corporeal diversity and distinctiveness. Many would not consider these developments to represent an effective resolution of the ageing that black bodies have had to 'weather'. There still is 'jeopardy' in having a black racialised identity in the USA. If this is less often realised in later life now, when various benefits associated with personal and occupational pensions, social security and Medicare have helped offset some of the earlier inequalities of working life, the effects remain both before and continue after the social protections of age are activated.

The impact of poverty, lack of education and poor housing on the quality of later life is undeniable; equally undeniable is the much greater likelihood that people of colour will have grown up in such adverse circumstances. But whilst such structural modelling of the adversities of the life course occupies sociological and social gerontological research, it is presaged upon and reinforces a model of docile ageing bodies that cannot but be other. This leaves, as it were, the sites of struggle over race and identity to other generations, and locates it in other life stages. Enabling bodily ageing to become a site of struggle not just for combating ageism but also racism is important. Enabling it to become an arena for differing ways of living longer is arguably equally important. Racialised identities can offer added opportunities for doing so. As more diverse forms of embodiment and self-care emerge, the hegemony of corporeality and the old binary oppositions of gender, 'race', able-bodiedness and age will necessarily be challenged. Linking ageing studies with ethnic studies, black studies and critical theories of race may prove a more exciting prospect for the social sciences than pursuing yet another attempt to test whether 'dual jeopardy', 'cumulative disadvantage' or 'age-as-leveller' better represents the truth about ageing and race.

Chapter 5

DISABILITY, AGEING AND IDENTITY

Of all the various forms of embodied identity, disability might seem to have the most in common with the new ageing. There seem obvious parallels between the disability movement's rejection of the idea of physical limitation constituting the basis for their embodied identity and the rejection within the cultures of the third age of corporeal weakness as a marker for later life. Yet such a coalition of interests has proved hard to realise, despite numerous calls for an alliance between older people's organisations and disability rights activists. This may be because both approaches have tended to pass over the subjective embodiment of both older people's and disabled people's lives, preferring instead to focus on issues of citizenship and civic rights. Another factor is the potential unease that such a coalition of interests might entail by implicitly acknowledging the body as a common 'flaw'. Addressing the body and its limitations might prove too uncomfortable, as it risks both groups being 'recaptured' by the modern institutions of health and social care from which they are still struggling to escape. However, an even more important factor in our view is the historical setting of the disability movement which emerged as one of the later 'new social movements' from the youth countercultures of the 1960s (Campbell and Oliver 1996, 46).

Like most of these counter-cultural movements, the embryonic disability movement rejected what it saw as the 'old fashioned' representation of disability maintained by modern society. The young disability activists, who started to emerge as participants in an identity based movement, shared the same desires for autonomy and authenticity, self-expression and the overthrowing of all the old, devalued identities as did their peers in the other already established new social movements. They sought to de-institutionalise 'care' and reject the existing focus on neediness, asserting, instead, the necessity of people with disabilities overcoming the 'disabling' structures of society in order to realise their own desires and express their own subjectivities. As with members of the other new social movements most of these young activists were intent on being young and certainly not on being associated with the old. A fusing of interests was therefore unlikely at the time. But young people, including disabled young people, do not stay young. The ageing of youth culture along with its cohorts of activists and supporters has begun to create a different form of engagement between ageing and disability than the one dominated by institutionalisation, but such engagement has been slow and difficult.

This chapter aims to explore the 'thinking through the body' that distinguishes the new disability movements from those that existed in the past; it will examine their contestation of the structuring and embodiment of impairment and assess the potential this creates for repositioning the relationship between ageing and disability. As with the notions of gender and race, the practices and narratives of those whose identities have been oriented toward their bodily differences – in this case disabled people – provide opportunities for re-thinking the corporeality of ageing and the dilemmas associated with its potential embodiment. While we are not alone in recognising this capacity of disability theory to offer new approaches to thinking about bodily ageing (cf. Minkler and Fadem 2002; Oldman 2002; Putnam 2002), realising such developments remains, for reasons we have alluded to, more difficult than might at first have been expected. Likewise, the ageing of those who formed the initial generation of disabled activists poses new challenges for how disability and disabled bodies are adequately represented. Ageing has been an 'absent presence' in disability activism and disability theory. The new ageing creates the conditions for a more explicit and extensive engagement.

The Making of Modern Disability

To understand the development of what has come to be known as the social model of disability and its positioning against the 'old fashioned' modernism of the twentieth-century nation state welfare policy, the disability rights movement needs to be put in an historical context. Doing so will allow us to better understand both the potential to engage with, as well as the conflicts of interest that arise from attempts to connect the narratives of ageing with those of disability. More specifically such contextualisation provides us with a standpoint from which we can examine the future potential of the disability movement to promote access, agency and engagement at all ages and not just for the non-aged.

The new disability movements have themselves begun to construct their own historical narratives concerning the position of people with disability in modern society (Mitchell and Synder 2003; Oliver 1990; Stiker 1999). They have argued that disability as a status, though existing 'in all communities throughout time' (Linton 1998, 4), only became a distinct source of identity within modern society. The industrialisation of Western nations in the nineteenth century saw the need for industrial wage labour and the growing geographical disjunction between home and work. Disability was identified primarily as an impediment to formal work carried out away from the home (Barnes 1997; Gleeson 1997). This process of identifying disabled people as 'unfit' for industrial labour saw the growth of institutional provision, the categorisation of types of disability and the development of training institutes to fit those selected for employment.

While the origins of the institutionalisation of people with disabilities can be traced back to the work of sixteenth-century Spanish monks who taught the deaf and blind children of aristocrats (Plann 2006), it was not until the eighteenth century that formal organisations and institutions were established across Europe to help blind, deaf and 'mentally impaired' children with education, training and support. Toward the turn of the nineteenth century, organisations for 'crippled' children began to appear (Borsay 2002, 106). It was not, however, until the late nineteenth century that specialist institutions for adults with physical or sensory disabilities came into being.

The majority of adults with physical or sensory disabilities were not to be found in institutions but amongst the 'outdoor' paupers of nineteenth-century society, eking out a living by begging or selling on the street. In England only a minority of the most impaired adults with disabilities were institutionalised 'en bloc', without reference to the particular nature of the impairment they had. Those who survived into old age, those who were unable to get around at all or to look after their own immediate needs were institutionalised in poorhouses and their associated infirmaries. It was through age, in short, that disability was institutionalised.

Things began to change after the First World War. Until then, adults with disabilities had received little specialist attention. While institutions providing teaching treatment and recreation for children with a range of physical and sensory disabilities were commonplace at the turn of the century in Europe and North America, once they outgrew their youth, people with disabilities were expected to make their own way through life, with no more support than might be offered to any other indigents. Amongst all the participating nations, the 'Great War' created a large number of young adults with physical impairments. In response, many Western governments established new charitable and professional organisations oriented toward the recognition and rehabilitation of adults with acquired disabilities. Large numbers of these young newly disabled people had suffered from locomotor injuries, which impaired their mobility, or from mental trauma (war neuroses), both of which prompted a focus on vocational rehabilitation. The sheer volume of disability stimulated the rise of advocacy organisations such as the Central Council for the Care of Cripples, set up in England in 1919 (Borsay 2002, 109), and the Disabled Veterans Association, set up in 1920 in the United States. The situation was similar in other countries. Stiker (1999) for example states that in France 'the origin of all work of rehabilitation is to be found in the problems raised by the redeployment and compensation of impaired veterans [from the Great War]' (Stiker 1999, 222, citing the work of Antoine Prost 1977).

The institutions and rehabilitation units that were set up during the early twentieth century focused upon men who had been injured or maimed by war, accident or work, typically ex-soldiers who had once been (and deserved still to be treated as) potentially productive workers. This period also saw the rise of the new 'therapy' professions – physiotherapy and occupational therapy in particular – each making their own distinct professional claim over the rehabilitation of these disabled, handicapped or injured ex-soldiers. While these developments were uneven and not easily sustained in the face of the economic problems of the inter-war years, they survived and after the Second World War they prospered as a more fundamental re-orientation took place in medical and surgical care for those disabled by traumatic injuries. Physical and occupational therapies now flourished as part of the new health care disciplines of rehabilitation medicine, and international medical rehabilitation bodies were established to cement the new sub-discipline within mainstream medicine.

Rehabilitation medicine has as short a history as the history of geriatric medicine, but it is one associated with less conflict and greater international consensus. The newly created World Health Organisation (WHO) established a section on rehabilitation as early as 1948. Various specialised hospital units were set up offering physical and occupational rehabilitation, some specialising in making and fitting prosthetic devices and developing specialised modes of transport, others emphasising sheltered workshops and re-skilling. These centres catered for young men blinded or made deaf by trauma as well as those immobilised by loss of limbs or neurological injuries. Unlike previous generations of disabled adults institutionalised because of their age or pauper status, these new generations of disabled adults were predominantly young men defined by their previous physical fitness, and in many cases by their courage and self-sacrifice. The old, 'ugly' face of disability, the unsightly ageing beggars that had been the focus of the 'ugly laws' enacted by various North American municipal authorities during the late nineteenth and early twentieth century (Schweik 2009) was transformed by the presence of these young, fit and disabled ex-soldiers. This young new constituency acted as a stimulus to the development of physical rehabilitation as a distinct branch of medicine, and led to a general re-organisation of medical and health care. Increased provision for those whose bodies had been damaged by war or work was extended to those disabled from birth or infancy, those with mental disorders and those whose impairments arose in the context of age associated illnesses and generalised infirmity. Within these new divisions of healthcare and welfare, those serving youth and the youthful body were the most privileged and although some were the historical precipitates of the previous institutional organisation for the poor, others were more distinctively modern products.

Postwar social policy toward disability maintained the separation between childhood, adulthood and old age (Jonson and Larsson 2009). In Britain, provision serving the needs of soldiers and those serving the needs of the aged infirm clearly privileged the former (Titmuss 1976), and despite some amelioration in the care of the aged this distinction was retained until the soldiers themselves had grown old. Rehabilitation medicine, no less than the subsequent disability movement, served the needs of the young, neglecting or confining the care of the aged and infirm to geriatric units where doctors and nurses sought to build their own distinctive 'rehabilitation units' that might compete with the units of mainstream (adult) rehabilitation medicine. But unlike the focus in the 'medical' rehabilitation units on the impairments of the disabled patients, geriatric rehabilitation units were focused on the need to 'unblock' beds in acute wards rather than as a means to equip their aged patients for 'independent living' (Pickard 2010).

During the postwar period it was British geriatric medicine that established itself as the leading voice of health care in old age. In doing so, it placed chronic illness, disability and infirmity at the centre of 'healthcare in old age'. Textbooks on geriatric medicine began to emerge, the first edited by the British geriatrician, John Brocklehurst, was published in 1973 (Fillit, Rockwood and Woodhouse 2010, 1). In this and similar textbooks, the emphasis was placed upon the distinctive complex of geriatric conditions that geriatricians had to deal with and the complex multidisciplinary service that was required to address them, including specialist day units and day hospitals designed to offer care without risking a potentially blocked bed. The 'rehabilitation' on offer in these services was located not in the specialist medical rehabilitation units set up during and after the second World War, but in hospital geriatric units whose inhabitants were caught between acute admission wards and the 'long term' care units of the old infirmaries. In geriatrics, it was not so much bodies as beds that defined the problem. Warren's model of the workings of a modern geriatric unit had been that of a 'central processing unit' admitting and quickly discharging older people 'out' to the community, to their old home or to new homes – residential homes, almshouses, or 'long stay annexes' (Warren 1943). Treating the infirmities of old age became a new branch of medicine whose legitimacy rested not upon the 'worth' or 'potential' of its patients as upon its success in unblocking beds blocked by old people (Millard and Higgs 1989). Disability in later life was less a status deserving of attention, more an obstacle to hospital efficiency. To justify this, the disabilities of these old patients were represented as made up of 'intrinsic' and 'excess' disability. The elimination of the excess disability became the aim of geriatric 'rehabilitation' while the infirmities that remained served as the passport to long term care.

In contrast, non-aged adult rehabilitation medicine was much more sensitive to the difficulties faced by people with disabilities. This new branch of medicine viewed disability primarily in terms of lack or absence – whether it was the lack of a limb or organ, the lack of physical or mental development or the general lack of functionality, especially locomotion. Making good this lack required a mixture of professional expertise and social welfare. Together this (hierarchically organised) partnership between medical and social expertise was seen to represent the best chance of relieving the individual tragedy of corporeal suffering. Disabled people were objects of care, but the object of that care had as its endpoint a transition toward the patient's increased, if still supervised self-governance. In contrast to the marginalised role of 'geriatric rehabilitation' within the postwar health care system, physical rehabilitation medicine sought not to empty beds but to rebuild lives.

The New Social Movements: People with Disabilities Speak Out

The new social movements that emerged in the 1970s provided a significant challenge to the postwar biomedical identification of disability with physical impairment, making more salient the distinction between having a disability and experiencing that disability (Putnam 2002). These groups' focus was less about redistributing health and social care resources – a continual issue for these institutions and their professional representatives – and more upon recognising their desires to be full participants in mass consumer society. These desires are typically the desires of youth and like most new social movements of the period, the disability movement was itself a movement of youth. Many of its principal leaders were either student activists or young unemployed men and women, keen to leave behind the paternalism of the past and direct their own way of living with their disability (Scotch 1989). Many of these movements were organised on college campuses and were oriented toward middle class youth in much the same way that other earlier counter-culture 'struggles' such as the Women's Movement and the Civil Rights/Black Power Movement had been (Hahn 2002). The disability organisations that had been set up during the first half of the twentieth century had sought to represent the interests of disabled people by concentrating primarily upon employment and economic issues, modelled upon labour movements and operating primarily as pressure groups (Barnes, Mercer and Shakespeare 1999). In contrast, the new disability movements of the 1970s expressed more personal concerns over authenticity, lifestyle, freedom and respect (Shakespeare 1993). The individual lives and experiences of those leading these movements were used to expose the oppression faced by all disabled people. At the same time, their narratives were used to illustrate the potential for transgression, such as that realised in the sit-ins and protests organised to pressure US President Carter's new Secretary of Health, Education and Welfare (HEW) into signing off the regulations to implement the anti-discrimination requirements of Section 504 of the 1973 US Rehabilitation Act.

Rehabilitation and readjustment were replaced by demands for full recognition of the rights of disabled people. They sought nothing less than full participation in the mass consumer society with which the majority of the able-bodied were engaged. Groups such as Deaf Pride, the Rolling Quads, and the Cripple Liberation Front saw their struggles to overcome marginalisation and exclusion as intimately linked with other liberation movements such as the Black Power movement, gay rights and the Women's Movement of the 1960s (Fleischer and Zames 2001). In order to draw upon the strongest collective influence, the movement sought to downplay individual differences in bodily sites of impairment, particularly rejecting any 'Cartesian' inspired distinctions between the vulnerabilities of the mind and those of the body. The position that people with disabilities shared – of disadvantage, disinvestment and disregard – was more important and more salient than any biomedical classification of their impairments and handicaps. In the United States, the 1973 Rehabilitation Act and particularly its Section 504 which dealt with employment discrimination, the use of affirmative action and the provision of civil rights to people with a disability, provided the framework that helped US disability activists in 1975 to form a cross-disability alliance known as the American Coalition of Citizens with a Disability (ACCD). In 1977, ACCD achieved its greatest success when the then HEW Secretary of State, Joseph Califano was finally pressured to sign off the regulations implementing Section 504 of the Act (Fleischer and Zames 2001). Focusing upon distinct corporeal sites and structures such as impairment or loss of a limb risked a return to the clinical gaze, and the dividing practises of institutional bio-social medicine. Joining forces across these sites, like joining with other social movements advocating a greater voice for minority groups in society, provided the new movement with a more powerful set of intellectual reference points as well as a common set of political goals and strategies of political activism (Johnson 1999).

These communities of difference created new forms of 'embodied' awareness, deconstructing the broader social construction of disability as a biomedical impairment and reconstructing it as an alternative position that emphasised the agency of disabled people, their rights and their desires. Explicit in this politics of the personal was an emphasis upon disabled people as oppressed social actors and the distinction between 'having a disability' and 'experiencing disablement'. Decentring the corporeality of physical impairments, the movement focused upon the recognition of distinction, the acceptance of difference and the civic rights of all citizens to participate on equal terms in the social and cultural world in which they live. The new disability movement spanned a variety of positions from the cultural politics of Deaf activists who sought to valorise Deafness as a distinctive ethnic sub-culture to people with spinal cord injuries seeking success and pleasure through sports, dance and the arts. Other elements within the movement continued to emphasise obtaining an adequate income, combating employment and housing discrimination and advocating a consumerist led approach toward accessing health and social care. At the heart of these movements was the 'social model' of disability that has provided much of the conceptual glue holding the various groups within the movement together, a model that has sought actively to replace a focus upon the corporeal with one located firmly within the social.

Decentring the Corporeal: The Social Model of Disability

Following in the wake of the new social movements of disability, disability studies emerged as an academic sub-discipline in the mid- to late 1980s. The academics staffing these departments and units drew their ideas and their inspiration from the positions that had already been articulated by the disability activists of the late 1960s and 1970s. Like them, their goal was both to improve the social and economic position of people with disabilities and to challenge the knowledge/power of the 'medical gaze', and its capacity to objectify and oppress people in the process of helping them. The discourse of the 'social model' of disability served as common ground for the disability rights movement and for the academic sub-discipline of disability studies, 'act[ing] as a litmus test for progressive disability politics and disability studies research within the Western academy' (Campbell 2009, 99). Although the interpretation of the meaning of the 'social model' of disability differs between Europe –particularly the UK – and North America its central premise, however nuanced, is that 'disability' arises not from the body but from the relationship of society and its institutions to its 'embodied' actors. Disability is not something one has – like a disease – but something one experiences, operating in the same way as racial prejudice or the hetero-normativity of sexual relationships.

The core of the social model developed by activist academics such as Victor Finkelstein and Mike Oliver in Britain (Finkelstein 1980; Oliver 1990) and writers such as Harlan Hahn in the USA (Hahn 1985, 1988, 1994) is that 'disability is the loss or limitation of opportunities to take part in the normal life of the community on an equal level with others due to physical and social barriers' (Driedger 1989, cited in Barnes 1991, 2). In short, the model makes the specific claim that it is the social institutions and social structures that 'disable' people with impairments. By changing the organisation of society disability can be altered or overcome. Understanding disability in terms of physical or biological limitations is, according to Abberley, akin to those sexist or racist ideologies that attribute a lower status to women or black people because of their corporeal limitations (Abberley 1987). As a result the focus upon bodily impairments encourages societal oppression and marginalisation of disabled people which in turn reinforces their poverty and their material and social disadvantage.

Such views supported a focus upon 'access' rights and challenged public attitudes towards, and assumptions about, the place of disabled people in society, as much as on achieving effective access to benefits and financial support. Some, such as Finkelstein, adopted a neo-Marxist approach and saw technological change as supporting the growing enablement of disabled people. He argued that much of the social disadvantages faced by people with disabilities arose as a direct result of the process of industrialisation, which demanded standardisation, mobility and manual skills from the workforce, thereby limiting the earning potential of disabled people. In a post-industrial society, technological interface developments could therefore transform the nature and extent of 'disability' in relation to both work and social relationships.

The widespread adoption of this model has seen the enactment of extensive national and local legislation across a growing number of countries, which has sought to achieve through the law the social inclusion of disabled people through increased provision of resources such as sign language support, public documents written in Braille, hearing aid loops in public settings, ramps and lifts in public buildings, adapted crossings and kerbs and public toilets with wheelchair access, raised seats and support bars, as well as anti-discrimination policies as well as practices designed to improve access to education and employment (Albrecht and Verbrugge 2003).

It has also contributed, directly and indirectly, to an emerging market for new enabling technologies that render disabled people less disabled, while making public and private spaces less constricting. Such developments include powered wheelchairs, automatic vehicle controls, computer based voice-assisted technologies, computerised control systems for domestic equipment, accessibility redesign of buses and trains, altered cinema, museum and theatre seating arrangements and automatic door openers.

Post-structuralism and the Social Model of Disability

Despite the influence of the social model of disability, the deliberate decentring of the body and the material nature of impairments has for some time been a source of unease. As Hughes and Paterson have pointed out, the sociology of the body and the sociology of disability have followed contradictory trajectories (Hughes and Paterson 1997), and while sociology was busy (re)discovering the body in the 1980s, the disability movement was busy distancing itself from it. The social model of disability viewed disability as 'socially produced by systematic patterns of exclusion that were [...] built into the social fabric' (Hughes and Paterson 1997, 328). This focus upon oppression and discrimination tended to marginalise the corporeal. As Michael Oliver has famously argued: disability 'has nothing to do with the body' (Oliver 1995, 4). Despite its relative success within health and social policy, the social model of disability has been accused of evading the subjective experiences of corporeal difference and impairment that people with disabilities contend with, and the alienation that arises from their bodies being positioned as 'other' within society (Thomas 2007).

The experience of 'otherness' has provided a second point of reference connecting the disability movement with other forms of identity politics, including the Women's Movement, Black Power and gay rights movements. People with disabilities are seen to share a similar position to those whom the state and society deem to embody weakness, instability, disorder or deviance (Hahn 1994; Oliver 1990). Consequently this has prompted the need once again to recognise that the personal is political. Within this 'post-structuralist' framework, people with disabilities are encouraged to value their embodiment as a positive 'difference' rather than focus solely upon achieving access as equally disembodied citizens to the 'public sphere'. This requires engaging in a 'discursive shift away from disability as deficiency to disability as a positively valued difference' (Gray 2009, 326–7). As part of achieving this, previous terminology used to discredit and devalue people with disabilities – such as 'cripple' or 'spastic' – has been re-appropriated by people with disabilities themselves, as acts of transgression that challenge the dominant meanings previously attributed to people's corporeal impairments (Mairs 1989; Milam 1983).

If the original social model is represented publicly by the impersonal symbols of stylised wheelchairs and disembodied ears, indicators of access rather than agency, the post-structuralist model re-directs attention to embodiment and the cultural enactment of physical difference. 'Repositioning' the disabled body by making salient its fears, hopes and desires, the post-structuralist model seeks to acknowledge both the inescapable subjectivity of the body and the significance that this has for ordering social relations. In Snyder and Mitchell's words, this model points toward re-introducing the disabled body 'as the more appropriate paradigm for a mutable (and one might add inherently vulnerable) humanity' (Snyder and Mitchell 2001, 386).

Crip Theory, Crip Practices

Within this more explicitly 'cultural studies' approach, disability moves from a position of structured inequality to one of 'alterity' or 'otherness'. Disability is reframed in the subjective terms of narrative and performativity, and people with impairments are cast as agents performing disability as one of many possible 'others'. '"Disabled" is not something one is, but something one becomes' (Moser 2005, 669). Following Foucauldian influences, this 'cultural studies' approach 'proceeds from a frame which figures disability as a representational system' supported by a variety of transgressive narratives, each of which offer alternative views of bodies that while different are still potentially 'desirable' (Campbell 2009, 170). Instead of focusing upon the structural constraints to social participation, this post-structuralist position concentrates upon disabled people as desiring and desired subjects, whose performances and narratives are limited more by their struggles to realise their personal desires than they are by the inaccessible nature of civic space. Within this framework, image and sexuality become important sites of agency, conflict and contestation – not just in terms of the sexual activities of people with disabilities but in terms of a broader engagement with individuals' sexualised identities and the art, fashion and media that shape and support such identities.

Theoretical concerns with performativity exemplified by the work of Butler and Shildrick and by Bakhtin's writings on the transgressive have been realised by writers such as McCruer (2006) and Snyder and Mitchell (2006), and in the practices of a number of disabled artists and activists who have sought to realise a kind of 'disability culture' that is distinct from the academic analysis and activism originally associated with the social model. Within this 'abject aesthetic', the bodies of people with disabilities become both object and subject, sharing in a common fascination with what might otherwise be deemed distasteful or shameful. Drawing in part upon 'queer theory', in part upon gender theory and in part on critical race theory, the vulnerability and instability of the disabled body is re-introduced as a universal element in the experience of human corporeality – in effect denying attempts to marginalise or differentiate the body of disabled people from other possible yet equally vulnerable bodies (Campbell 2008; McCruer 2006; Mitchell and Synder 2006; Shildrick 2005).

So called 'abject art' has sought to establish a poetics of bodily waste, as part of the desire not simply to shock, but to challenge the very idea that human relationships acquire the kind of 'normative' perfection that rids them of their incomplete, messy nature. People with impairments posing nude or being photographed or painted nude, choose to 'perform' their disability other than as a member of 'the deserving poor', the halt and lame, society's faithful but flawed followers. In doing so, they invite a response that can move from disgust to desire, from repulsion to attraction, as the flawed body becomes both 'model' and 'object' serving, as a contrasting corporeal authenticity set against the air-brushed flawlessness of conventionally unreal models of beauty.

Examples of this transgressive 'othering' of beauty, range from the actress, Playboy model and lecturer Ellen Stohl to athlete, actress and model Aimee Mullins, famously owner of 12 pairs of prosthetic legs. Mullins' prostheses have served not only to project her as an athlete and model, but also have acted as representations themselves of a designer ethos that replaces clinical with athletic or aesthetic functionality (Pullin 2009). Similarly, if more prosaically, the 'rights' of disabled people for a sexual life have been championed by a number of disability-based organisations where there is a joining together between the traditional perspective on 'access and independence' associated with the disability rights movement and the cultural subjective concerns of the post-structuralists. Viewing a person with disabilities as both a desiring subject and an embodiment of desire has lead a number of activists to draw attention to the limitations as well as the possibilities for sexual pleasure that are available to people with disabilities.

Tuppy Owens, a British activist and writer, founded the Sexual Health and Disability Alliance (SHADA), with the aim of bringing together health professionals, people with disabilities and others to foster links between sex and disability. She began her work as a publisher of erotica, trained as a sex therapist in the 1980s and set up the charity The Outsiders as a dating and partnering agency for people with disabilities. Her work linked health and social care professionals with disabled people to foster improved attitudes and access to 'healthy sex' for disabled people. As writers such as Wilkerson have noted, in coming to terms with sexuality, its problems and its promises, disabled people confront the sense of shame and guilt that is associated with failing to meet the sexual standards of 'heteronormativity'. Their experience of shame and abjection links them to other men and women such as those with homosexual desires or those able-bodied people for whom sex remains a desired yet difficult enterprise (Wilkerson 2002).

The need to confront the potential for abjection and shame attached to sexuality and to bodily impairment provides a major theme in the disability studies literature. While post-structuralist approaches have sought ways of celebrating corporeal diversity and of universalising bodily difference, the new narratives of transgression attached to sexuality, subjectivity and bodily impairment have re-inserted the experience of internal personal struggle into the social theorising of disability. Rather than emphasising only the positive opportunities of choice implicit in the idea of alternative performances of disability such as 'the super crip', these writers address the constraints on performance, the experience of shame and the distress created by the corporeal limitations of the body and the sense of 'ill-being' that this can engender. It is to this theme of theorising vulnerability and suffering in disability studies that we now turn.

Ill-Being, Vulnerability and Universal 'Suffering'

Forming yet another element in the post-structuralist model of disability, a number of writers with and without a disability have begun to explore the corporeality of experienced impairment and the suffering that it occasions. As Tobin Siebers has noted, the disability rights movement and its social model has challenged the corporeal representation of the body by 'provid[ing] insight into the fact that all bodies are socially constructed – that social attitudes and institutions determine far greater than biological fact the representation of the body's reality' (Siebers 2001, 737). Yet, as he notes, more recent autobiographical accounts of living with various bodily impairments have begun to bring a new 'realism' that seeks to re-appropriate bodily experiences not as part of a celebratory transgressive aesthetic but as part of the 'crude reality' of life, illness and suffering. This narrative 'return to the body' does not mean a simple return to medical discourses of and about disability. Siebers refers to the new writing about disability as an attempt at demythologising ideas of 'disability as advantage' (Siebers 2001, 745) whilst not kicking away the supports of the conceptually limited social model of disability, nor dismissing entirely the cultural stance adopted by the post-structuralist writers. Instead this new writing brings to bear new representations of the corporeal as both narrative and performance, linking them to theoretical ideas about the body that have been developed by second and third wave feminism and the decentering of traditional social theories associated with 'queer' theory and other 'subaltern' studies (Seidman 1998).

Hughes notes that 'ideas about frailty and vulnerability in disability studies [...] were banished by the rise of the social model in the 1980s and 1990s' (Hughes 2009, 401). Focusing upon society's structural barriers and the agency needed to overcome those barriers, he suggests, led to the 'fleshy issue of impairment' being neglected. Post-structuralist feminist writers such as Rosemarie Garland-Thomson, Elisabeth Grosz and Margrit Shildrick have sought to reconnect with the wounded, the monstrous and the abject elements of disability and impairment, but, accepting Hughes' point, there remains in much of this queer and/or feminist theorising an element of abstraction, of reification and even of voyeurism that elides the corporeal specifics of impairment with the looser generalities of gender, sexuality and their performance as 'display'.

Liz Crow delivered a powerful critique of the 'silence' within the disability movement over bodily impairment when she wrote:

> Many of us remain frustrated and disheartened by pain, fatigue, depression and chronic illness [...] many of us fear for our futures with progressive or additional impairments; we mourn past activities that are no longer possible for us; we are afraid we may die early [...] we desperately seek some effective medical intervention; we feel ambivalent about the possibilities of our children having impairments; and we are motivated to work for the prevention of impairments. (Crow 1996, cited in Wendell 2001, 23)

An uneasy relationship, Wendell points out, exists between disability activists and the notion of chronic illness. It is, she argues, easier to advocate for disability pride than to advocate for pride in illness and impairment. By promoting images of the 'able' disabled, those less able to 'conform to an inspiring version of the paradigm of disability' are rendered failures in properly embodying its distinction. Such failure to be positively disabled acts as a threat to narratives that stress the social oppression and disadvantaging of disabled people. Perhaps improving access and independence are not the only (or even not the most important) issues for people with disabling illnesses or impairments. 'Solidarity', she points out 'between people with chronic illnesses and people with other disabilities depends on acknowledging the existence of the suffering that justice cannot eliminate' (Wendell 2001, 31). The youth culture in which so many of the new social movements flourished valorised autonomy, choice, pleasure and self-expression, and represented the various embodiments of youth as equally important sites for personal and political development. Set against this youthful energy and optimism, time can seem be an enemy and age a source of limitation. Just as critics of the 'successful ageing' paradigm have argued, such a movement can serve as much to marginalise the unsuccessful majority as promote the well-being of the 'ableist' minority.

The importance of providing a space for suffering for people with impairments has also been emphasised by Rita Stuhkamp. She is at pains to point out that 'intangible suffering continues to exist and there is no answer to it' (Stuhkamp 2005, 712). The dilemma between the personal experience of corporeal suffering and the civic struggle of the oppressed to assert their rights and gain 'social' entry, while resisting the ever present objectifying gaze of the normative other, is not confined to those with one or more disabilities. It has obvious connections with the dilemmas facing people in later life, whether or not they experience themselves as disabled. It is in essence the dilemma of maintaining a lifestyle that is conscious of, but yet not constrained by, the limitations of the corporeality upon which it must to some degree rest.

Integrating Age and Disability Studies

Promoting a positive model of corporeal difference without marginalising corporeal limitations and personal suffering is a dilemma common to the discourses of positive ageing and disability studies. Yet ageing has often been sidestepped by the disability movement, perhaps because it is thought of as 're-introducing' the idea of limits, a notion which distracts from the aim of achieving equalised access and an assertive presence for people with disabilities as desiring subjects. Whatever the reason, ageing and old age have been problematic for disability movements. The temporality that defines ageing contrasts with the 'atemporality' associated with the social positioning and representation of disabled people. Although there is increasing interest in the history of disability and disability organisations, the contextualisation of disability has been set against social, not personal, time scales. Idealised models of disability stress both its lifelong nature and its unchanging presence – where change is located primarily in social histories and personal journeys. Even when disability is contextualised by reference to the life course, the focus remains static, as if children with disabilities remain forever children, working age adults forever of working age while old people remain old and largely silent.

Repeated calls have been made to link the disability movements of the 1970s and 1980s with the concerns of older people who have disabilities, however, these calls have so far proved more or less ineffective (Oldman 2002). Peter Townsend, one of the first sociologists to draw attention to the potential for linking together issues of later life with those of disability, pointed out how, throughout the 1960s, policy toward the disabled was 'still largely governed […] by the source, rather than the effect of disability' (Townsend 1973a, 113). This, he argued, militated against the best interests of older people whose disabilities are 'generalised and tend to merge with the limitations associated with particular conditions' (Townsend 1973b, 101). Yet in some ways Townsend missed the point. He suggested that there was 'a failure fully to acknowledge disablement among the elderly' (Townsend 1973a, 97), a claim reiterated by Oldman when she writes that later life studies pay little attention to disability (Oldman 2002). Arguably the position is the complete opposite. Gerontology and geriatrics are drenched with disability and disablement. The textual links and institutional connections between old age and disability are extensive and point exclusively in one direction – from 'becoming' old to 'becoming' disabled. The reverse is much harder to contemplate, and what is most noticeable about Disability Studies is the relative absence of ageing and a general neglect of the transition from 'becoming disabled' to 'becoming old'.

Incommensurable paradigms of disability contribute to this neglect. Within gerontology disability has a different meaning from that which is commonplace in the world of disability studies. There, 'people with a disability' are the principal subjects of attention, their actions those of social agents striving for visibility and a voice. 'People with a disability' are generally not old – though some do acknowledge that people with bodily impairments are now living long enough 'to enter the ranks of old age' (Putnam 2002, 799). Old people, on the other hand, are commonly seen as being or becoming disabled as part of their own agedness, with age dominating their qualifying for such a 'becoming'. Numerous reports indicate how the numbers of people with potentially disabling conditions are assumed to 'increase substantially in coming decades' as 'aging baby boomers […] fuel this growth' (Iezzoni and Freedman 2008, 332). But while 'people with a disability' are now accorded more respect by ceasing to be 'disabled people', old people are rarely reframed as 'people of a certain age'. Old people and disabled people share a common position in terms of a public standard of functionality or health, but the meanings invested in age and disability, the capital to be extracted from their commonality and the exclusions, limitations and pain associated with each position vary substantially.

From the start, gerontology has been preoccupied with reifying the disabilities of age, measuring them through a variety of composite indices (Pickard 2011). Since its origins in the 1940s, a stream of publications from gerontology has led to innumerable indices of disability such as the Barthel Index (Mahoney and Barthel 1965); Townsend's Index of Incapacity Scale (Shanas et al. 1968) Lawton and Brody's Activities of Daily Living (ADL) and Instrumental Activities of Daily Living (IADL) scales (Lawton and Brody 1969) and Katz's Activities of Daily Living Scale (Katz et al. 1963). Whilst these indices have served as important sources of academic and professional capital, with each research group preferring the use of its own particular favourite instrument, these 'disembodied' versions of disability fail completely to convey what disability may mean to older people themselves, what struggles they conceal and what shame they hide. Disability measures remain determinedly third person accounts defined by the limitations observed, but never by those that are felt or struggled with. People of working age are expected at least to help define their disability status through completing or being assisted to complete official forms which address them in the second person, and can expect to be rewarded for doing so by receiving whatever allocated benefits and resources their scores entitle them to. By contrast, the ascertainment of disability in later life is little but a process of 'othering', supporting professional practice and determining resources accruing to services, but rarely representing individuals' experience of corporeal limitation in a way that can be used by the older person for their own benefit.

Such disjunctures between 'people with disabilities' and 'old people' make the integration of positions and perspectives a difficult proposition. While representing oneself as 'disabled' provides a potential site of agency and entitlement for those who are not old, adding an identity of agedness, unlike for example those associated with gender, race or sexuality, restricts more than it enhances the space within which the embodiment of disability can be presented, practiced and re-presented. For older people, in contrast, successfully eschewing the status of disability increases their chances of performing merely as 'not young', but without being named and shamed as positively 'old'.

Technology, Ageing and Disability

If there is one arena however that demonstrates the possibility of enhanced embodiment for people who are 'not young' and/or 'not able-bodied' it may lie in the development of technologies for somatic enhancement. Even as geriatric and rehabilitative medicine are beginning to recede from the landscape of medical care (Claussen 1997; Grahame 2002) other branches of medicine and surgery are growing in size and influence, and offer an alternative perspective as providers of 're-abling' or 'rejuvenating' services to older people adversely affected by disability. One such specialty, orthopaedics, rose to prominence upon the treatment and rehabilitation of the crippled child (Cooter 1993) and flourishes now as a provider of hip and knee replacements that successfully mobilise hundreds of thousands of people over the age of fifty (Ibrahim et al. 2010).

Other branches of medicine have also inserted themselves into later life, such as dermatology, ophthalmology and plastic surgery. Like orthopaedics, their aim is less to contain or colonise later life but to release older people from the limitations, shame and suffering associated with the impairments of their ageing bodies. While geriatric medicine has become increasingly 'international' and its once concise textbooks re-issued as gigantic tomes anxious to be seen not to neglect any potential medical, social or psychological aspect of ageing (cf. Evans et al. 1992; Fillit, Rockwood and Woodhouse 2010; Soriano et al 2007), its source of distinction has become limited to defining, defending and managing the boundaries of a fourth age framed by a disembodied yet pervasive state of dangerous disability or 'frailty', a narrative of marginality more profoundly 'other' than the normative otherness of everyday ageing (Gilleard and Higgs 2011b; Grenier 2007). This re-positioning of geriatric medicine from a concern over excess disability to one over immanent frailty frees up disability in later life to become more easily connected with the disability of those not yet 'not young'. Unshackled from the undifferentiated 'othering' gaze of geriatrics and gerontology, disability can at last be confronted and negotiated at all ages under similar terms and conditions.

Addressing the corporeal nature of disability in this way becomes part of democratising the life course. Blindness, deafness, lameness or haltness can be understood and addressed at any point in the life course and the desire for corporeal enhancement or embodied equivalence made to matter equally at each and every point. Such arguments go beyond conventional ideas of 'impairment' or 'disability', and raise more general questions about the acceptability of all corporeal limits to wholeness and the significance of chronological age as a legitimate source of exclusion. Should the correction of a particular visual or hearing impairment in later life be afforded similar treatment as the more general desire not to have to have one's senses dimmed? Should laser correction be used to correct only 'ageing' eyes or should it be applied universally so that all adult eyes possess an ageless visual acuity? Should cochlear implants be confined to those who have never benefited from hearing or should they be made available to anyone wishing to enhance their hearing? Should adults be free to choose to exchange their limbs for a carbon fibre prosthetic that would enable them to run longer and faster? Or should such options be available only to young amputees? And if so, when exactly does 'young' pass its sell by date? The possibilities of aspirational medicine raise new concerns over the boundaries of human corporeality in ways only beginning to be glimpsed. Technology unites at the same time as it divides; whichever way, it is creating new spaces for debate within both disability and ageing studies that need to be carefully pursued.

At any age, corporeal imperfections can be redefined as the 'fractured terrains' of a 'multi-sectional market' that thrives upon difference and the endless desire for new and improved identities, lifestyles and social spaces (Mitchell and Snyder 2010, 191).

A market for enhancement and for distinction co-exist, if at times uncomfortably, with the bio-politics of the modern state and its strategies of self-governance. This governmentality is not without its own difficulties as its 'regulatory spiral' (Beck 2007, 685) seeks to keep up with the new opportunities opened up by technology and biomedicine. The task is to match the freedom of diversity with an awareness of its potential negative consequences. The marketing of strategies for corporeal augmentation and reduction that are promoted in some post-structuralist models of disability foregrounds issues of vulnerability, and makes the struggle against being marginalised central to the understanding of 'disability'. But like all new social movements, the disability rights movement is also capable of engaging with a consumer oriented capitalism that has learned to embrace and indeed incorporate counter-cultures into its activities (Boltanski and Chiapello 2005; Heath and Potter 2005). Could such developments be extended to address the challenges posed by the impairments of later life? Clearly they can and there are already many examples, from the provision of hair transplants to the sale of fashion-house designer spectacles, from HearWear style hearing aids to electric all-terrain scooters, from dental implants to bilateral cochlear hearing implants, from hip and knee replacements to cosmetic tattooing. As Graham Pullin has pointed out in *Design Meets Disability*, appliances, prostheses and enhancement technologies can be seen as either distinguishing/privileging bodily differences/deficiencies or supporting a more general desire for personal betterment (Pullin 2009). While the near universal appeal of technologies such as the mobile phone can be used to support people with hearing impairments, an exclusively designed mountain-bike wheelchair can also be used to distinguish the (disabled) athlete from the (disabled) couch potato. In this recognition that all desire to be embodied actors on a corporeal stage, to be better than our bodies were born to be, makes designing for enhancement a market that excludes only those who cannot afford it. The fact that not all are equally likely to succeed in this enterprise is, of course, the other side of the coin and reinforces the experience of the transience of people's lives and their inherent corporeal vulnerability.

Conclusions

We have outlined how disability has come to form an embodied identity with the potential to contribute to thinking otherwise about embodiment in later life. Within the disability movement, two broad approaches toward the body can be identified. The first seeks to decentre the body as a site of distinction, focusing instead upon issues of access and engagement. Within this narrowly 'social' model, attempts to draw attention to the body as the site and source of particularised social differences are discouraged, and the focus placed upon achieving material change in the lives and opportunities of people with disability, through local and national political activities and lobbying. The second approach seeks instead to re-imagine the embodied nature of disability, combining its universalising qualities of vulnerability and imperfection with the privileging of distinct forms of embodiment, where 'shame will no longer structure our wardrobe or our discourse' (Linton 1998, 4). Although both structural and post-structuralist models of disability have achieved much of relevance for older bodies, disability studies and the disability rights movement still marginalise issues of age and ageing. In doing so, they tend to assume an unchanging essentialism in the identity of disabled people allowing social, but not personal, change to render identity contingent. At the same time, as geriatric medicine shifts to consolidate its resources upon the idea of 'frailty', gerontology remains tied to the biomedical model of disability and dysfunction where disability still operates as an index of insufficiency and predictor of adverse outcomes. It is a property of others; an objective status of an otherness that is misrepresented as 'ageing'; an otherness to be coped with.

What it means to struggle, tentatively and unaided, to cross a room; to lose the taste for good food as eating with ill-fitting dentures becomes increasingly uncomfortable; what it means to feel tired and dizzy after walking ten steps up the theatre stairs; in short all the various individual struggles and contestations over being identified as an old, disabled other, scarcely find a voice in the gerontological literature. The ageing body is defined while its subjectivity is denied by gerontology. For all its post-structuralist flourishes and its dour strategic demands for recognition, disability studies have at least created openings that ageing studies have so far failed to exploit. What is needed is for a less essentialist narrative to emerge within disability studies, that acknowledges the changing and unstable nature of disability, and that embraces a position that rather than belittling or rejecting the idea of embodiment instead seeks to explore and expand it, through technology, culture and self-care as well as through welfare policy and practice. It would be a mistake to ignore the obstacles that exist in creating a unified 'movement' between older people and people with disabilities. Neither group will necessarily benefit. But a common desire for betterment and a shared realisation of vulnerability and corporeal transience may yet serve as a bridge.

Chapter 6

SEXUALITY, AGEING AND IDENTITY

Earlier chapters have explored the embodied identities of gender, race and disability and how these different engagements can transform our understanding of ageing and its embodiment. The post-sixties' cultural environment, we have suggested, re-oriented social relations around the body while also facilitating the commodification, segmentation and fetishisation of the body through lifestyle marketing (Heath and Potter 2005). These developments problematised the bodily binary oppositions such as man/woman, black/white and able-bodied/disabled. With the opening up of second modernity and the ageing of those cohorts involved in its features, the binary opposition of 'youth' versus 'age' also began to unravel. Ageing, and bodily ageing in particular, was represented through a more diverse and contested set of narratives and practices which were oriented less towards realising a particular version of 'old age' than to not becoming old. By asserting the continuing relevance for 'performing age' of the various narratives associated with able-bodiedness, gender and 'race', alternative ways of ageing could be constructed that could not be easily reduced to the old narratives of decline (Gullette 1997).

Societal concerns surrounding sexuality and sexual orientation also provide an equally important terrain where a confrontation between the binary narratives of youth and age is witnessed. More than other forms of embodied identity, identities that privilege sexual preference and sexual practice can be seen to position themselves against the conventional embodiment of age. Youthfulness has long been associated with sexual desire; age with its decline. If continuing to perform as a sexual being in later life seems a transgression of age, performing as an aged homosexual person seemingly represents a double transgression, of both age and of sexuality. Within this matrix of age and sexuality, the ageing homosexual individual doubles the risk of failure, first by not being able to maintain in later life a lifestyle embodied by the distinctiveness of his or her sexual preference, and secondly by failing to affirm age within a gay or lesbian identity. Such personally positioned identities therefore risk collapsing into an abject, neutered old age. While such risks are by no means absent in the relationship between age and gender (or race or disability), they become much more salient and challenging when the relationship between identities embodied through sexual orientation has to be negotiated in the context of age.

Sexuality involves both a narrative of identity and a performativity of practice. The link between these two reveals an important thematic bridge throughout this book, namely the fluidity of the relationship that exists between embodied identities and embodied practices. Thus far, we have examined how the 'contested' embodiment of gendered, disabled and racialised identities serve as vectors disrupting and disturbing the narrative of bodily ageing as decline. We have also noted how corporeal ageing serves a similar, reciprocal function, destabilising the 'un-aged' identities of gender, race and disability. Sexual activity whether conceived as practice or preference has long been deemed relevant in representing and understanding bodily ageing. However, this understanding has been achieved more through the exercise and expression of sexual activity than through its role as embodying a distinct social identity.

Unlike sexual practice, sexuality as a gendered partner-preference is a distinctly modern source of social distinction (Foucault 1990a; Halperin 2000; Weeks 1985). It has consequently had less time to affect the various realisations and representations of bodily ageing. Arguably, it is only in its late twentieth/early twenty-first century framing that sexual partner choice has emerged as a source of embodied identity in later life. This relatively narrow time frame limits the possibilities for sexuality to engage with ageing as an embodied identity or lifestyle. Faced with the assumed incommensurability of sexual activity and ageing, the problematising of the relationship between sexual orientation and age is both more acute while lacking in precedent and practice.

As in previous chapters, we will begin this chapter with a historical perspective on sexuality as an embodied identity and explore its relationship with age. We will focus primarily on the emergence of modern 'homosexuality', the circumstances that saw the construction of this identity and the subsequent gay and lesbian movements that emerged within the counter-cultures of the 1960s. With this in mind we will explore the consequent engagement and confrontations with ageing by 'gay liberation' and the various gay and lesbian movements that developed in what has been described as the post-Stonewall era. The final sections of the chapter engage with developments connected to the emergence of 'queer theory' and its impact on ideas of embodiment and identity. Specifically it will engage with notions of 'outing' alternative understandings of ageing that mainstream heterosexual culture has seemingly either ignored or paid less attention to.

Sexuality Becomes Identity: The Making of the Modern Homosexual

By drawing attention to the possibility that sexual behaviour, like the body, could confer an identity, Foucault's work on the history of sexuality re-orientated the way the humanities and social sciences approached the body and sexuality (Foucault 1990a). Cocks (2006) has argued that it is only in the modern era that 'we can say that we have 'a sexuality' as the prime essence of selfhood […] through the rise of bio-power in its various forms […] placing […] heterosexuality along a spectrum of various types of behaviour' (Cocks 2006, 1212). Following Foucault, before the modern era sexual acts were understood by reference to their legality, their civility or their moral acceptability and were not seen as constitutive of some distinct aspect of human individuality. Procreative heterosexual intercourse provided the only accepted and acceptable model; as the antinomy of such practices, the act of sodomy was the archetype of uncivilised, unconstrained and immoral sexual behaviour. Only as the nation state established its new disciplinary 'bio-powers' with the creation of police forces, criminology, forensic medicine and psychiatry were distinct sexualities identified. Through these means, Foucault claimed, sexuality began to define individuals and not simply individual practices. Halperin (2000) points out that in this sense, the naming of same-sex sexual preference as 'homosexuality' represented a 'modern construction, not because no same-sex sexual acts or erotic labels existed before 1869 when the term 'homosexuality' first appeared in print, but because no single category of discourse or experience existed in the premodern and non-Western worlds that comprehended exactly the same range of same-sex sexual behaviours, desires, psychologies and socialities […] that now fall within the capacious definitional boundaries of homosexuality' (Halperin 2000, 89).

The extent to which such 'sexual identities' were the specific product of modern sensibilities is still debated (e.g. Boswell 1991). What is less contestable is that the late nineteenth century naming of 'homosexuality' as a identifier applicable to both genders of persons sharing same-sex 'behaviours, desires, psychologies and socialities' (Halperin 2000) laid the foundations for innumerable 'personal discoveries' that enabled men and women, previously confused by their sexual desires, to articulate a more distinct sense of who and what they were. The modern narratives of 'sexual identity' that were created in this way led to the disruption of the simple binary opposition of gender. In its place, sexual identity established a more complex, fourfold categorisation, one which divided gender (male and female) by sexuality (heterosexual and homosexual). This broader categorisation seemed at first to capture within its matrix the totality of modern sex and sexuality.

This public naming of homosexuality made the criminalisation of homosexual acts matters of active political debate. If people engaged in same-sex acts because of who they were, rather than what they were, medical and non-medical advocates began to argue that it made little sense to treat such behaviour as the expression of deliberate criminality. While drawing upon 'pathology' as the lens through which homosexuality or 'sexual inversion' was identified, the late nineteenth and early years of the twentieth century saw the beginnings of a public advocacy for 'homosexual rights', complementing as it were, the 'first wave' of the sexual revolution. The impact of two world wars and their associated bodily discipline closed off, or at least severely limited, this emerging debate. It would take the broader currents of the second sexual revolution and the confluence over sexual liberty across the new social movements to draw to a close the modernist imaginary of (male) homosexuality.

Gay Liberation and the Sexual Revolution of the 1960s

With the publication of the Kinsey Reports after the Second World War (Kinsey, Pomeroy and Martin 1948; Kinsey et al. 1953) sexual behaviour was described through formal systems of measurement and quantification and in so doing they became the first 'census' of sex. In the process of such quantification, the modernist binary division between 'heterosexual' and 'homosexual' started to break down, suggesting instead a new 'dimensionality' of sexual preference. The essentialism that had dominated the early forensic discourse of homosexuality also seemed to be in need of revision by a much less rigid categorisation of sexuality and sexual preference. According to Kinsey's research: 'nearly half of the population [...] has had sexual contacts with or reacted psychically to individuals of their own as well as of the opposite sex' (Kinsey, Pomeroy and Martin 1948, 616). Under these circumstances, he argued, homosexuals and heterosexuals were 'merely' the extremes in a much more plastic human sexuality than had previously been imagined in mainstream society. The widespread publicity that the Kinsey reports received renewed calls for the decriminalisation of homosexuality and encouraged some men and women to 'come out' with their homosexuality. In the United States, however, the process of 'coming out' was temporarily suspended during the McCarthy era as a postwar American witch hunt began for communists and homosexuals 'hiding under the bed'.

By the 1960s, the politics of McCarthyism were widely discredited. Movies began to portray sympathetically the lives and lifestyles of homosexuals (*Advise and Consent* 1962; *The Detective* 1968; *Victim* 1961; etc.). At the same time, most major US cities had begun to see a successful, if still ghettoised, homosexual scene, where it was safe for homosexual men to meet up, cruise, mingle and have sex. It was in one such setting that perhaps the most significant event took place that triggered the counter-cultural 'gay liberation' movement. The Stonewall riots of 1969 took place outside the Stonewall Inn in New York which was a bar in which gay men from a variety of social backgrounds would socialise. Following a police raid characterised by a particular brutality towards the clientele of the bar and those in the neighbourhood, the gay community reacted by staging a riot. As the first organised protest by homosexuals against police brutality, the Stonewall riots provided the impetus for the creation of Gay Liberation and Gay Pride. Leaders of the gay liberation movement sought to position homosexual men and women as another socially marginalised, oppressed minority, akin to the position that other ethnic or racial minority groups occupied (Valocchi 1999, 60). This 'positioning' of homosexuality as an oppressed minority community soon entered the social sciences reflecting the integration of the counter-culture within academia at that time (Robinson 2006). In a key 1968 article entitled 'The Homosexual Role', the English sociologist and feminist, Mary McIntosh argued that 'it is not until he [sic] sees homosexuals as a social category rather than a medical or psychiatric one that the sociologist can begin to ask the right questions about the [...] homosexual role and about the organization and functions of homosexual groups' (McIntosh 1968, 192). This appropriation of homosexuality as a social rather than as a medico-pathological construct provided the grounds for a new discourse around identity and community that was elaborated by several of the 1960s' 'sexual revolutionaries'.

Gay liberation and lesbian feminists embraced their new social identities through a variety of 'collective action frames' (Valocchi 1999, 60). These included the positive valuing of homosexuality as an identity (gay pride), claims for the liberatory potential of homosexual sex (gay liberation), identifying the oppressiveness of the dominant 'heterosexism' permeating the organisation of society and social relations (gay and feminist consciousness) and the location of this oppression in the state, the family and popular culture (gay activism). But as Valocchi has pointed out the links that were made with other new social movements of the 1960s as well as the older social movements such as organised labour in the search for a 'unity of difference or oppression' were not easily sustained. Soon two routes emerged in the direction taken by the various gay and lesbian rights movements. One route, expressed most forcefully in the Gay Pride 'sub-cultural' approach, celebrated the distinctiveness of a homosexual identity and/or lifestyle. This approach particularly helped stimulate and was supported by the consumerist 'capture' of gay culture. The other, less travelled, but more overtly political saw itself as linked to a broader coalition of other, no less marginalised minorities who placed themselves in opposition to the powers that dominated modern society. This approach, initially more critical of the consumerist incorporation of gay culture, 'lost out' on the streets if not in academia, to the narrative of 'gay is good; buy it'.

Sub-cultural and counter-cultural strategies alike saw sexual activities, like other embodied practices, 'embedded in social scripts' that could become sources of personal identity because of their inextricable engagement in the social organising and policing of inter-personal relationships. The habits and practices of the body were political strategies that required 'boundaries and techniques to enforce those boundaries' (Valocchi 1999, 66). This 'politics of the personal' discourse espoused by the women's rights movement (Rowbotham 2011, 15) argued that, however arbitrarily these boundaries of gay and lesbian identity were constructed, they were needed in order to support and stabilise the still fragile gay and lesbian communities that were emerging at that time. Despite setbacks during the 1980s HIV/AIDS pandemic, homosexual communities continued to expand, while developing new ways of thinking and acting that cross the homosexual/heterosexual divide.

This crossover between gay and heterosexual identities has refashioned mainstream culture. These crossover practices have been commodified and marketed in much the same way as the crossover practices of other counter-cultural movements of the 1960s have (Heath and Potter 2005). As well as impacting upon the visual importance of men 'looking good' and hence increasing the demand for 'male' self-care (Luciano 2001, 153), the crossover of practices has worked the other way, through the attainment of heterosexual 'family' rights for gays and lesbians, in areas such as adoption, assisted reproduction, marriage and partnership rights. These legal breakthroughs have enabled gay and lesbian citizens in various countries to become almost equal citizens in a multicultural, multi-layered second modernity. At the same time, being unmarried or remaining single as well as maintaining serial partnering have become acceptable heterosexual lifestyle choices. While these changes can be located within particular twentieth-century cohorts, such 'crossover' developments have begun to extend their influence over the whole of the adult life course, changing the meaning of later life for homosexual and heterosexual people of both sexes.

The initial demographic base for these changes – as it was for many other social movements of the 1960s – lay among the youth. It was young people who on the campuses, in the clubs and bars sought sex and the security of belonging (Berger 1984). Some commentators of the time saw homosexuality as a social pattern of sexuality that was mostly expressed by teenagers and young men. McIntosh, for example, argued that homosexuality was a social construction, an identity formed within and largely confined to a particular stage of life. Drawing upon Kinsey's cross-sectional data, McIntosh wrote that 'as they grow older, more and more men take up exclusively heterosexual patterns' (McIntosh 1968, 190). This 'youth' bias she suggested was reinforced by the importance of sexuality in framing youthful identities. The emphasis upon sexual identity and youth has continued. Reviewing recent research in this area Heaphy, Yip and Thompson have noted how 'the growing research on lesbian and gay lifestyles is predominantly concerned with youthful experience' (Heaphy, Yip and Thompson 2004). While homosexuality has its own life history it is still one that pivots around youth, retaining a significant generational gap that limits the 'age-integration' of homosexual communities even in the post-Stonewall period (Boxer 1997, 189).

In the last decade of the twentieth century, the focus upon youth began to change as the post-HIV/AIDS epidemic 'epidemiology' of sexuality witnessed a decline in the perceived youthfulness attached to homosexual identity. At the onset of the epidemic, the average age of homosexual men contracting and dying of AIDS was between 21 and 34. Over the next two decades, the average age at death rose substantially. In Australia, over three quarters of the gay men who became HIV positive in the mid- to late 1980s were under the age of 40 but by the mid-2000s, over half were middle-aged or older (Murray, McDonald and Law 2009, 84). By the time effective retroviral treatments became available, HIV was no longer a disease confined to young adulthood. In the West, at least, the homosexual community came to terms with mortality and by the end of the twentieth century it was beginning to come to terms with ageing.

Changing views and experiences of 'being' and 'becoming homosexual' have come about both through systems of cohort replacement and over time within cohorts themselves. There has been growing acknowledgement that homosexual identity and homosexual lifestyles extend and persist well beyond the confines of youth, informing people of different ways of growing up and growing old (Fredriksen-Goldensen and Muraco 2010; Slevin and Linneman 2010). Reflecting this process of cultural change, a literature and ethnography has started to appear which addresses issues of adult development and ageing among gays and lesbians. It is to this new literature that we now turn.

The 'Grey and Gay' Literature

As death rates from AIDS climbed inexorably throughout the 1980s, intimations of mortality spread through the (male) homosexual community. For many sexually active gay young men, reaching old age seemed a limited rather than a limiting prospect. Prior to the AIDS epidemic several accounts of gay men facing ageing had been published, mostly framed around the stereotype of a strongly 'youth' oriented gay culture and the all too abject position this implied for the 'ageing queen' (Allen 1961; Bennett and Thompson 1980; Harry and DeVall 1978; Kelly 1977; Kimmel 1979; Minnigerode 1976; West 1967). As AIDS made a gay old age less likely, the early interest in the problem of ageing within the gay (male homosexual) community seemed to decline (Boxer 1997).

By the 1990s however, as more HIV positive men survived into and beyond mid-life, reaching old age began to have something of the cachet of 'success' that 'successful ageing' was having in the heterosexual community. Research on gay and lesbian adult development and ageing became resolutely more positive, even 'transgressive'. Although homosexuality and 'ageing' still went largely unaddressed in the biomedical sciences literature (Snyder 2011), 'queer ageing' was beginning to influence gerontology and ageing studies (Hughes 2006). Papers began to be published which destabilised the taken-for-granted nature of categories such as heterosexuality and homosexuality as writers sought to develop a distinctly 'queer' perspective in gerontology not only by challenging the 'old' folk tales of the lonely old queen in society, but also by asserting the 'open' and contested nature of both sexual identity and age (e.g. Pope 1997; Harrison 1999; Peacock 2000; Grossman, D'Augelli and O'Conell 2001).

While the development of gay identities had initially privileged youth and often treated ageing gay people and lesbians as representatives of an old-fashioned and no longer wanted group, the ageing of the post-Stonewall 'baby boom' cohort presented a new and different challenge, of staying gay while growing grey. Male homosexuality began to be viewed as a 'modifying agent' in the adult life course, a different kind of ageing (Drasin et al. 2008). Previously, youth had been idealised within the male homosexual community and older homosexual men were perceived to be 'cast out' from this privileged age category. The result was that they (middle-aged gay men) ended up experiencing a premature and lonely old age (Allen 1961; Gagnon and Simon 1973; Hoffman 1968; West 1967). Although empirical support for the 'premature ageing' hypothesis was limited (Kelly 1977; Kimmel 1979, 1980), it retained an iconic significance for providing one of the first examples of sexual identity-based difference in the organisation of the adult life course. Previously hetero-normativity had dominated models of the life course. The alterity of homosexuality exposed it as more contingent, implying that homosexual men acquired the identity of 'old' at a chronologically earlier stage, and labelled as old corporeal signs that in the heterosexual world were used to indicate 'male maturity' (Fox 2007).

Even if the idea of the 'limited life expectancy' of active, engaged homosexuality has been challenged, it expresses a contingent reality about time and age. A preference for relationships with younger men for example was found more often among 'pre-Stonewall' older cohorts of gay men than was the case for older men born later (Harry and DeVall 1978). Disengagement from gay sub-cultures has been found to be more common amongst older cohorts than younger ones (Gray and Dressel 1985, 86–7) while middle-aged and older gay men have been reported more likely to seek out younger partners when they are not part of the 'gay scene' community (Harry and DeVall 1978). While this particular approach to 'queering the life course' may now seem a little anachronistic, the exploration it represented of the ordering of gay and lesbian life courses served as an early blueprint for more general questioning of the hetero-normativity of contemporary models of adult life course development.

This questioning of the hetero-normativity of adult development and ageing has been extended into other arenas, including issues of 'age and identity development', 'age and sexual practice', 'age and anti-ageing consumerism' and 'age and social relations'. Research into homosexual 'identity formation', for example, has challenged the universality of Eriksonian theory of 'identity formation' (Erikson 1963, 1980), by locating the acquisition of a homosexual identity at a much later age than the period of adolescence to which Erikson had originally assigned it (Drasin et al. 2008). At the same time this heterosexual/homosexual difference seems equally contingent, as there is also evidence that male homosexual psychosocial development itself demonstrates a marked 'periodicity', with members of pre-1950 birth cohorts 'coming out' at later ages than their age peers from more recent, post-1950s birth cohorts (Drasin et al. 2008). Compared with the heterosexual community, chronological age seems a weaker marker of significant change in the personal and social identity development of gay men who find themselves 'doing at 48 what most people do at 23' (Herdt, Beeler and Rawls 1997, 240).

The second challenge that viewing ageing through the lens of homosexuality provides is the issue of sex in later life. Although ageing has traditionally been associated with a decline in sexual activity, expression and desire, this has mostly been read as a decline in the frequency of sexual intercourse 'negotiated' in the context of a longstanding monogamous heterosexual relationship. Those heterosexual men and women who are without a longstanding partner in later life typically show a decline in sexual activity (DeLamater and Moorman 2007; Reece et al. 2010; Herbenick et al. 2010). Having to seek a sexual partner outside the hetero-normative domestic sphere of married life seems to demand more agency, more deliberation, and perhaps more uncertainty over what kind of sex might occur and how often it might happen. Conventionally as individuals got older there is a transition toward a more 'sexless' sex life, particularly for those without marital partners. In contemporary circumstances, however, the individualised and less exclusive homosexual sexual partnership provides an alternative model for aging differently from that of heterosexual married life.

Because of the limited nature of large scale comparative studies of sexual activity amongst older single and partnered homosexual and heterosexual individuals these hypotheses remain conjectures. Given the centrality of sexuality to identifying as gay or lesbian, there may be a greater pressure for homosexual men and women to continue being sexual beings in later life, than is the case for the 'default' heterosexual community. In support of this conjecture, research suggests that there is relatively little change in either the number of sexual partners or the amount of sexual activity that gay men experience from their twenties through to their late sixties (Gray and Dressel 1985), while research looking at same-sex partnering amongst both men and women suggests that this may not be the case for women who do show evidence of a decline with age in the number of same-sex partnerships experienced over the last year (Butler 2005). However, Butler's analyses also revealed that there was an overall increase in the number of women having same-sex sexual partnerships over the period 1988–2002, suggesting that both young and old lesbians are expressing their sexuality with a greater degree of freedom than before, even if they express their sexuality this way less often with age. Certainly the relative lack of age-associated decline in sexual partnering and related sexual activity among older homosexuals contrasts with the sexual practices of older male and female heterosexuals (Reece et al. 2010; Herbenick et al. 2010). The hypothesis that sexuality amongst older gay men and, more recently, amongst older lesbians is more actively expressed than among older straight men and women has at least some indirect empirical support. Arguably, how large or distinct such differences are, is, perhaps, not the key point. What is significant about same-sex sex, at any point in the life course, is that it is intrinsically more diverse and perhaps also more self-consciously practiced than heterosexual sex. In this sense, gay and lesbian sex might more fully embody the values of choice, autonomy, self-expression and pleasure said to characterise the 'habitus' of the third age (Gilleard and Higgs 2011a; Higgs and McGowan 2012) than heterosexual sex, through perhaps at the price of an increased fear of being overtaken by 'old age' (Fox 2007; Schope 2005).

Part of the reframing of ageing within the gay and lesbian community, it has been claimed, is that it 'encounters older people not just as bodies [...] but also as erotic beings [...] [leading to] a celebration of the erotic in oldfulness' (Hughes 2006, 56). Such revisioning of the erotic raises the question of whether older gay men are also more likely to buy into the consumerist framing of age and sexuality and whether, in contradistinction, older lesbians are less likely to do so. After the AIDS/HIV pandemic passed its peak, an emerging gay market was identified that was 'estimated [in the USA] as encompassing between 14 and 25 million men and women' (Haslop, Hill and Schmidt 1998, 318). As Wentzell has pointed out: 'the American 'gay niche market' [...] developed in the 1990s in concert with the expansion of gay-targeted media [...] which expanded, becoming more sophisticated – and less sexualized – and attracting mainstream advertising' (Wentzell 2011b, 110). Unlike other 'oppressed' identities, the identities of sexual preference were rarely framed as being over-determined by the relations of production. Instead gay and lesbian communities have been identified with consumption, and, as the consequence of their liberation from the economic confines associated with the male breadwinner household, seen to be 'endowed with significantly above average discretionary spending power' (Haslop, Hill and Schmidt 1998, 315). Research conducted into the gay market indicates that this particular community of consumers values highly notions of 'freedom', 'self-expression', 'community', 'individualism', 'hedonism' and 'diversity' (Haslop, Hill and Schmidt 1998, 323).

How far consumerism also mediates the relationship between gay culture and ageing is difficult to judge, and whether this engagement is more evident than it is in 'mainstream' heterosexual culture is debatable and probably contingent upon gender. The hypothesis that older gay men are more engaged with the practices of self-care while older lesbians are less engaged with them seems one worth pursuing. Several writers have argued that older gay men continue to perform as 'erotic' or 'hedonistic' beings longer and later in life than their straight peers. Halperin, for example, writes that contemporary queer culture:

> Far from producing practices of freedom, has simply promoted new forms of discipline and constructed even more insidious procedures of normalization [...] as well-socialized lesbians and gay men spend a lot of time – and more tellingly money – acquiring the requisite T shirts, muscles, haircuts, tattoos, dietary habits, body piercings and so forth [...] reducing politics to a consumerist lifestyle. (Halperin 1995, 112)

In a way, this rueful account echoes Angela Davis' comment about black politics and hairstyles noted in chapter 4. But much of what Halperin excoriates is a particularly 'masculinist' gay culture. The question of whether older lesbians engage with the market as much as, or much less than, gay men is open to further inquiry. It may be argued that they do not because lesbians of all ages less often frame their erotic identity through the enhanced embodiment of 'femininity'. Whatever may prove to be the case, these questions illustrate the value of studying the difference different sexualities may fashion in their various embodiments of ageing.

Until recently, conventional research on sexual activity in later life has tended to ignore people with non-heterosexual identities and it is not yet possible to determine whether Hughes' notion that gay culture 'celebrates the erotic in oldfulness' is evidently the case, or whether it is selectively the case for men but not women, or indeed whether sexuality does lead to different ways of embodying age. There is some evidence, for example, that a stronger orientation towards the body, a preference for relating to partners and peers rather than to kith and kin and a sub-cultural emphasis upon youth and appearance is more typical of gay sub-cultures than it is of lesbian communities (Schope 2005). As contemporary gay sub-cultures have expanded, Schope claims, they have become more youth-oriented and body-fixated. 'Older lesbians', Schope found, 'are more likely to be accepted at lesbian social […] events than older gay men are at gay events […] [because] older lesbians, less burdened by challenges to their self-esteem, have changed how lesbian society […] perceives the aging process' (Schope 2005, 34). Older gay men may thus serve as icons in consumerist 'third age' cultures and support the ideals of 'successful ageing' (Friend 1990). In contrast, older lesbians may choose to invest more of themselves and their bodies in family or family-like relationships, providing 'mothering' or 'grand-mothering' roles within the lesbian community that reinforce rather than reframe traditional models of gendered ageing while minimising or making less salient the corporealities of ageing (Orel and Fruhauf 2006).

Set against the individualised body work that some gay men continue to pursue in later life, gay and lesbian communities may serve as alternative social structures that provide a collective setting in which members can retain a sexualised but less corporealised identity throughout their adult lives. If family and kin relationships serve to sustain the gendered roles and identities of heterosexual family members throughout their adult lives, without explicit reference to their individualised bodies, active engagement within gay and lesbian communities might serve a similar function. This re-shaping of 'family' and 'social relations' in later life provides a fourth theme in reframing ageing through a non-heterosexual lens, where the body, its corporeality and its embodiment are perhaps less salient – whilst being less open to negotiation and the practices of freedom that Foucault wrote about in his later years.

For many older gay and lesbian individuals, the social ordering of their age and gender by family relationships has been, if not absent, then much weaker than is the case for their straight peers. Homosexual identities are often self-consciously defined *against* those that were forged within their families of origin (Muraco, Le Blanc and Russell 2008; Sears 2008). At the same time, family, in the conventional sense, is not without significance for gays and lesbians. Studies indicate that about 14 per cent of gays and 28 per cent of lesbians in the USA are parents while a larger minority have family ties typically associated with heterosexual marriage – like in-laws (Black et al. 2000). Here too, cohort differences render such generalisations contingent. In one Australian survey, no homosexual men in their twenties were married or had children, while 21 per cent of those in their mid-forties were married and 32 per cent had children, rising to 25 and 50 per cent respectively for those in their mid-sixties (Jorm et al. 2003). Assuming that part at least of these chronological age differences are cohort differences, this study suggests that kin are becoming less of a tie for increasing numbers of gay men. Similar trends are evident for homosexual women. Only 5 per cent of 20-year-olds were married in this survey, and 9 per cent had children; while 19 per cent of those in their mid-forties were married and 46 per cent had children; with figures of 33 and 50 per cent for those in their mid-sixties (Jorm et al. 2003).

Projecting these trends forward might imply that gay men and lesbians will be increasingly likely to remain childless and unmarried in later life. However, the very recent rise of civil partnerships and gay and lesbian couples adopting or conceiving children through alternative means may prove a counter-balancing influence. Even so, gay and lesbian marriage/civil partnerships may be confined to a minority within a minority, for some time to come and the more limited kinship ties surrounding the adult life course of gay men and lesbians may continue to place greater demands on the active construction of an embodied identity than is the case for those in more traditional family settings where moral rather than corporeally based identities are sustained. Several writers in the 1960s and 1970s described the relative 'rolelessness' of single ageing male homosexuals which they thought contributed to 'premature' ageing that was discussed above (Weinberg 1969; West 1967). Prior to Stonewall this may well have been the case, as older homosexual men and women found concealing their sexuality easier as they aged into companionate marriages within a heterosexual household. Current mid- to late life gay men and lesbians are perhaps the first generation to be in a position fully 'to live out gay lives' (Muraco, LeBlanc and Russell 2008) and to follow more fully an alternative life course trajectory. Those reaching adulthood in the post-Stonewall era have grown up and are growing older within non-traditional 'family' settings shaped by and oriented toward a 'homosexually' embodied identity. It could be argued that this creates new possibilities for later lifestyles that are less strongly attached to youthful ideals of forever performing 'gay', permitting instead an alternative, 'queerer' way of ageing.

The presence and extension of gay and lesbian cultures and their role in reconstructing the social networks of the family of origin has both benefits and costs. In the absence of the normative framework that families typically create around age and gender, gay men and lesbians may live their lives 'less aware of the ageing process' (Heaphy, Yip and Thompson 2004, 885). But, if entry to and continued membership of homosexual communities is contingent upon the ageless 'performativity' of homosexuality, the instability of partners and chosen kin, coupled with 'the limiting conditions of the body' that ageing can bring (Gilleard and Higgs 1998), might enhance the risk of not being able to continue enjoying sexual intimacy and, more importantly, to retain a 'queer' identity in the absence of sex within a community that, unlike families, requires the continued presence of sexuality as embodied practice as the grounds for continued community membership.

Queer Theory and Ageing

In demonstrating how ageing problematises sexual identities as much as sexual identity problematises ageing ones, we now turn more explicitly to the perspective of 'queer theory'. Drawing upon the ideas of Derrida and Foucault, queer theorists challenge the particular binary distinctions associated with sex and sexuality – and by extension, those associated with gender, able-bodiedness, and 'race' (Seidman 1997). By acknowledging that each term in these binary pairings (gay, black, women, disabled etc.) implies and demands its opposite (straight, white, men, able-bodied etc.), the idea of homosexuality is seen as ever 'present' even in nominally heterosexual discourses and practices, just as the idea of blackness is ever 'present' in white discourses and practices. Instead of treating sexuality as an essentialised identity, queer theory sees it, and all other dichotomised forms of embodied identity, as masking more fluid, multi-layered sources of contingent differences.

Queer theory argues that it does more than just recognise the importance of multiple differences in the way, for example espoused by proponents of 'inter-sectionality', and instead confronts more directly the contradictions of every form of identity politics. As Seidman has pointed out:

> The American culture of eroticism contributed to the rise of sex as a basis of self identity. As sex was valued for its expressive pleasurable and communicative aspects apart from marriage and love, individuals were able to focus on particular sexual pleasures [...] with questions of identity and normality moving into the center of social conflict. (Seidman 1997, 218)

The result, for queer theorists was the establishment of communities of identity around homosexuality which have morphed into models of a quasi-ethnicity, fostering a separatist cultural politics within gay-male and lesbian-feminist communities. According to Seidman, while direct conflicts over gender were avoided by this division of identity labour, issues of race and class (and disability) were effectively ignored. In addition, the very notion of a unitary sexual identity came under assault and 'the very discourse of liberation with its notion of a gay subject unified by common interests was viewed as a disciplining social force oppressive to large segments of the community in whose name it spoke' (Seidman 1997, 128). As a result, queer theorists began to call for the destabilisation of identity in sexual politics, replacing it with a view of identity as a 'relation of difference' rather than something located by its corporeal base – what Seidman calls a shift from the (late modern) politics of identity to the (postmodern) politics of signification (Seidman 1997, 132).

If the roots of queer theory thus lie in conflicts within the sexual politics of homosexuality, the question arises of what might queer theory contribute to ageing studies? Two useful lines of argument may be suggested. Firstly, age can be viewed more as a position of difference rather than a deviation from a youthful norm – a state of being 'not youthful' rather than 'full of age'. Secondly, queer theory can link with other kinds of post-structuralist thinking, around 'gender' (such as Judith Butler and Elisabeth Grosz), 'race' (such as Henry Louis Gates, Paul Gilroy and Cornell West) and 'disability' (such as Robert McCruer and Margrit Shildrick), in seeking to destabilise any assumed essentialism around the identity-conferring aspects of corporeality, including those conferred by the corporealities of age.

Recognising that people are not 'at base' either black, gay, disabled, or old, but become so under particular sets of historical circumstances and institutional structures is one of the more important contributions made by queer theory. Within this post-structuralist framework, understanding the corporeality of age allows for an understanding of the many social structures, practices and narratives within which 'old' and 'young' are constructed and emerge as significant sources of social difference. 'Queering age', in this sense, provides a potential analytical strategy for understanding issues around embodiment rather than offering a totalising solution to the problem of understanding 'age and ageing'. It helps researchers recognise that the corporeal (and non-corporeal) aspects of ageing may have different meanings in different contexts and times (Seymour 2008). 'Queering the ageing body' adds complexity and contingency to the variously 'embodied' circumstances of age. In a sense it reinforces the turn towards more flexible and contingent 'third age' habitus rather than attempting any closure by 'fabricating' a revisionist 'croning' of old age (Ray 2004).

On the other hand, drawing on 'queer theoretical notions of "embracing shame" and the abject', as Sandberg has suggested, it may also be possible to rethink the positivist framing of later life as 'productive' or 'successful' and view it instead as an expression of aspects of 'vulnerability' and 'abjection' that have resonance for all of humanity (Sandberg 2008, 120). Such an approach bears similarities to that discussed in the previous chapter on disability and the post-structuralist turn toward the body as a site for transgression. By revealing what is otherwise hidden (through tropes such as drag queens and older body builders) these transgressive forms succeed in destabilising the social relations that serve to fix ageing into a process of 'becoming old'.

Bodily ageing presents a challenge to the possible ways of performing sex and gender as much as sex and sexuality do to performing age. While the social contexts that serve as reference points for the various practices and narratives of embodiment are made more complex by examining them through a 'queer' lens, the perspectives adopted by queer theory may also serve to sharpen the distinctiveness of age compared with other forms of embodied identity. While most individuals spend their lives within the singularity of one term within the binaries of gender or race, no-one spends their life occupying the singularity of age. Age contrasts the singular structuring of the life course through gender and race with the contingencies of time. Age embodies ambiguity and relational difference within subjective experience as much as, and perhaps more acutely than, in social relations. While queer theory has tended to view identity as a difference located primarily, if not entirely, within social relations (being straight requires that others not be) age contains/incorporates difference within the person, through the experience of having become other than what one has been.

By seeking to de-stabilise the marginality and 'abjection' attributed to the ageing body, queer theory has challenged as much as it has celebrated the positivity of the new ageing and its various third age cultures. However, there is another side to this balance sheet, because in locating 'otherness' primarily in the context of social differences, queer theory has ignored (as, indeed, do other 'social constructivist' accounts) the 'othering' that arises from the processes of self-alienation that ageing makes possible, the alienation of sense of self from sense of the body achieved by the stability of social institutions contrasted with the instability of the corporeal. While such 'ontological' alienation may not in the end prove resolvable, the self-reflexivity that queering age promotes may offer researchers a key way of understanding the instabilities and indeterminacies of the personal as much as they are able to make sense of those of the social and political.

Conclusions

Physical ageing has long been gendered; it is now becoming sexed. As men's and women's lives have lengthened, the opportunities and expectations for ageing differently have grown. Retaining a sense of gendered distinction and the potential to remain a desiring sexual being are central elements of contemporary 'third age' cultures (Katz and Marshall 2003). For sexual minorities who have experienced in their own lifetime a progressive reduction in the oppressiveness of their sexuality, the freedom to continue to perform as gay men or lesbians in later life seems an important outcome of the 1960s' cultural ferment. The observation that Viagra and similar medications designed to enhance or restore male sexual functioning seem to be consumed more often by gay than by straight older men only reflects such privileging, particularly when set against the past policing of the non-normativity of gay sexuality (Romanelli and Smith 2004; Wentzell 2011a). Similar points may apply to the use of cosmetics and anti-ageing preparations by older men and the relative importance of their continuing to look good in the sense of remaining 'sexually attractive'. For older lesbians sexual intimacy in later life might prove a less conflicted issue than for heterosexual women, if the pressures of performativity in sex do not compromise their relationships to the degree they seem to do for heterosexual couples.

Traditional ideas about the 'folly' of remaining sexual in later life have been replaced by new expectations of being 'forever' sexual. It is too early to tell whether a premodern form of oppression is being replaced by a postmodern one. Whatever else, the effect of the sexual revolution is unlikely to be reversed. The benefits of providing heterosexual and homosexual men and women with greater opportunities to remain gendered, sexual beings for a lot longer and in less stereotyped ways are not to be gainsaid. However, if sexual activity is reified into a 'new normativity' of embodied sexuality, choosing always to be 'other' may prove of limited value in liberating later life.

Chapter 7

SEX AND AGEING

In the last chapter we explored sexuality as an embodied identity that acquired new social and political purchase in the wake of the 1960s' sexual revolution. The ageing of the post-Stonewall generation – and the impact of the AIDS/HIV epidemic – influenced the subsequent gendered construction of age and ageing within the gay, lesbian and bisexual communities. One consequence has been queering/questioning the corporeal essentialism of 'heteronormative' ageing; the other a greater reflexivity expressed about issues of 'age' and 'sex' that has become evident inside and outside the gay and lesbian communities. Re-interpreting gender and sexuality as forms of embodied identity, has led to sex becoming an 'embodied practice', fashioning the identities both of gender and of sexual orientation at the same time as influencing the ideals of a healthy lifestyle and of ageing well (Elders 2010).

Sexual performance and the embodied practices related to it have been central to the 'identity' conferring nexus of sexuality. While gay and lesbian sub-cultures have not just been about sex and sexual partnering, without sex, sexual identities are separated from the key element of their embodiment. One of the challenges in maintaining a gay or lesbian identity throughout adult life is consequently how to continue to represent oneself and to see others represented as potential sexual partners in a more demanding way than was traditionally the case in the heterosexual life course. This has the result both of 'queering' age as a de-gendered, de-sexualised identity or status, while challenging the essentialised ageism evident within gay and lesbian communities. While gay and lesbian culture and gay and lesbian communities have been important in 'revisioning' the relationship between sex and age by challenging the traditional assumption that when age is in, sex is out, queer theory further challenges the apposition itself.

Examining the relationship between sex and ageing, we now shift our focus from a concern with embodied identities in later life to a concern with embodied practices. The former has been concerned with identities and lifestyles based around socially significant, shared sources of bodily difference where those sources have been conventionally associated with marginalisation and oppression. We have argued that the new social movements associated with identity politics created alternative lifestyles whose subsequent evolution over the life course has helped shape the new ageing. Many of the processes by which these developments re-positioned embodied 'minorities' from the margins to the mainstream occurred through particular body-oriented narratives and practices that Foucault has termed 'practices of freedom' or 'technologies of self-care' (Foucault 1982, 1988). Amongst such practices, sex has become an important example, being deployed not just for personal pleasure but as a source of alternative narratives and practices that sustain and strengthen various embodiments of identity. However privately they may once have been realised, sex now involves a set of bodily practices that are more clearly oriented toward society and the achievement of social distinction.

As a consequence of the sexual revolution of the 1960s sex moved out of the private realm and began to inform and shape the public sphere. This reflected a more general trend where embodied practices or forms of 'body work' that were once associated with 'personal' care and the routines of private life became aspects of public culture. Sex was now part of a healthy lifestyle symbolising freedom, autonomy and pleasure. The subsequent evolution of this idea to the point where sexual practice became an essential constituent of successful 'healthy' ageing has represented a remarkable transformation of the previous narratives and practices about age and sex. It is not so long since 'ageing well' required the opposite – either abstaining from or performing sexual intercourse as little as possible (Acton 1867; Carpenter 1859; Reveille-Parise 1854). To contextualise this shifting positioning of sex in later life we need to revisit the history of this relationship.

Sex and Ageing from the Pre-modern to Modernity

In much of the pre-modern period, sexual activity in later life 'was viewed as immoral, inappropriate and negative' (Covey 1989, 99). It was policed as much by comedy and ridicule as it was by invocations of sin and damnation. The comedic contrast between older people's desire for sex and their unfitness to perform provided a major theme in classical, renaissance and early modern theatre (Ellis 2009). By violating the civic and moral position of old age, lecherous old men and women were used for their transgressive potential rather than as models for 'successful ageing'. Within the literature of ancient Greece and Rome, older men attracted ridicule for their impotence to realise their sexual desires while older women elicited disgust for attempting to assert themselves as sexual beings (Falkner and De Luce 1989; Falkner 1995). Not only was sex deemed inappropriate to the virtue of old age, it was thought also to contribute directly to 'premature' ageing, jeopardising aspirations for a happy and successful old age by using up the 'radical moisture' sustaining life. Many renaissance treatises on 'successful ageing', for example, advised older men to refrain from or restrict their sexual activity in order to attain a long and healthy old age (Gilleard 2013).

To age well was to age without sexual desire. The virtuous old were expected to present themselves as, if not asexual, then at least untroubled by sexual desire (Paleotti 1506). To be ensnared by sex in later life was both derisory and immoral. In such a context, questions of sexual orientation were largely irrelevant, adding nothing to the master narrative that age and sex shouldn't mix. While sexual relationships with the same sex were not always condemned in the pre-Christian West, and while there seems at times to have been a degree of acceptance of same-sex relationships, particularly between older and younger males, this acceptance did not create any cultural contradiction in the positioning of age, gender and sexuality within classical Greek or Roman society. In neither culture, for example, is there evidence that sex with young men was promoted as a kind of 'rejuvenant' for older men or women.

For women, sex with young men was condemned and/or ridiculed. Sex with young women, on the other hand, was sometimes viewed as rejuvenating for older men, but more commonly it was treated as an inherently comic encounter, revealing the older man's absurdity and frailty.

As Foucault noted in the introduction to his *History of Sexuality*, the conversion of Europe made sexuality problematic for all ages (Foucault 1979), while the civic and moral value attributed to men and women who avoided performing sex rose in comparison. Age acquired a new authority in part because it was seen as liberating the individual from sexual desire and sin. Senior churchmen were selected on the basis of the spiritual capital of their agedness. Although the humanism of the Renaissance would begin to challenge the political and cultural authority of aged men, age remained spiritually and politically 'untoppled' by these challenges (Minois 1989). In short, throughout the pre-modern period, aged men retained their power, their *patria potestas* (power of a father); sex more than any other activity risked compromising this, by inviting ridicule in old men's claims to power. They were better off without it.

With the enlightenment, scientific thinking became a more significant element in popular culture. New discourses emerged that would eventually reshape the attitudes of the wider population concerning sex and its connections with old age. Foucault described the rise of science in the early eighteenth century as the moment when the unitary discourse of sex and sexuality broke down into 'a multiplicity of discourses produced by a whole series of mechanisms operating in different institutions' (Foucault 1979, 33). This fragmentation, he suggested, led both to a 'quietening down' of concerns over heterosexual monogamous sex and an increased preoccupation with and scrutiny of what constituted 'natural' and 'unnatural' sex and its 'peripheral sexualities'. This division is perhaps one of Foucault's own making – certainly it was not backed up with any evidence. Other writers have, however, provided backing for a change in thinking about sex and gender occurring during this period. In particular there was a decline of the long held view that there was fundamentally just one sex, with men and women representing superior and inferior versions of it (Laqueur 1990; Oudshoorn 1994, 6).

The rise of physiological science 'sometime in the eighteenth century' made the 'two-sex' model an accepted fact (Laqueur 1990, 149). As a result, the difference between men and women was now seen to extend beyond their genitals and their role in sexual reproduction to encompass each and every part of the body. Medical research became pre-occupied with women as 'different'. The search to find the seat, the essence of 'femininity', finally ended when Virchow discovered it was not to be found in the womb but in the ovaries (Rothman and Rothman 2004, 24). This shift in perspective represented the ultimate triumph of physiology over anatomy. It created the foundations for a new way of looking at the human body that emphasised its plasticity and its capacity to be changed – eventually empowering men and women to turn their bodies into 'a means of self expression, for becoming who we would most like to be' (Davis 1997, cited in Rothman and Rothman 2004, 23).

Physiologists such as Acton and Carpenter were amongst the first to outline the 'normal life course' of sexual function, from childhood to advanced life (Carpenter

1859; Acton 1867). Carpenter suggested that adult (male) sexual power began around ages 14 to 16 but 'is not retained by the male to any considerable amount, after the age of 60 or 65 years' (Carpenter, 1859, 846). Acton argued that full sexual maturity occurred much later, in a man's early twenties, while concluding with Carpenter 'that sexual power is not retained by the male to any considerable amount after the age of sixty or sixty five' (Acton 1867, 265). Acting in contradiction to this natural life course, Acton warned, 'must sooner or later tell its tale. In some its effects assume the form of hypochondriasis, followed by all the protean miseries of indigestion; in others of fatuity; in the more advanced stages paralysis or paraplegia comes on accompanied by softening of the brain' (Acton 1867, 265).

Sexual power was seen as a kind of capital that needed carefully to be built up before being cautiously expended – reflecting the rise of industrious capitalism and men's needs to retain their vital force and spend their capital in the most effective and productive manner. Physiologists in Europe and America ended up as advocates of a Victorian productivist morality that saw 'manhood' strengthened the more the body was controlled. Sexual expression was a matter of growing concern and age became particularly important in the 'policing' that took place over its boundaries. The new physiology re-circulated the pre-modern 'humoral' belief that man had a stock of vitality that needed to be stored with care during childhood and youth, and would eventually run out with age. It recommended 'manly' constraint and continence at the beginning and at the end of the lifespan. But in seeking to serve such moral ends, it would also create the tools that would undermine its own position and lead to a very different understanding of sex and ageing in the twentieth century.

Sex, Ageing and Modern Medical Hygiene

The longstanding condemnation directed toward sexual expression in later life was placed on a more scientific footing as sexual expression – particularly male orgasm and seminal emission – were proposed as causes of 'excess' senility and 'premature' ageing (Acton 1867; Carpenter 1859; Reveille-Parise 1854). But as physiology divorced itself from the constraints of anatomy to pursue its interests in the body's 'internal secretions', its increasingly experimental turn led the way to a reconceptualisation of the relationship between age and sex. This was epitomised in the work of Charles-Édouard Brown-Séquard, Claude Bernard's successor to the chair in medicine at the Collège de France, and considered by many to be the founding father of endocrinology. On the basis of observations on men and other male animals' sexual functioning, Brown-Séquard hypothesised that the testes contained some substance besides semen that was responsible for 'giving strength to the nervous system and other parts' (Brown-Séquard 1899, cited in Rothman and Rothman 2003, 134). By the mid-1880s he had begun a series of 'rejuvenation experiments' on dogs and rabbits, injecting old dogs with extracts made up of the blood and crushed testicles of guinea pigs and observing the effects on their appearance and behaviour. In 1889, at a meeting of the Société de Biologie in Paris, he announced that he had successfully rejuvenated himself by 'mixing small quantities of distilled water with blood taken from the testicular veins of young and healthy dogs [...] [and] semen and juices from their crushed testicles' (Haycock 2008, 169). Dismissed in many quarters as an ageing charlatan, his work on rejuvenation was enthusiastically pursued on both sides of the Atlantic. One such enthusiast was the Russian Serge Voronoff. Voronoff began by taking slices of testes from young rams and goats and grafting them onto the testis of older animals. By 1921 he had extended this work to humans, grafting slices of chimpanzee testicle onto the testicles of a 74-year-old Englishman, one Arthur Liarder (Haycock 2008, 177). 'Before' and 'after' photographs of Liarder were used to illustrate the effectiveness of his work. In his book, *Rejuvenation by Grafting*, he claimed to have performed almost 1000 such operations, arguing subsequently that through this process of resexualisation/ rejuvenation 'senile old age (could be) practically eliminated' (Voronoff 1927, cited in Haycock 2008, 178).

By the time Voronoff (and others) were grafting youth into old men's bodies, further developments in endocrinology had demonstrated that spermatic fluid could be differentiated from another 'male fluid' that was discharged internally not externally. This finding defined maleness as a quality conferred by sources separate from men's fertility. This male fluid was produced not by the tissues that produced sperm but by the testes' interstitial tissue, the Leydig cells. It was the inner secretions of these cells, not his sperm, that made a man a man. From this point on the model of a 'spermatic economy' began to collapse. The desirability of saving up one's sperm and spending it down carefully no longer mattered. It became possible instead to seek ways of increasing the male fluid as a means of restoring men's health and power. This route was first followed by Voronoff's contemporary and rival in the race for rejuvenation, Dr Eugen Steinach, a well-established, middle-aged Viennese professor and research director at the Physiology Unit in Vienna's Institute of Biology (Benjamin 1945).

Steinach's work had first concentrated upon the determinants of sexual identity. He sought to change the sexual characteristics of guinea pigs by removing the sex glands of one sex and implanting those of the opposite sex. This work was followed by human experimentation, first by trying to 'convert' homosexual men into heterosexual men by castrating them and then replacing their testes with other presumed heterosexual men's undescended testicles. In 1920 he published the first results of his research on ageing, claiming that he had achieved the 'rejuvenation' of ageing male rats by permanent ligature of the *vas deferens*. Drawing on the distinction that had recently been made between spermatic and interstitial tissue, he argued that by sealing off the *vas deferens*, through what we would now call a vasectomy, the amount of spermatic tissue would decline, causing the amount of interstitial tissue to increase and thereby restoring a new found strength and vitality to 'prematurely aged men' (Steinach and Löbel 1940). For Steinach, as for Brown-Séquard and other advocates of 'organotherapy', sex was now 'the most obvious root [of ageing] because it is the root of life [and] just as it produces physical and psychic maturity [...] so it is responsible for the withering of the body and gradual loss of vitality' (Steinach and Löbel 1940, 24). Rather than sex being a cause of men's ageing, it was offered as its cure.

Controversy followed Steinach, as it had Brown-Séquard and others before him. The prospect of the indefinite prolongation of life 'by a series of Steinach operations' was mooted (Michael Schmidt, *Time Magazine*, 30 July 1923, cited by Haycock 2008, 182). Hundreds of ageing men, including, it is said, Sigmund Freud, came to Vienna to receive the Steinach operation. However, the medical establishment were quick to condemn Steinach's work, not least because it seemed to spread the idea that old men could regain a youthful sexual performance as a consequence an idea that not so long since had been seen as both immoral and unnatural. More germane, perhaps, was the failure to find any empirical evidence that vasoligation lead to any proliferation of the interstitial Leydig cells in the testes – the process that Steinach claimed was responsible for increasing male hormone production which then leads to 'rejuvenation'. Nevertheless, despite the criticisms of the medical establishment, a number of researchers across Europe and North America began pursuing the idea of a potential 'revival' of male powers in later life through means of the external stimulation of the 'internal secretions' – albeit stressing the mental and physical gains in power that could be achieved, and downplaying, in professional circles, the idea of regained sexuality (Haycock 2008, 184–5).

Steinach seems to have been genuinely hurt by the hostility of his critics. In the late 1920s he turned his interest from men to women, researching female sex hormones and their potential for what he called female 'reactivation'. With help from the Schering Corporation he managed to produce a 'purified highly potent' female sex hormone that the company named 'Steinach's Progynon' (Benjamin 1945, 439). This served as the base from which the first synthetic female sex hormone would later be manufactured and which would lead eventually to both the female contraceptive pill and hormone replacement therapy. In the meantime, interest in male sexuality, the idea of a male climacteric and the rejuvenation of male sexuality declined (Watkins 2008) and by the 1960s, women's sexuality had taken centre stage.

The 1960s' Sexual Revolution: Women on Top

The precise periodising of the sexual revolution remains a contested subject but there is general agreement that important changes in sexual activity, sexual expression and sexual attitudes occurred from the late 1950s through to the early 1970s, in North America and in European societies (Hofferth, Kahn and Baldwin 1987; Petigny 2004). This change incorporated a number of cultural, social and technological influences, including the desegregation of workplaces during and after the Second World War, the influence of Freudian and neo-Freudian ideas about the societal importance of sex (particularly evident in marketing and the media), the statistical data collected on 'normal' sexual behaviour by Kinsey and his associates and widely reported in the media, the growth of coeducational colleges, the rise of various counter-cultural movements and their links with an expanding consumer culture and, as noted earlier, the development and marketing of the contraceptive pill (Allyn 2000; Cook 2007).

Sexual liberation – the freedom to have whatever sex one wanted, with whoever one choose to have it with – was linked through popular culture to the civil rights movement, the women's liberation movement and other related liberation struggles. Having sex was not just personal, it was political. It helped make the body increasingly oriented toward the cultural and social. Sex was to be seen and was no longer regarded as obscene. Three features help define this revolution in attitudes and behaviour. First, the assertion that sexual activity and the expression of sexual desire are at one and the same time critical elements of self-expression, as well as providing a corporeal source of identity and selfhood; second, that sexual pleasure is a necessary, legitimate and affirmative component of life – a 'natural' phenomenon that turns unhealthy when repressed; and third, that acceptance of oneself as an active sexual being meant, for women, a liberation from their role as housewife and mother and for homosexuals – gays and lesbians – a liberation from the stigma, marginalisation and criminalisation associated with same-sex sex. Sexual expression was self-expression; it represented authenticity and freedom from what one author at the time called the apparatus of 'repression/oppression' (Marcuse 1969). While there were contradictory processes contained within these positions, as there are in any revolutionary position, sex as a vehicle for expressing personal agency provided the common theme underlying all these narratives. Whether women were liberated or just oppressed differently by the sexual revolution, it was still important that they should experience not just sex, but good sex; and good sex was sex between and amongst equals (Dell'Ollio 1973).

The sexual revolution was not confined to the frequency of or tolerance for a wider range of sexual activity. Popular culture conveyed the sense that sex was newly invented by the youth of the 1960s. Old sex was replaced by new sex and new sex was better, freer and infinitely more self-fulfilling. It became part of the radical sell. Sex had been known to sell goods and services well before the 1960s, of course, but what was distinct about the new sex of the 1960s was its permeation across so many domains of popular life, in popular music and dance; in books and films; in clothes and fashion and in the rise of venues where sexual relationships could be established – in colleges, coffee bars, clubs, cinemas, dance halls, etc.. Sex as a consumerist habitus was increasingly realised through a set of places, practices and relationships where young unmarried people spent their free time and developed their sense of identity, self-esteem and self-expression.

Men and women over 30 years of age were not untouched by the sexual revolution. After the Second World War marriage was increasingly viewed in a 'companiate' form and the quality of the sexual relationship used to judge the quality of the marriage (Friedan 1963; Giddens 1992). For the young and the 'young at heart' the quality of their sexual relationships became subject to a more reflexive form of self-scrutiny. Women's magazines once dominated by cookery, clothes and cleaning began to include sections on personal 'relationships'. Agony-aunt columns discussed problems of 'intimacy' while men's magazines provided a mixture of soft pornography with technical details on how to improve their and their partner's sex life; and on top of all that was the new feminisation of ageing and sexuality.

The hormones making up the contraceptive pill had been synthesised just before the Second World War. Their development and manufacture as a medium of healthcare for already healthy people, however, did not begin until the 1950s. The contraceptive pill, based upon the work of the controversial biologist Gregory Pincus and the support of the longstanding women's activist Margaret Sanger, was first licensed in 1960

(Oudshoorn 1994). A number of factors have been proposed to explain the timing of the pill's manufacture, but its singular importance lay in two areas – first, the control it gave women to regulate and separate their own heterosexual behaviour from the domestic sphere of sexual reproduction; second, the fact that the pill was the first physiological method of contraception that in effect mimicked the menopause by rendering women of child-bearing age temporarily and reversibly 'aged'.

The other major development in the commercial production of synthetic hormones had the opposite effect, rendering post-menopausal women 'forever feminine'. Robert Wilson, gynaecologist and author of *Forever Feminine* was one of the first promoters of the idea that hormone replacement therapy could act as a lifelong means of helping women remain desirable – and desirous (Wilson and Wilson 1963; Wilson 1966a). Prompted by such medical advocates, the pharmaceutical industry was keen to expand its sales using a new marketing strategy that drew directly upon the new 'women's liberation' rhetoric to suggest that taking HRT was itself a liberating practice (Roberts 2007). As the preoccupation with the male climacteric and men's ageing declined, the menopause began to rise in significance – as a solvent of personal identity and symbol of age's ruthless 'de-gendering'. Roberts cites psychiatrist David Reuben's depiction of the menopause as the time when 'a woman comes as close as she can to being a man [...] not really a man but no longer a functional women' (Reuben 1969, *Everything You Always Wanted to Know about Sex*, cited by Roberts 2007, 121).

In short, the sexual revolution of the 1960s saw interest in ageing men wane along with attempts at masculine rejuvenation while interest in protecting women from ageing blossomed. The 'forever feminine' woman was liberated not just from the constraints of her economic and social position but from the cultural ordering of her life course, whether by men or by nature. As both sexuality and gender became more fluid identities, ageing began to be represented as an obstacle to be overcome, as the product of old habits from which women needed to be liberated. The ageism that existed in the society of the 1960s – the preference for the new over the old, the young over the aged – was used to sell the idea of a more plastic view of sex and sexuality, the impact of which was eventually to change views about ageing and sex.

After the Revolution: Sex Grows Old

The practice and narratives surrounding sex and gender expanded within and across successive postwar birth cohorts, and sex and sexuality in later life were changed in the process. There was a progressive rise in the numbers of people of all ages reporting different, formerly deviant, sexualities; a rise in cohabitation; increases in multiple family formations across the life course; more people than ever before experiencing divorce and/or separation; more people living alone but with partners; and a decline in long term, lifetime marriages. Public representations of sexual activity were no longer confined to hard or soft pornography, while pornography itself became incorporated into mainstream culture. Sex and the expression of one's sexuality became social virtues, indicators of emotional physical and mental well-being. Sexual expression became a right to which all are entitled, to the point that those unable to access sexual partners because of their age, disability or personal misfortune were considered to have 'unmet needs' that health and social care services should at least consider, if not meet (Appel 2010; Oriel 2005).

Just as sexuality came to define the good life, so it also came to define active, productive or successful ageing. A number of doctors and gerontologists began to argue that lack of sexual interest and activity in later life was determined less by biological changes than by 'social taboos' and persisting social strictures affecting the sexual lives of old people (Loughman 1980, 182). Butler and Lewis (1976) and Felstein (1974) were among the first to write popular books advocating sexual liberation in later life. The pre-modern view that sexual decline was the consequence of the progressive spending down of sexual vitality was replaced by the view that it was the result of falling hormone levels. This modern model was soon supplemented by a new focus upon psychological well-being and its links with sexuality. With the emergence of the new sexology and the iconic work of Masters and Johnson, sexual function came to be seen as much a matter of mental attitude and personal relationships as it was of sexual physiology. A woman can reach orgasm at any age, Masters and Johnson claimed, provided she is regularly and properly stimulated (cited in de Beauvoir, 1977, 386). All sexual problems could eventually be resolved and sex for all achieved through the efforts of good sex doctors and good therapists like themselves.

As the new 'sexology' of the 1960s was adapted for the over sixties, the foundations were laid for the twenty-first century's mantra of 'sex for health and pleasure throughout a lifetime' (Elders 2010, 248). Liberal ideas about sexuality gradually extended across all adult lifestages, making 'sexual freedom' and 'sexual experimentation' no longer the monopolies of youth or the exclusive domain of men. Secular trends in reported sexual activity provide evidence indicative of a pattern of change in sexual activity across the life course. In direct contradiction to the views of the Victorian physiologists, sexual intercourse now starts earlier and lasts longer, adults report more sexual partners and sex is expressed through a wider variety of practices than before (Turner, Danella and Rogers 1995; Bajos et al. 2010).

Sexual activity in later life is now more common than it was in the 1960s and 1970s (Beckman et al. 2008; Gott 1994; Bajos et al. 2010). Such generational change was anticipated even in the 1960s. Writing in the *Journal of Gerontology*, Eric Pfeiffer and his colleagues suggested 'it is quite possible that the dissemination of information about sexual behaviour in the present generation will materially influence the patterns of sexual behaviour in future generations' (Pfeiffer, Verwoerdt and Wang 1968, 198). Current trends have proved them right and an increasing 'sexually active life expectancy' can be anticipated to continue for some time to come (Lindau and Gavrilova 2010). Surveys of Swedish 70-year-olds, conducted between 1971 and 2001, indicate more positive attitudes toward sex and more frequent sexual activity amongst the more recent cohorts (Beckman et al. 2008). Figure 7.1 illustrates this secular trend, with the number of older men and women both reporting more sexual intercourse over this period.

It is not just the Swedes who have sex more often in later life. Rates of intercourse for Americans in their sixties are higher now compared with those reported thirty years ago and it seems probable that the secular trends observed in Sweden apply generally

Figure 7.1. Secular changes in frequency of sexual intercourse among Swedish 70-year-old men and women (data derived from Beckman et al. 2008).

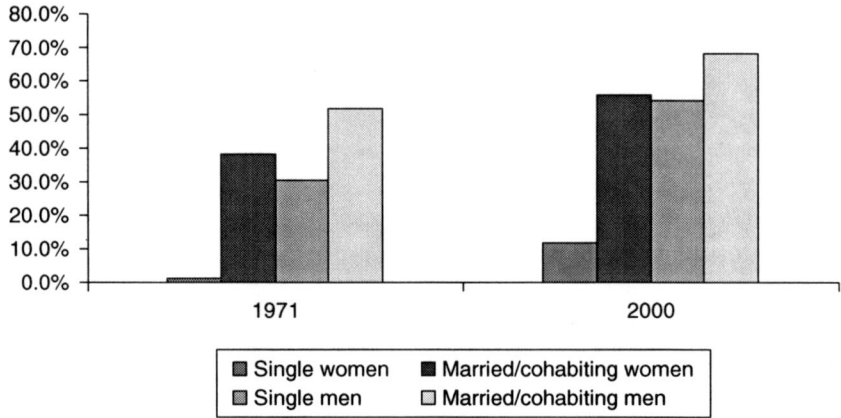

to other developed societies. Within this changing context, the significance of intimate 'partnerships' in maintaining sexual activity in later life still seems as true now as it was in Kinsey's time (and no doubt before). As Figure 7.2 illustrates, while married people aged over sixty are less likely to have intercourse than married people in their thirties, they are more likely to do so than single unattached people are, at any age.

While the occurrence of vaginal sexual intercourse in later life might be considered to represent the continuity of 'conventional' sex, other data indicate that more 'adventurous' approaches toward sex can be observed in later life, including more frequent oral and anal sex and increasing use of sex toys such as vibrators. Although definitive data are lacking, trends toward expanding sexual experience seem to be influencing the sexual behaviour of adults at all ages. One recent internet study, for example, examined the

Figure 7.2. Frequency of sexual intercourse by age, gender and partnership status – US National Survey, 2009 (from Reece et al. 2010; Herbenick et al. 2010).

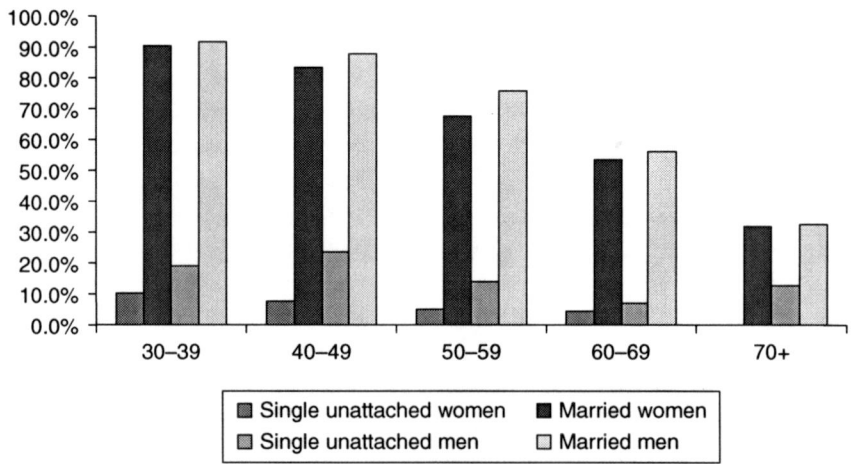

Figure 7.3. Frequency of giving oral sex by age, gender and partnership status – US National Survey, 2009 (from Reece et al. 2010; Herbenick et al. 2010).

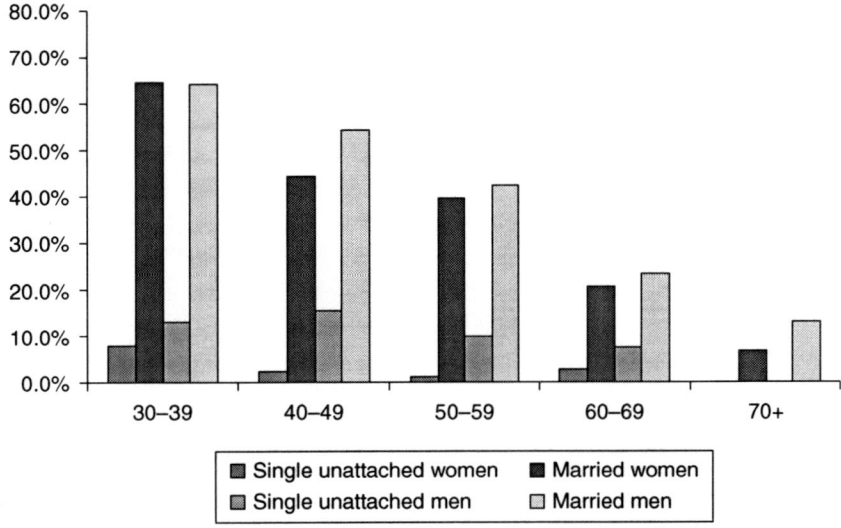

frequency of the use of sex toys (vibrators) and found no evidence of age/cohort differences in a national sample made up of 18 to 60-year-old US women (Herbenick et al. 2009). Epidemiological data on the frequency of oral sex, however, suggest there are age/cohort differences in the prevalence of giving and receiving 'oral' sex in the last 90 days, with age/cohort and partnership status equally limiting such experiences.

As sexual activity has become incorporated into the new 'active' ageing paradigm, the lack or decline of sexual activity in later life has itself become problematised. This can be seen as yet another outcome of the 1960s' sexual revolution and particularly the work of Masters and Johnson who helped establish the new vocabulary of 'sexual dysfunction'. The limited success of sexual dysfunction clinics in restoring clients' active sex lives has become apparent in subsequent decades. This caused a shift in emphasis away from a primary psychotherapeutic orientation aimed at personal liberation to one based upon pharmacological and/or medical enhancement (Hawton et al. 1986; Hawton, Catalan and Faff 1992; Heiman 2002). These new techniques initially ranged from pharmacotherapy with yohimbine (Reid et al. 1987), use of antidepressants (Kurt et al. 1994), testosterone patches (for men and women), and vacuum constriction devices (Cookson and Nadig 1993) all the way to artificial implants to eliminate male impotence (Furlow, Goldwasser and Gundian 1988). Outcomes remained poor (Jarow et al. 1996). The breakthrough came in the 1990s, with the introduction of Viagra as a specific pharmacological treatment for erectile dysfunction. Originally developed as a treatment for high blood pressure, the little blue pill's impact upon male sexual performance led to a patent being drawn up in 1996 for its use with sexually dysfunctional males. Licensed by the US Food and Drug Administration in 1998, Viagra became one of the world's best-selling pharmaceuticals, finding a market among heterosexual and homosexual men of all ages (Fisher et al. 2006).

As this market grew, studies of sexual activity re-oriented themselves toward a new population health agenda. Since Viagra was licensed, numerous surveys on the 'prevalence' of erectile dysfunction have been conducted (Blanker et al. 2001; Laumann, Paik and Rosen 1999, Laumann et al. 2006; Nicolosi et al. 2003; Richters et al. 2003; Simons and Carey 2001). These studies then expanded to include 'female sexual dysfunction' drawing upon a similar population health perspective, covering the prevalence of an increasing number of what have been framed as potentially 'remediable disorders' (Anastadias et al. 2002; Basson et al. 2003; Hayes and Dennerstein 2005; Kadri, McHichi and McHakra 2002). A public health campaign soon followed to 'dissolve the vicious circle of "speechlessness" [that] makes a pleasurable and satisfying sexual relationship impossible in later life' (Hartmann et al. 2004).

With the introduction into the American Psychiatric Association's revised DSM-IV (APA 2000) of a new disorder, hypoactive sexual desire disorder or HSDD, the mass market for sexual health promotion has expanded still further. Researchers have now begun to call for the 'expansion and revision' of female sexual disorders within DSM-IV (Basson et al. 2003). New categories of dysfunction have been added, such as that of sexual desire/interest disorder or SDID, focusing less on personal 'interest and fantasies' and more on a reduced responsivity to one's partner. Studies have begun to examine whether these disorders too could be framed as 'age associated illnesses' (Hayes et al. 2007), with research suggesting that while one (HSDD) may fit the label, the other (SDID) may not (Botto et al. 2011). The marketing of this medicalisation of age associated disorders of sexual expression offers is evident. As one epidemiological study points out: 'in 2000 there were more than 42 million [US] women older than 50 years. Given our estimates of low desire and HSDD prevalence, at least 16 million women aged 50 years or older currently experience low desire and approximately 4 million are distressed by their low desire' (West et al. 2008, 1447).

Clearly there is more business to be had. For both men and women, the declining importance of sex and sexuality traditionally associated with bodily ageing has been challenged, if not overturned. Sex has won a larger place in public culture and gained a new status as an index of health and well-being across the life course, while the quest for sexual variety in later life has grown more insistent (Woloski-Wruble et al. 2010). New pharmacological and leisure technologies have created opportunities to expand sex as a major leisure pursuit in later life. At the same time these changes have created new expectations and with it the potential for new forms of oppression – the demand to be forever sexual – for men and women. There is a shared expectation that men and women should remain sexual beings into later life, even if the expectation is expressed differently for both genders. The same can be said for older homosexual men and women. While one can argue that there is more scope to construct individual narratives and take individual decisions about the significance of one's own sexuality and of one's own bodily ageing, this increased reflexivity comes at a price. The opportunity for choice creates the requirement to choose and in doing so risk the consequences of making the wrong choice. While having sex once risked overturning the authority of age, not having sex now risks overturning the claims of 'successful' ageing.

Conclusions

Physical ageing has long been gendered and now it is thoroughly sexualised. In traditional, pre-modern societies bodily ageing was less marginalising for men than for women, particularly among the elites. In modernity, the body's capacity to perform – whether that performance involved civic duties, labour or various forms of governance – became the central issue for men's ageing. For women, issues of appearance and the appropriate performance of 'gender' were always more central. While for both men and women bodily ageing has always posed a degree of threat – whether from its capacity to obliterate the distinctions of gender, the pleasures of sex and the power of authority or from its significance as harbinger of illness and disability – it has also been represented as a kind of relief; a haven from the ceaseless efforts of adult life and relationships, including the pressure to remain forever sexually accessible, forever sexually functional and forever sexually attractive. For the most recent cohorts of older people, however, that haven has become harder to reach as the longer term impact of the sexual revolution has made sexuality a key element in personal well-being and self-expression throughout adult life. By removing the 'taboo' against performing sex in later life, new taboos risk being erected that treat any ageing of sex as a form of sexual dysfunction and reinforce age as a source of disease. Sexual inactivity can no longer be viewed as part of successful ageing in the way it once was. Now it is framed as indicative of dysfunction disease or disorder. Failure to perform sex at any time in adult life signifies either a physical impairment – whether of desire or of performance – or form of social handicap – of loneliness or isolation – or both. As de Beauvoir once noted, traditionally, 'age provides alibis' to lowering one's own standards or, more often, to pre-emptively quashing others' demands – for love or labour (de Beauvoir 1977, 318). Second modernity suggests that now no part of adult life provides such hiding places.

As aging well involves continuing to express one's physical and psychological vitality and engagement with the world – not so much performing as a young person as no longer following the 'old' conventions of 'natural ageing' – sexuality becomes a site of personal and cultural conflict. Older people need to balance the pressures of 'not being old' with the equally salient pressure to 'be one's age'. These contrasting pressures are further refracted through gender and the unstable requirements of masculinity and femininity. How men and women learn to perform age – as men and women – and how they resist, reframe or ignore 'being old' is no longer a universal, embodied and engendered transhistorical dilemma. These new conflicts over gender, sexuality and age are becoming more salient for people entering and making their way through later life as a result of the social and cultural changes that were set in motion during the long 1960s. As women's identity 'as women' has become less closely linked to reproduction, child rearing and unpaid domestic work, ageing and later life have become if anything a more distinct 'phase' of life, linked more closely than before to the common identity conferred by retirement (one shared with men), as workers and producers of goods and services, whose virtue and value is determined as much by the wages they once commanded as the children they once raised.

At the same time that retirement has become a common site of identity and lifestyle for men and women, the body has developed as a more salient point of reference in identity and lifestyle formation throughout the whole of adult life. The body and the uses to which it is put – embodiment in short – now competes with its previous reification in the productive processes. This struggle over embodiment and the blurring of the corporeal reference points of what constitutes masculinity and femininity can be seen as part of a general de-standardisation of the reference points that constitute everyday life. Within late modernity, the reified wage value of the male worker and the corporeal value of the female consumer have lost much of their gendered definition, in later as in earlier adult life. Growing old without acting or appearing old is not a novel idea, but it has become a more common goal as the opportunities and expectations increase for men and women to realise a new, more agentic, ageing. Retaining a sense of gendered distinction by remaining a sexual being is a central element of contemporary 'third age' cultures even as the terms of those distinctions are changing (Higgs and McGowan 2012). For sexual minorities who have experienced a progressive reduction in the oppression of their sexuality, the freedom to continue to perform as gays and lesbians seems important. But whatever role sex and sexuality may play in shaping and sustaining a sense of self, in later life, as at other times, choices still have to be made. Choosing not just with whom but how to perform as a sexual being has become part of the new ageing.

Chapter 8

COSMETICS, CLOTHING AND FASHIONABLE AGEING

Although the signs of a long life are inscribed on the body, it is through age not longevity that such signs are read. Wrinkles and grey hair provide the text that says a body is growing old. Whatever fortunes may or may not arise from living longer, most people prefer to avoid being read as 'old'. The fear of looking old is every bit as great as the fear of being old and while the latter may be open to contestation, corporeal evidence of agedness seems to lie outside the authority of the self, turning the body into a text read by others through the dominant narratives of decline (Gullette 1997). While other visibly embodied identities such as disability, race and gender once lacked personal authority second modernity has undermined these narratives of marginality and otherness, and women, black, gay and disabled people have acquired new forms of embodied authority enabling them to attach to their bodies more valued sources of social and cultural distinction. Age has not yet achieved this resonance, despite the fact that these other, alternative voices are now finding themselves experiencing their own, distinctive ageing. It seems as if, for many among these new cohorts of people 'ageing differently', another strategy is being deployed, one that resists one's identity and lifestyle being overtaken by age.

In short, it seems that these emerging embodied identities are beginning to challenge or simply sidestep the older masculine, heterosexual white narratives of age, decline and neutralisation. These processes of not becoming old were a major theme in the previous chapters on gender, race, disability and sexuality. When, in the last chapter, we moved our attention from identities embodied otherwise than by age to address the practices through which these otherwise embodied identities are realised, we turned from a concern with ageing bodies being *read* as other, including being read as other than old, to a concern for bodies *performing* as other, including performing other than as old. Drawing upon the seventeenth-century English philosopher Francis Bacon's fourfold categorisation of practices and disciplines that address the 'good of the body', we explored what he called 'the sensuous sciences' in establishing coordinates for the new ageing. We were concerned with how ageing bodies perform as still desiring adults, still sexualised and still seeking intimacy with others. Sex and sexuality served as a bridge between the embodiment of 'not old' sexual identities (gay, lesbian, heterosexual) and the performance of embodied sexual practices that support and sustain that identity. In this and the next two chapters we will address other practices aimed at the good of the body. Performed primarily as forms of self-care and self-fashioning, they are also oriented, directly and indirectly, so as not to be read as the performances of a body that has become old.

Part of what Bacon placed under the rubric of 'sciences for the good of the body' might now be described as 'body work'. Along with sex, these practices are associated with and oriented towards aspects of embodiment, lifestyle and identity other than age, including the identities and lifestyle defining one's sexuality, gender, ethnicity and/or 'able-bodiedness'. Because such practices incorporate these other aspects of the body, and because they are associated with identities and lifestyles removed from representations of age, they can convey meanings that are at odds with, or ignore, 'age' and consequently become forms of resistance in later life, repositioning otherwise embodied identities as performing 'against' age.

To date such body work practices have been given little credit within the social sciences as significant forms of socially mediated agency. Rather, they have been treated as the 'ephemera of a consumerist society' (Crane and Bovone 2006). This has been unfortunate since they reveal the possibilities and the limits whereby the corporeality attached to particular forms of embodied identity can be either enhanced or undermined. This is the case whether the identity concerned is that of gender, race, able-bodiedness or, by extension, old age. The emphasis in this chapter is on 'appearance management' and its capacity to problematise the polarisation of age and youth. By appearance management, we mean those body work practices regularly performed in order to fashion the appearance of the body, typically through the use of cosmetics, self-care products, fashion and clothing. In the remaining chapters, we will examine other body work practices that focus upon achieving a more lasting impact on the body through exercise and an orientation to the achievement of fitness. All body work practices serve and support a diverse set of lifestyles and identities which may or may not make salient the issue of ageing. Body work represents a polysemous set of practices which are often particularly ambiguous in their orientation towards age. Whether directed toward maintaining appearance or function, most body work seeks to achieve a socially mediated internal status, independent of any particular embodied identity that is framed variously as one of well-being, self-esteem or, in Bacon's terms 'virtú'. The objective of most body work is thus neither the realisation of a particular status, nor the expression of a particular identity, but rather the reaching of an internal state in which identity and lifestyle serve as the social context, the means rather than the ends. In this sense body work expresses the desire for a 'forever' feeling, of goodness, of worth, of satisfaction, perhaps, in some way, even of self-realisation. As such it is inextricably linked with the passing away of time, the impermanence of all bodily configurations and the instability of the self-image.

Appearance Management and the 'Technologies of the Self'

Most embodied practices concerned with 'appearance management' are enacted through the body but mediated through a variety of social and cultural lenses which structure our self-care, self-expression and self-improvement. Most are thoroughly imbricated in consumption and social distinction, sumptuary practices that are capable of being attacked and criticised for breaking social rules or challenging the structure of power by presenting one's body as some body that one is not. Creams, dyes, grooming products, lotions, make up, powders, perfumes, soaps and so forth constitute distinct technologies of body work that were once designed for the elite to 'improve' their appearance as only the elite were deemed entitled to do so. During the course of the twentieth century, access to technologies of self-improvement and self-care was extended to, or appropriated by, the 'masses' and as these practices extended, so they became 'mass practices'. Now, as the practices of the majority, they have become less open to the kind of moral critique directed to those who thought themselves the better part of society, to the point that those who do not use these products or carry out these activities risk becoming themselves the criticised and uncaring minority.

These points apply equally to clothes and fashion as they do to cosmetics and self-care products. As Entwhistle has pointed out 'the very personal act of getting dressed is an act of preparing the body for the social world, making it appropriate, acceptable indeed respectable and possibly even desirable' (Entwhistle 2000, 7). Beyond the deliberate individual act of dressing, however, it is equally important to remember that the clothes that are chosen are themselves the products of design, revealing as much about the market's structuring of social relations as they conceal it. The social reflexivity of cosmetics, self-care, dress and fashion is revealed in the deliberations over their design, their production and marketing, as well as in their selection and purchase. In a society distinguished by consumerism and the promotion of consumerist agency, clothing and cosmetics play a key role in embodying identity. This centrality represents a marked shift from the concerns of first modernity where fashion like most consumerist behaviour was seen as little more than the peripheral indicators of class and the display of 'distinction' (cf. Simmel 1957; Veblen 1953). Whereas dress, makeup and hairstyle were judged at the time as highly structured indicators of social position, their mass production as well as the associated 'democratisation' of their use from the mid-twentieth century onwards saw much of this social structuring break down. The over-determining roles of class and necessity have been replaced by the individualised wardrobes of the consuming majority. What is noteworthy is that perhaps the first arena in the fashion and cosmetics industries where the breakdown of the barriers of class occurred was in the consumption behaviour of postwar youth and their growing demand for self-expression within the various youth sub-cultures of the 1960s.

Our concern here is how practices that were first developed as 'mass practices' by and for the youth of the postwar period have since re-oriented themselves around age and particularly around 'not becoming old'. It is not just a matter that retired people are overtaking youth in their discretionary spending power; nor is it that youth no longer sells. But fashion and style are less and less an exclusive pitch and ageing fashionably, as well as fashions for all ages, are making age a more explicit feature in the sales and marketing of the fashion industry, in much the same way as anti-ageing creams and hair dyes have become ubiquitous features of cosmetics sales counters. While in previous centuries it is not difficult to find various remedies for achieving a young pretty complexion, for preventing skin wrinkling or combing out grey hairs, the mass production and mass consumption of such products within the beauty and fashion industries are a distinctly modern phenomenon. Geared toward a youthful mass market, these products are now increasingly segmented by age. To understand how these industries have helped model ways of 'ageing without becoming old' we turn toward their initial appearance in the market, when modernity itself was still young.

Self-Care and the Beauty Industry

In the heady days of 'becoming modern', distinguishing between the enthusiast and the eccentric was not easy. Among the biographies of the beauty industry, the various pioneers, rogues, villains and cultural innovators appear almost indistinguishable from one another (cf. Brandon 2011; Haiken 1997). Cinema and the mass media helped create the precursors of a celebrity culture, as images of beauty and glamour reached out from the billboards, cinema screens and magazines to an eager and increasingly affluent mass public. During the early decades of the twentieth century, aspirations of personal betterment were rising amongst all classes and, in America, as much within African American communities as amongst the white majority (Chambers 2006). Stimulated by the rise of mass culture, the cinema and the entertainment industries and by developments in the chemical, electronic and oil industries, the early twentieth century saw the beauty industry establish itself in Europe. In 1909 a German hairdresser and wig maker, Karl Nessler, developed the first electronic 'perming' machine. Hans Schwarzkopf, a German chemist, invented the first modern hair shampoo in 1903, while a French chemist, Eugène Schueller, created 'L'Oréal' as the first 'safe' hair colorant in 1907. In 1901, the Prussian chemist and entrepreneur, Oscar Troplowitz patented Nivea as the first cold cream facial, which would become the foundation of the massive Beiersdorf Corporation.

Although most of the pioneers of modern cosmetics were white men, a number of enterprising women made important contributions. Elizabeth Arden and Helena Rubinstein established their own beauty salons where they successfully manufactured and marketed beauty creams and skin colorants. In the USA, Madam C. J. Walker and Annie Turnbo Malone set up their own companies selling hair and beauty products to a largely African American customer base (Jones 2010, 48–65). Faced with rising levels of female employment and income, increased leisure for both men and women and the cultural stimulus provided by the cinema, cosmetics were becoming an accepted ritual of daily urban life. At the same time, the highlighting of makeup and hair styles in the cinema close up provided opportunities to display new fashions in facial cosmetics, hair styling and hair dyes.

Even so, the beauty industry remained a relatively small business accounting for estimated worldwide sales of some $70m (Jones 2010, 366; Peiss 1998). After the First World War, the centre of the industry shifted from Europe to the USA. Here a mass market for cosmetics had already begun to emerge, spurred on by the country's increasing affluence and urbanisation, the rise of Hollywood, and the growing popularisation of beauty through pageants, competitions and advertising (Jones 2010). Although the Depression disrupted progress, it proved only a temporary setback. By the time of the Second World War cosmetics had become an established mass product, so much so that they were considered a wartime 'necessity' by the American military. Even the British government decided that beauty products could 'no [longer] be considered as luxuries enjoyed by a privileged few, but must be considered in the same category as cigarettes, sweets and beer and similar accepted necessities of a modern standard of living for the mass of people' (Jones 2010, 136).

In mid-century America, and in Europe, cosmetic use became part of a culture of femininity 'no longer seen as suspicious for its potential to mask the true women underneath and also in general dissociated from prostitution and loose morals' (Black 2004, 35). Like fashion, hairstyling and makeup was becoming part of the democraticised culture of postwar consumer society. The turn toward the body as a site of social esteem increasingly equated well-being with attractiveness and youthfulness. Elizabeth Haiken quotes a 1956 'Glamour Book' in which the author calls upon its women readers to unite in becoming 'young in thought, feeling and appearance' (Dache cited by Haiken 1997, 145). Throughout the heady postwar decades, cultural and technological change witnessed the rapid domestication of modernity. TVs and telephones, vacuum cleaners and washing machines, electric cookers, built in wardrobes, record players and electric razors, soaps, creams and shampoos, 'do-it-yourself' hair dyes, electric hair curlers and hair stylers became central elements in fashioning the postwar lifestyles of the middle classes. Just as clothes were becoming cheaper, enabling the majority of the population to expand their personal wardrobes so an increasing range of mass produced beauty products went on sale at prices affordable to the consuming public.

During this period, the cosmetics and self-care industries found themselves experiencing 'a record of growth [...] which has been virtually without parallel elsewhere in the economy [...] in the post war years' (North 1963, 39). As television replaced the cinema as the source of mass acculturation, TV advertising amplified the penetration of 'the look' as a potent signifier defining and determining valued lifestyles. United within an ever changing process of market segmentation, the viewing masses were eagerly transformed into a consuming public. Sales of magazines devoted to fashion, make up, fitness and food rose. Even for those who could scarcely afford it the mass media were still busy creating a cultural imaginary based around youth and beauty, and social, cultural and political change seemed omnipresent in the 'long 1960s' (Marwick 1998).

Only the old were left behind, a demographic group placed outside the market, granted 'mere survival and nothing more' (de Beauvoir 1977, 276). In 1962, a *Life Magazine* survey of 'Expenditure Patterns of the American Family' revealed that those aged 65 and over were least likely to have made a major expenditure on durable goods, least likely to have taken an expensive vacation (costing $100 or more) and least likely to have spent money on manicures, massages and slenderising treatments (Wells and Gubar 1966). But within this most impoverished age group, there were already signs of an emerging 'leisure class' (Michelon 1954). Despite its marginalisation through the 'long' 1960s' incessant celebration of youth, age would re-emerge in the 1980s as a significant, mid-life market segment for the 'youthed out' cosmetic and self-care industries.

By 1968, the beauty industry was one of the world's largest market sectors, spending more money on television advertising than almost any other industry and providing the highest profit margins of any industry apart from alcoholic drinks (Jones 2010). In a climate of increasing affluence, rapid social and cultural change and the inter-generational fracture of the 1960s 'revolution', cosmetic enhancement of one's appearance became an acceptable ideal. Fashion models such as Jean Shrimpton and Twiggy became stars in their own right, as did Donyale Luna, 'the first black model to become an international star' (Keenan 1977, 173). The turn to the body was evident across multiple fronts, creating new consumers, fostering new identities and establishing new sites of distinction. The body had become a powerful source of distinction, an expression of authenticity and a means of liberation for the individuality buried beneath the old clothing of class and the cloying conventions of the past. That, at least, was 'the rebel sell' exemplified by the 'Biba girl' who 'did what she felt like at that moment and had no Mum along to influence her judgement' (Dyhouse 2010, 112).

Despite criticisms from the conservative right and the radical left (Hansen, Reed and Waters 1986), the beauty industry continued to blossom. Young middle and working class women saw their future investing in their appearance and the accompanying 'beauty work'. According to the industries' advisors the rising demographic of baby boomers, a national emphasis on youth and youthful appearance, rising levels of women's education and increasing numbers of working women, together with increased leisure, continuing urbanisation and expanding retail outlets, would lead to a stable and growing demand for toiletries and cosmetics projected into the 1980s (Karo 1967). By 1973 'one half of the total fragrance, eye shadow and sun care products, 60% of the mascara and 80% of the shampoo' consumed in America was accounted for by women in the 18–34 age group (Jones 2010, 189). In Europe the young, too, were the target audience. Their desires and aspirations increasingly drove the fashion and beauty industries. The prewar centralised, seasonal production systems of fashion were changing into faster, more responsive systems of mass production and the cosmetic and self-care industries were quick to follow suit. Young men were also becoming customers. By the mid-1960s, while there were only a few hair dyes available for men, over 25 different hairsprays, 170 types of razors and over 300 colognes were marketed to men in the USA alone (Karo 1967).

Estimated global sales of self-care products rose from $460 million in 1950 to some $14 billion by the mid-seventies (Jones 2008). As the sub-cultural styles of 1960s evolved into the 1970s' search for 'authenticity', the market responded swiftly by increasing the diversity of its products, marketing natural and organic products (Heath and Potter 2005). Up until the 1980s, age-dominated systems of segmentation meant that cosmetic sales continued to target customers in their teens and twenties. While there was some growth in male toiletries and cosmetics (symbolised by the 'glam' rock bands of the early seventies) and toiletries and cosmetics that were tailored toward 'ethnic minorities' (symbolised by the black model 'crashing through the color bar' (Keenan 1977, 173)), the emphasis remained upon being '*young* gifted and black'.

Youth Meets Age: The Rise of the Cosmeceutical Generation

By the 1980s, the bodies of this 'revolutionary' generation were beginning to show signs of ageing. For this group, with its deep acculturation into the consumerist habitus of the postwar era, this did not mean abandoning beauty work. New markets and new cosmetic products were emerging that catered for a new consumer demographic, mid-lifers and the 'young' aged. An important stimulus to this growth was provided by the development in the 1980s of 'cosmeceuticals'. Albert Kligman had pioneered the use of the term to describe cosmetic products with biologically active ingredients purporting to have additional medical or drug-like benefits beyond those of simply skin moisturising (Kligman 1993). While traditional cosmetics had been mostly face powder and compacts, whose use was based on common domestic practices, these late twentieth-century developments moved cosmetics from colouring, shading and smoothing to targeting the physical texture and appearance of the skin (Draelos 2008, 628). In the process the line between medicines and cosmetics became blurred. The first 'trials' of topical anti-ageing skin creams began to be reported (Kligman et al. 1986; Weiss et al. 1988a, 1988b). They were favourable.

Without the benefit or need of clinical trials, the beauty industry kept on growing, its profits swelled by the demands of the mid-life baby boomers. Procter & Gamble's beauty revenues rose from $13m in 1950 to $630m in 1977 to $2.3bn in 1989; L'Oréal from $11m to $803m to $3.7bn; Beiersdorf from $7m to $571m to $2bn; and Revlon from $19m to $810m to $2.4bn (Jones 2010, 369–71). A new anti-ageing aesthetic was emerging. L'Oréal, Estée Lauder, Avon and Beiersdorf began spending increasing amounts of money on basic research into the anatomical and metabolic determinants of skin structure and applied research designed to establish reliable measures of skin texture, colour and thickness. Within this new culture of 'aspirational science', various vitamins, coenzymes and polyphenols were introduced into skin cream products, to counteract collagen depletion and degradation associated with skin ageing. These ingredients were supplemented by the use of cell regulators such as retinol, polypeptides and growth factors designed to stimulate collagen synthesis and/or reduce wrinkling through their muscle relaxant properties, producing a growing range of 'anti-ageing' creams and lotions (Kerscher and Buntrock 2011).

Initial marketing of anti-ageing products to those who were becoming conscious of their own ageing proved so successful that the industry extended its concern with managing the bodily signs of ageing to people who might otherwise still be considered 'young'. From the turn of the twenty-first century, people in their twenties and thirties were recommended to begin the 'prophylactic' use of anti-ageing products as the industry further developed its segmentation of the market, developing products 'for each generation' to help them stay young looking and attractive (Euromonitor International 2011). While there is a general correlation between chronological age and the consumption of anti-ageing skin care products, studies have demonstrated that factors other than chronological age play an important part, with people's 'anxiety over ageing' being more influential in determining consumption of anti-ageing products (Muise and Desmarais 2010). Since objective and subjective indices of attractiveness in later life have not been found related to the use of anti-ageing preparations, the desire to consume such products must spring from motives other than the desire for mere attractiveness (Graham and Kligman 1984). Perhaps there is a belief, expressed by one cosmetic dermatologist, that 'the quality of aging [is] important [...] to remain good looking and young [...] [and] to maintain good health' (Serri 2008, 589). Looking after one's appearance, it seems, has become integrated into a broader agenda of 'successful' ageing. According to a report in one trade journal:

> The largest growth [in cosmetics] is coming from anti-aging creams, home microdermabrasion kits and wrinkle remedies. One reason for the growth is a diversification of distribution channels, which now include upscale and mid-tier department stores, specialty stores, spas, supermarkets, chain drugstores, mass merchandisers and Internet retailers. But demographics are also widening beyond the 40-plus woman, with men in their twenties and teens showing interest. (*International Cosmetic News* 2006)

While several writers have argued that the pressure to appear 'attractive' and/or 'young' and/or 'slim' – in short the pressure to engage in beauty work – is much greater for women than for men (Cruikshank 2003; Calasanti and Slevin 2001; Hurd-Clarke and Griffin 2008; Wolf 1990), the evidence from the market suggests that what Sontag called the 'double standard' of ageing may be having a little less purchase than it once had.

Makeup, Masculinity and Maturing Markets

American consumers spent $4.8 billion on men's grooming products in 2009, according to Euromonitor International, doubling the amount of 1997. Among the fastest growing men's segments is skin care – the use of non-shaving products like facial cleansers, moisturisers and exfoliants. Behind these purchasing decisions, consumer research has revealed similar motivations amongst men and women for looking good and not looking old. Thus, one cross-national study examining men's consumption of cosmetics found that the most significant motivation for buying cosmetics was the desire to look good/attractive and the wish not to look old (Souiden and Diagne 2009). Nevertheless, as Coupland (2007) has shown, marketing of anti-ageing messages to men is new and fraught with difficulties and contradictions. Adverts may approach the topic indirectly, emphasising the value of 'not looking tired', the need to 'take care' because of today's stressful/busy lifestyles, or as a way of 'fighting back' against ageing (Coupland 2007). While some degree of evident ageing is acceptable amongst older men, showing signs of 'having lived' (Coupland 2007, 58), men are now spending 'more mirror time' as a legitimate means of supporting rather than undermining a mature but masculine self-image.

The commodification of masculinity is more a phenomenon of the 1980s than the 1960s. Some of the first 'beauty salons' for men were opened in the 1980s in Japan (Miller 2003) but they have since become commonplace in countries as diverse as India and Ireland, Belgium and Bangladesh, as the market for male self-care and male appearance management products have 'taken off' (Ahmed 2006; Khan and Tabassum 2012). By the end of the first decade of the twenty-first century, the sales of male cosmetic products in the USA reached nearly $5 billion, while in the UK sales increased by over 800 per cent, with those specifically targeting the over 50s increasing by over 400 per cent (Hill 2008; McDougall 2012; Newman 2010). As the male market for toiletries has grown so too has acceptability of 'anti-ageing' toiletries amongst both straight and gay mid-life men. Some industry sources claim that while the male market is some '15 years behind' the female market it is catching up fast. Figures quoted by US market analysts claim that up to 25 per cent of men now use facial skin care products such as cleansers, exfoliants, eye products and anti-aging serums and creams (McDougall 2012).

Men's concerns with ageing, however, are less focused upon their faces but tend instead to emphasise their overall body shape – with ageing associated with developing a paunch and the loss, thinning or greying of their hair. Concerns over wrinkles and 'ageing' skin seem to bother them less (L'Oréal 2010). Workouts are more 'acceptable' in disciplining the ageing male body than cosmetics or clothing, although future cohorts of mid-life men may have differing perspectives. But whatever the form taken by these variously embodied practices, increasingly they are oriented toward the external rather than the internal state of the body – whether those externalities are represented in terms of gender/masculinity, ageing or health.

Self-care practices aimed at fashioning appearance are not confined to 'cosmetics'. While we shall discuss the embodied practices of exercise and fitness in the next chapter it is important to note here that men and women's 'cosmetic' practices extend beyond makeup, self-care and toiletries. Studies of indoor tanning, for example, have found that while older people are, as a group, less likely to use tanning beds, men over 65 years of age are no less likely to use them as women of that age (Heckman, Coups and Manne 2008; Dissel et al. 2009). In contrast, older men are much less likely than women to seek to manage their appearance through the active mediation of body workers, such as beauty therapists, manicurists or pedicurists. One reason, perhaps, is the socialisation practices associated with these forms of practice. Research on the beauty salon indicates that it functions as a source of gendered support and sociality, and self-care is experienced as much in the relationships between customers and practitioners as it is through the procedures and products themselves (Solomon et al. 2004). Such intimacy is rarely sought or experienced by older men even at the barbers, reducing their exposure to self-care practices as socialised forms of 'embodiment' and making decisions to embark upon late life body fashioning perhaps more intense and more unforgiving.

Body Workers and Body Work Places

Body work has become an area of increasingly 'professionalised' employment. Although hairdressers and beauty therapists have been part of the beauty industry for over a century, the period after the 1960s saw a rapid increase in the number of self-care workers, not just those working in hair salons and beauty parlours, but also those in health spas, nail parlours and other related professional self-care services (Black 2004; Willett 2000). Within these usually gendered 'homosocial' settings, beauty work practitioners provide a range of services, as well as teaching new self-care practices and drawing customers' attention to 'new-on-the-market' self-care products. The gendered nature of these settings defines 'beauty work' as women's work. The beauty salon has been described as a place 'where women cherish female companionship, exchange information, share secrets, and either temporally escape or collectively confront their problems and their heartaches' (Willett 2000, 3). Adding to the sense of being 'cared for', special 'me time' services are often offered to customers, young and old (Black 2004).

Beauty salons have always accommodated customers with a range of ages, even if they have maintained formally and informally distinctions of gender and race. They are now incorporating anti-ageing products and anti-ageing procedures alongside their traditional practices of facials, eyebrow shaping, manicure and pedicure, including services designed specifically to remove or reduce the signs of ageing, such as 'minimally invasive' procedures like Botox injections, micro-dermabrasion, epilation, and the use of facial fillers. The beauty salon's engagement with women's 'ageing' and 'age resistance' has been explored by Furman (1997) and by Hurd-Clarke (2011). The former concentrated upon a particular beauty salon, defined by the age, gender and ethnicity of its clients while the latter addressed age associated beauty work conducted in salons as well as in individuals' own homes. Both authors demonstrate the ambiguous position that age presents within such settings, in terms of promoting or defending one's attractiveness, self-image and social standing. They illustrate how these women subject themselves (and their peers) to a gaze, which to varying degrees objectifies their body as 'old' and 'past it'. Arguably it is through their experience of treating age as a shared threat that enables these women to negotiate its contradictions. Black has also pointed out how this process of 'negotiation' can be facilitated by the 'beauty worker' who can be seen as 'normalising' the experience, especially when she is someone with whom the client can identify (Black 2004, 46).

Accommodating beauty work with age raises the question of how and why, despite expressing clear dissatisfaction with their ageing bodies, the women interviewed nevertheless persisted in their beauty work (Hurd Clarke 2011, 61). It has been described as a position of apparent 'double consciousness' – performing 'femininity' through beauty work, while still actively embodying age. The contradictory position in which visiting the salon puts these women is clear to many of these research subjects. The existence of similar others, and the identity and intimacy developed with the practitioners seems to make 'being past it' a shared, ironic position that comforts what otherwise may be a more lonely confrontation with corporeal age.

Does a double standard of ageing confine contemporary older women to the gendered habitus that they helped create in the heyday of their youth and desires for self-expression? Are women baby boomers consequently more enmeshed in these conflicts than their mothers? While it is difficult to know whether there are any cohort differences in expectations and opportunities to 'resist' ageing through beauty work, it could be argued that such expectations and opportunities have increased for older women now. What is also changing is the reluctance of many 'contemporary' older people to acquiesce to outdated ways of performing beauty work. Evidence that this may be so can be found in a recent UK study of older people and their experience of visiting the hairdressers. One of the respondents is reported as saying: 'Tuesdays were the days to avoid going to the hairdressers because it's pension day. Pensioners' days are the ones to avoid. Everyone comes out with the same hairdo' (Ward and Holland 2011, 301). Such hairdressers were seen not as mediators of self-care, but as agents imposing self-care through a 'uniform' pensioner's hairdo. This led to the customers feeling as if they 'were like peas in a pod. The style was a perm on top and shingled at the back' (Ward and Holland 2011, 302). Another respondent, speaking of the way two mobile hairdressers worked, described the outcomes as 'stereotyped' but then wondered 'if it's because that's what old people want or are they just accepting that because that's what's offered?' (Ward and Holland 2011, 302). These authors emphasise the importance of the co-production of appearance that emerges from these encounters, suggesting that 'hairdressers reinforce the message that while younger consumers may pursue an image as a mode of distinction, older people are required not to stand out' (Ward and Holland 2011, 303).

As self-care product choices and the performed practices of self-care become more various, the practitioners of beauty work and the subjects of beauty work are likely to be involved in more extensive processes of negotiation around ageing and its appropriate embodiment. 'Compulsive beauty' and its associated 'body panic' are not confined to ageing persons; they are activated in and through other embodied identities, such as gender and ethnicity. Increasing the choices of how to look fit, healthy and attractive may make not choosing to do so even more difficult to express as a choice. The double consciousness of performing age and performing beauty is felt more often and acutely by women than by men, but what research into beauty work places shows is that women can also negotiate these contradictions as a shared experience: facing a common foe. If beauty work is becoming less tightly gendered, the question arises of whether men can also draw upon sufficient 'homosocial' resistance to navigate the dual consciousness of ageing and not becoming old.

Dressing Up Democracy

Like cosmetics, clothing and fashion are practices oriented as much toward gender and ethnicity as toward age. A similar story can also be told about the emergence of 'fashion' as a youth-oriented, 'democratising' element in postwar consumerist society. Unlike cosmetics which has gradually accommodated and indeed embraced the opportunities of ageing in consumer society, the clothing and fashion industries have found such accommodation harder to achieve, perhaps because age served as such a powerful marker in transforming and democratising them. During the 1960s, Lipovetsky argued, '[f]ashion began to connote youthfulness; it had to express an emancipated life-style, free of constraint, relaxed with respect to the official canon […] a promotion of an age-based code imposed on everyone in the name of the increasingly compelling code of individualization' (Lipovetsky 2002, 100). After the monopoly the war effort imposed on the textile industries and the post war rationing of clothing, the 'make do and mend' mentality of the various war generations was transformed by a new 'postwar' generation who were growing up with time and money to spend. The consumerist habitus of the new youth sub-cultures helped shape 'the emergence of the 1960s throwaway, consumer society [where] short-lived fads became the norm, clothes were disposed of long before they were worn out and a youthful image was suddenly desirable' (Mendes and de la Haye 1999, 158). The juxtaposition of youth and fashion that was first promoted in the 1920s was fully realised as a mass phenomenon in the 1960s when fashion was transformed from a class to a youth aesthetic (Lipovetsky 2002, 88–9).

The 'long 1960s' marked the point where the fashion practices of the elite, however constituted, were overtaken by the activities and style of those closer to 'the street'. Popular music and its sub-cultures helped to set the scene. Each new band and popular singer sought distinction not only in the music they played, but in the way they looked. Hairstyle and clothing became complementary elements in pop culture. Surrounding the popular musical scene were entrepreneurs like Mary Quant who, with her partner and husband, created the first 'boutique' clothes shop, Bazaar. The formality of the traditional shop was replaced by the casual atmosphere of the new boutique. Here buying clothes was fun, pop music played continuously and the customers saw themselves mirrored in the style and manners of those serving them. In such settings, the boutique owners could 'keep pace with the movement of the very volatile, quickly changing youth market in a way that was impossible in the big store' (Ewing 2005, 185) as fashion moved from class differentiation to 'collective selection' (Blumer 1969).

In 1960s' pop culture, youthful clothes, designers, models and photographers mixed with equally youthful actors, singers and musicians of the 'pop' world in the embodiment of a new form of celebrity. The boundaries between popular and high culture became blurred. New styles and patterns of clothing were influenced by developments in contemporary 'op' and 'pop' art. The working- and middle-class youth wanted to be as fashionable as they could while the youth of the upper classes were as inclined to imitate working-class dress and fashion styles as they were to access their own styles of dress. What all sought to achieve was a generational distinctiveness, setting the colourful, informal and idiosyncratic styles of youth against the mass produced uniformity of dress that made the old and the middle-aged ciphers for an old fashioned, class conscious conformity. This process of 'informalisation' became one of the key cultural tropes of the time (Wouters 2007).

These differences were not confined to outward appearances. Changes in dress style were happening on the inside. Underwear, clothing normally invisible from the social gaze, provided another source of generational distinction. Mini-skirts made stockings, corsets and suspenders unsuitable; they also drew attention to underwear as a source of erotic interest. Several fashion writers have argued that until the 1960s underwear served primarily a functional role in providing comfort and hygiene (Entwistle 2000; Wilson 1985). The 1960s made underwear 'sexy'. The young women of the time became the main customers for tights and coloured bras, knickers and patterned pants, selecting them as much for their look as much as for their function.

The possibilities of this kind of consumption were realised through three particular material developments. The bra was modified through the introduction of artificial fibres that increased the potential for colouring, patterning and styling it; stockings suspenders and corsets were replaced by tights, first made from wool, but only becoming popular when nylon and other artificial fibres were used in their manufacture; and the arrival of the mini-skirt that made underwear visible and capable of a fashioned display. Men's underwear underwent its own more silent revolution. The prewar era of union suits, long johns and singlets was replaced by elasticised pants, 't-shirts', briefs modelled after the jockstrap, and introduced in the 1940s as 'Jockey' briefs. Although most of these changes took place before the Second World War, the needs of war meant that they were effectively 'held off' until war was over. From the 1950s, t-shirts, jockey shorts, boxers and briefs were mass produced, elastic was added to cotton to provide a better and more comfortable fit and posters advertising men's pants and vests began expressly to present the man in underpants as 'glamorous' and even 'sexy'.

A generation of young men and women grew up wearing underwear distinctly different from the undergarments that their mothers and fathers, grandmothers and grandfathers had worn. By the end of the 'long 1960s', the women still wearing corsets and stockings were old fashioned and the men still wearing long johns outdated. The young working man's collar and cuffs disappeared as did the flannel trousers and the cloth cap; amongst the middle classes the striped shirt, suit and trilby hat were replaced by new casual clothes for work, with more flamboyant ties and shirts. Hats disappeared as sources of class distinction. Floral patterned shirts, denim jeans, pointed shoes, boxer shorts and jockey briefs served as the new uniform of leisure when going out to the cinema or dance hall, the coffee bar or night club. In the 'bar', 'pub' or 'working man's club' the unreconstructed older working class men would still congregate, dressed distinctively and differently, the residue of a past and soon-to-be forgotten era. In the 'long 1960s', clothes became a key marker for a new and distinctive generational divide.

Fashion and the Changing Life Course

The ageing of 1960s' youth undermined the very age segmentation system that these cohorts had helped establish. By the mid-1980s, the 1960s youth were approaching middle age, reaching the chronological ages of those earlier cohorts whom they had once been exhorted to ignore or disregard. Few were ready to abandon the investment in clothes and fashion that had made them once feel so distinct and so not old. Fashion obviously changes; democratic fashion changes even faster. The habits of fashion such as building and discarding a wardrobe on the basis of style rather than suitability were now woven into the habitus of a generation. Time alone would not undo such generational habitus.

Thus, as they aged most women did not replace their tights and revert to wearing 'old fashioned' stockings, nor did they trade their bras and briefs in and return to wearing corsets and suspenders. Ageing men did not give up their boxers and briefs to go back to wearing long johns or 'union suits'. The changes in fashion that had taken place in the 1960s continued to change, but the demise of such 1960s and 1970s period items as high collared floral shirts, bell bottom trousers, black and white 'op art' dresses and white plastic boots did not lead to their representation as an old fashioned old age; instead they maintained their distinctiveness of youth and acquired the capacity to be recycled as 'retro-wear' suitable for both past and present youth to wear, ironically and in a way that previous, less democratic fashions could not (Jenß 2004).

Jeans and t-shirts exemplified the democratisation of fashion for both men and women. Once the clothes of soldiers and working men, they had become, in the 1960s, the iconic style of all classes, ethnicities and genders. Even when they became the clothing of choice for those no longer working, they did not lose their 'radical' appeal. These and other generationally defined items of clothing retained their appeal long after the generational schism they signalled had passed. This is the case with tights. Once confined to radical, mini-skirted youth, tights are now worn by women of all ages. Like the ubiquitous 'UK size 12' dress they seem to accommodate women of all sizes shapes and ages. In contrast, the decline of the hat and the headscarf still marks that clear generational divide, symbols of past lives which have never since been taken up as later life wear.

While growing up means larger sizes, growing older has no simple corporeal trajectory. While it leads, arguably, to a greater heterogeneity in body shape, ageing does not lead to any inevitable 'down-' or 'up-sizing'. What the increased heterogeneity associated with ageing has meant is a growing dissatisfaction with the rigidity of sizing systems for ready to wear dress, skirts and tops (Goldsberry, Shim and Reich 1996; Holmlund, Hagman and Polsa 2011, 109). While the relationship between grading, sizes and the physical anthropology of the human body has never been more than approximate (Schofield and LaBat 2005), the criteria that have been used for sizing have been based around the physique of developing bodies or young grownups, whose bodies are generally less varied than those in later life. What are perceived to be age related changes may better be viewed as age associated diversity in body shape. As existing systems of allocating clothing sizes have become more individualised and more idiosyncratic over time, varying not just by country but by retail outlet, there is more reason now for people of all ages to shop around to get a decent fit. Attempts to re-base sizing systems on twenty-first-century data have and are being made, but the standardisation of clothing once aspired to in the 1940s and 1950s has melted away. Stores increasingly use the idea of 'size' as a signifier of generalised desires rather than of specific dimensions.

The age-based segmentation of the market that shaped fashion's earlier democratisation privileged youth. Such age segmentation, however, has proved no more sustainable than the earlier privileging of class. Evidence from the mid-1970s onwards makes clear that older women are as fashion conscious and want to shop in high fashion stores as much as younger women (Martin 1976). They are as interested in dressing well as younger women (Reynolds and Wells 1977). Recognition of age associated changes in corporeality set against the new age invariance in embodied fashion consciousness has led clothing retailers to downplay age as a source of segmentation. Instead life-stage, cohort or generational segmentation has been emphasised, particularly in the USA where the baby boomers or the 50+ demographic have been identified as 'sophisticated consumers with money to spend [...] [who are] mobile, interested in consuming, respond to changing trends and are advertising literate' (Haynes 2004, cited in Reisenwitz and Iyer 2007, 202).

Although fashion stores still make implicit use of age categories in their display and selection of clothing, and although clothing choices are still sensitive to age effects, the age ordering of fashion has become subject to so many contingencies that retailers express relatively little concern with age-based market segmentation. Increasingly they seem to be acting under the belief that it is the consumers who segment the market rather than the other way round (Danneels 1996, 43). The segmentation system created in the early mass consumer society now seems as outdated as the earlier sizing systems. One of Danneels' retailer interviewees suggests as much when s/he states that: 'the segmentation system is gone. Older people become younger, younger people grow older. It used to be more extreme but now segmentation fades' (cited in Danneels 1996, 46). The clothes industry has shifted increasingly from 'lifestage' toward 'lifestyle' although, as Julia Twigg has noted, lifestyle 'cannot be separated wholly from issues of age' (Twigg 2012, 12). Fashion is and remains age conscious but it is no longer designed to exclude.

Conclusions

While cosmetics and cosmeceuticals are intended in varying degrees to 'improve' bodily appearance, fashion serves a more polysemous function. Just as hegemonic feminist views of cosmetic surgery as oppressing or constraining women have begun to be challenged, so have such views about fashion. Postmodernist fashion, it has been claimed, does not offer women 'a specific identity (but) assumes a variety of possibly contradictory identities' (Crane 2000, 207). Among these contradictory and inconclusive messages, an ageing appearance has been inserted as a kind of optional lifestyle upon which fashionable clothes can (still) be hung. Even if still outweighed in sheer numbers by young models in their teens and twenties, models of older men and women have become more present in the pages of fashion and lifestyle magazines, where they are distinguished by their grey or silver hair but not by their cut or their wrinkles.

The dressed body is not dressed by age nor is it dressed for age. Clothing and dress are cultural products that mediate between our corporeality and the world beyond the body. Within this type of cultural mediation, ageing has become a more significant influence upon fashion. As fashion has become democratised, for the majority of adults, clothing has come to be as much about fashion as about wear. Within this more fashion conscious world, the lengthening of a life does not pose the same constraints it once did – whether in terms of wear or of simply accumulating 'old' clothing. Discarding one set of clothes for another is no longer dependent upon their being worn out; changing one's wardrobe is perhaps less regular than changing a person's makeup or hairstyle, but it is more commonplace than before. Once it was the privilege and pleasure of the young, now the very changeability of clothing can help divert attention from the change that corporeal ageing presents. It is not so much a matter of staying young as outsmarting age. Fashion offers ways of keeping up appearances that neither denies, nor masks agedness; it dresses age up, makes it part of a performance that can be conducted by individuals of any age, gender, race or sexual identity.

Of course, the decoupling of age, status and fashion is not so absolute. But the relationship has become more ambiguous and widening models and markets have multiplied choice across all ages and stages of life (Mumel and Prodnik 2005). While there are various fashion advisors who suggest key elements in staying smart and ageing fashionably, such as the cut, colour and fabric (Palma 2008), the presence of corporeal impairments can still serve as major constraints. It can be difficult to negotiate the uniformity still presented by the shape, size and styling of clothes and footwear. Shoes in particular can be difficult to select if the wearer suffers from swollen ankles, bunions, arthritic joints or fallen arches (Naidoo et al. 2011). Other conditions may prevent the person from dressing themselves without help or assistance from another person. Gerontological research is full of studies of functional impairments and disabilities, but it is difficult to find much written about how people can, and do, strive to remain fashionable and keep up appearances when corporeal limitations are present. Since such conditions are not confined to any particular age, however, the work of disability activists can be extended not just to gaining access to social and cultural resources like the cinema or public transport, but in becoming better able to choose to dress fashionably and smartly.

Reflecting such possibilities is the development of 'fashionable' or 'aesthetic' prostheses. Here, fashion and design are brought to bear on the production of prosthetic devices that enhance the appearance as well as the function of people – of all ages – with an impairment or disability (Pullin 2009). While the transgressions of a disability aesthetic have been shaped around the transgressions of young 'rebellious' bodies, the scope for fashionable prostheses goes beyond youth and sexuality to embrace conceptions of 'ageless' beauty and 'ageless' functionality. The scope that the disability model offers for the 'cultural re-symbolization' of disability (Eiseland 1994, cited in Garland-Thomson 2002, 23) is still quite narrow, steering a course between 'the conventions of sentimental charity images exotic freak show portraits [...] or sensational and forbidden pictures' (Garland-Thomson 2002, 23). Ageing and its representation as an arena for fashion is perhaps rather less constrained, but, as ever, such tailored approaches risk marginalising age-associated disabilities just as disabled fashions can risk marginalising age. Prosthetic aesthetics are less constrained as the fashion possibilities of glasses as 'eyewear' has shown. Extending these ideas to 'ear ware', 'chair ware' and to other supports and prostheses is one obvious direction for a growing market.

Cosmetics like clothing can be seen as an arena of embodied practice that is determined principally by fashion and fit. But cosmetics too can be extended to 'cosmetic therapy' which has been shown to improve older people's self-esteem (Graham and Kligman 1984). Just as it is possible to turn cosmetics into a system that marginalises older people through pensioner hairstyles and outdated products, so it is also possible to turn such practices towards re-socialising older individuals to a more gendered sense of self and a more distinctive sense of later lifestyle. Even care assistants can be re-branded as self-care technicians to become active co-producers in disabled people's own fashioned subjectivity.

Chapter 9

FITNESS, EXERCISE AND THE AGEING BODY

In Chapter 9 we turn from the body work associated with cosmetics, self-care, dress and fashion to a consideration of fitness and physical exercise and their role as forms of body work directed toward 'not becoming old'. While physical activity has conventionally been associated with youth, changes over the last half century have seen exercise and fitness become not only commodified, but also incorporated into the new discourses of ageing. Among the many factors that distinguish exercise from other body practices is its engagement with the idea of fitness as both an interior and exterior virtue. In its attention to both the internal self and civic virtue, physical exercise has long been part of the care and cultivation of the self. Alongside medicine, cosmetics and the 'sensual arts', it formed part of the quartet of human sciences addressing what the philosopher Francis Bacon described as 'the good of man's body' (Bacon 2002). Of course, this is not to claim that such sciences have not changed over time. In contemporary society, exercise has become a more 'individualised' and a more 'fashioned' aspect of lifestyle through which social distinction is sought and interpreted. It may be over-stretching a point to claim that this may represent a continuous link with the regimes and practices that promote health, functioning and beauty known by Galen as *gymnasia* (Galen 1997). These regimes were described as activities of 'child training', creating the conditions of health fitness and beauty in youth. This particular age orientation lasted up to the mid-twentieth century, but by the latter part of the twentieth century exercise had become an all-ages activity of leisure. Unlike the individualistic practices associated with fashion and cosmetics, physical exercise contains an important dimension of promoting the agentic nature of social citizenship (Lupton 1995). Its role as a public good has become a central motif in the widespread public health campaigns that articulate the message that health and fitness are virtues to be cultivated at all ages and amongst all groups, a necessary part in the endless war against the ills of 'indolence' and the diseases of affluence (Campos 2004). The contemporary pursuit of fitness in later life thus elides the 'youthful' individual desire to do better and be better with the 'mature' virtue of not becoming sick, fat, idle or old.

The criticisms directed toward cosmetics, clothing and fashion as signs of an effete and effeminate vanity doomed with time to failure are rarely voiced against exercise and the pursuit of fitness. The links established in youth between health, fitness and beauty have not been dissolved with age. Unlike the pursuit of 'looking good' or even 'looking attractive', pursuing an ageless fitness finds general approval – providing of course it is directed toward public virtue and not personal good. As we saw in the previous chapter, because of their use as sources of personal enhancement, cosmetics and fashion deployed at any age have always stimulated gendered complaints but especially so if practised in later life. While time might condemn all body practices at some point to failure, the lack of success in achieving ageless health and fitness (though not beauty) through exercise is not seen as reflecting the kind of *'mundana vana gloria'* ethos that the failure to succeed in cosmetics and fashion does. Exercise retains a determinedly 'masculine' virtue, at all ages, even if it is no longer the exclusive concern of male bodies, just as fashion and cosmetics retain their role as 'feminine' vices even if they are no longer only a concern of women.

Ageing and Exercise: From Avoidance to Participation

As noted above, although the virtuous pursuit of exercise has a long history, its extension into later life is of relatively recent origin. The elision between fitness, exercise and successful ageing has become a distinctive feature of contemporary society. Going back two thousand years, Cicero argued that in later life great deeds are done by thought, character and judgement, not through strength, physique or swiftness (Cicero 1971, 220). The renaissance physician, Zerbi advocated extreme moderation in both sex and exercise, suggesting that old men should exercise by regimes that 'are gentle, soft and light' such as 'being carried about, or riding [...] being rocked on water or in a cradle, by standing, lying or sitting in a boat in a port or on a river' (Zerbi 1988, 111). This advice was repeated by later renaissance writers such as du Laurens and Ferdinandi who also proscribed too frequent or too strenuous exercise in later life. While du Laurens advocated ball play and 'foot walking', he thought: 'old folke must content themselves with moderate exercise for fear that the little naturall heat which they have should be spent' (du Laurens 1599,189). To this end he also recommended: 'frications or rubbing of the parts [...] beginning at the armes and from thence to the shoulders, backe and breast, from thence we must goe downe to the thighes and rise up again from thence to the shoulders [...] [leaving the head, which] must be the last which must be combd and trimd up every morning' (Ibid.). In short, throughout the premodern era exercise was treated as a minor element in 'productive' or 'successful' ageing and if undertaken a clear preference was shown for the more passive forms of massage over active exercise, and light and gentle exercise over more vigorous exercise likely to raise the pulse and make the body sweat.

Such views continued to hold sway into the early twentieth century. Patricia Vertinsky quotes a Dr Wainwright, writing in a 1900 issue of *The Medical Record* to the effect that 'the aged should undertake no violent exercise whatever [save only] gentle exercise involving slow steady movements' (Wainwright 1900, cited by Vertinsky 1991, 77). Such attitudes remained prevalent even in the 1930s and 1940s. They were encapsulated in the writings of another 'modern' US doctor, Peter Steincrohn. Author of numerous medical self-help manuals, Steincrohn wrote a booklet entitled *You Don't Have to Exercise: Rest Begins at Forty* (1942) in which he emphasised the importance of rest and leisure for the 'over-stressed', 'over worked' middle-aged man. Muscles, he said, were for the young. Men over 40 should avoid assaulting their 'creaking joints' and 'beat up circulatory systems' with anything more vigorous than a bit of gardening, golfing and, maybe, a little light sailing (Luciano 2001, 58). A similar wariness of exercise was evident in mid-century Britain. As John Benson has noted 'during the first half of the [twentieth] century the middle aged were advised – and seemed to accept – that they should wrap up well and be careful not to overdo it' (Benson 1997, 128).

Much of the early physiological research on ageing and exercise was oriented toward assessing older men's fitness for work rather than their capacity to live longer and better (cf. Åstrand, Åstrand and Rodahl 1959; Botwinick and Shock 1952; Dawson and Hellebrandt 1945; Barry et al. 1966). Chief among the twentieth-century physicians advocating active exercise in later life were the practitioners of postwar geriatric medicine. Marjorie Warren in particular became famous for her 'activation' of old people when she found herself in charge of the British prewar institutions for the chronic sick (Warren 1943). While her approach can be seen as extending the earlier Victorian tradition of providing public resources to promote the health and leisure of the labouring masses, exercise within the hospital was as much about getting old people up and out as restoring their health, let alone rejuvenating or prolonging their lives.

A public health tradition that had arisen in the mid-nineteenth century as part of a general concern for public sanitation and a concern with the general fitness of the nation under conditions of industrialisation, urbanisation and a newly professionalised militarism. Most concern was directed at overcoming the outbreak and spread of infectious diseases as well as regulating working conditions of women and children during this period. However, as Edward Higgs has observed, the Victorian state and its municipalities also began to play an active role in promoting and regulating the leisure and character of the masses (Higgs 1983, 141). Public libraries, public baths and public sports grounds were established as resources for active healthy leisure and the means for improving the capacities of the nation, while controls were extended over undesirable leisure activities such as betting and gambling, circuses, music halls, amusement parks and the use of animals to provide 'sport' and entertainment. Whilst the latter were viewed as sources of potential harm to public health and moral well-being of the masses, the former were associated with the promotion of the public good.

The 'new callisthenics' whose origins lay in Scandinavia and Germany, was imported as part of this new ethos and began permeating British and North American schools, youth organisations and the military during the late nineteenth and early twentieth century (van Hilvoorde 2008). The focus on physical exercise in adulthood was given particular emphasis in Britain by the military recruitment campaigns during the Boer War when recruits were found to be ill-equipped for the rigours of mass warfare (Searle 1971). The experiences of the First World War further reinforced this focus on adult physical health and its idealisation within the education and military systems. The 'martial physique' demanded of future soldiers was echoed in the new images of masculinity provided by the cinema and by the end of the Second World War, Luciano has argued, the US ideal of men's adult body image had changed. While early twentieth-century cinema had idealised the reassuring manly plumpness of the nineteenth-century 'Gilded Age', Hollywood in the mid-twentieth century turned toward slim, muscular, youthful bodies instead (Luciano 2001, 20). Concerns over national fitness were articulated between and after both World Wars. Schoolchildren and youth were targeted in particular and youthful fitness became part of the overt political ideology of countries such as Germany and the Soviet Union. In Britain various national fitness programmes were developed to ensure that schools and colleges provided better 'Physical Exercise' (PE) lessons. But after the age of 18 or so, people were 'expected to fend for themselves' (Luciano 2001, 56).

The concern with fitness was not just a concern of policy makers and military strategists. Historically there had long been an interest in fitness as an end in itself. Van Hilvoorde has argued that the 'postmodern' practices of fitness which have become predominant today have their origins in the late Victorian ideals of manly physical exercise and sport (van Hilvoorde 2008, 1308). He traces three elements in this process: the development of a physical anthropometry that set standards for the shape, size, symmetry and performance of the fit and ideal body leading to the associated development of manuals and rules for achieving this; the creation of the spaces and equipment that gave a material focus for practising physical exercise and fitness; and the popular showmanship that helped stimulate the public fascination with what bodies could become. While the 'commercialising' aspect of the latter can be contrasted with the nation-building aspect of the former, both elements were equally present at the beginning of the twentieth century. Although they coalesced in the cultural ferment of the 1960s, they did so in contradictory ways. School sports and school callisthenics, fitness, workouts and body building lost any appeal for the 1960s youth as they were identified with the regimentation of the older generation. Conversely, while young men were cultivating their sense of fashion, young women were beginning to embrace the idea of actively looking after their own bodies, a theme clearly reflected in the 1970s Boston Women's Health Book Collective handbook, *Our Bodies, Ourselves* (BWHBC, [1973] 1984). The new feminism challenged the old masculine ideals of fitness.

Prior to the 1960s, collective and national exercise and fitness programmes had overwhelmingly focused upon men – as actual or future workers and soldiers. During the nineteenth and early twentieth century, women, like the elderly, were advised against any but the gentlest forms of exercise. Exercise was thought to risk 'damaging' women's reproductive capacity while in later life 'aging women were perceived to be invalids in need of care, lacking the necessary vital energy to participate in onerous daily activities' (Verinsky 1991, 77). Women were generally prescribed 'a combination of rest and gentle exercise [...] to prolong health and equilibrium as far as possible' (Vertinsky 1991, 78). Throughout the late nineteenth and early twentieth century, medical literature was used to constrain young women's participation in certain sports education and the majority of sports (Vertinsky 1987), as well as to prevent older women's enjoyment of exercise.

What changed? The introduction of exercise into women's lifestyles took place in the wake of the women's movement and the demand for women to 'think through the body'. As men were turning away from the martial display of fitness and physicality in favour of looser lifestyles and fashion, the women's movement began to engage with an idea of fitness that in some ways broke with the past – one that van Hilvoorde has described as 'a culture in which people motivated by a mix of cosmetic and medical concerns voluntarily and deliberately engage in physical exercises' (van Hilvoorde 2008, 1320). The rise to prominence of 'cosmetic and medical' concerns enabled a less narrowly gendered culture of fitness to emerge, one that contrasted the imposition of collective routines designed to render bodies fit for war and work with regimes to make bodies whole, healthy and attractive. This refashioning of fitness established a culture of exercise that was less rigidly gendered, more flexible in its practices and goals, and oriented away from collective goals toward a broader and more individualised set of psychosocial outcomes. It was realised through some specific developments of the time – jogging as a non-youth oriented form of exercise (Bowerman and Harris 1967), aerobics as a form mixing dance and exercise, but based on the aerobic system guiding exercise practices (Cooper 1970) and the new 'body workout' designed to achieve muscle tone and muscle definition without the old connotations of masculine 'body building' (Chapman 1994).

Jogging Alone: The Individualisation of Exercise in Contemporary Society

A youthful focus upon body building was still being promoted by Charles Atlas in the 1950s and 1960s. According to Benson, it was not until the late 1960s that exercise emerged, at least in Britain, as a desirable goal for the mass of middle-aged and older people (Benson 1997, 128). Attention began to move towards the middle-aged with the introduction of jogging, aerobics and the body 'workout' which became mass phenomena by the 1980s. The removal of the old prohibitions on women of child-bearing age or older from exercising, the middle-ageing of the 1960s' 'baby boomer' generation and their concern to stay young, and the continued expansion of a somatic society in which images of the body proliferated as signifiers and stimulants of desire made exercise and fitness lifelong concerns. Glassner has argued that fitness is quintessentially a postmodern condition where the appeal of fitness products and practices offer 'the opportunity to disenthrall [one's] self from the perceived shortcomings of everyday life in modern culture – in particular from constraining dualities such as expert versus amateur, self versus body, male versus female and work versus leisure' (Glassner 1989, 182). According to Kagan and Morse, over 20 million Americans took part in aerobic dance-exercises in 1986, 'the vast majority of them women' (Kagan and Morse 1988, 164), with almost one-third making use of video-cassettes. The most popular tape was one produced by the 1960s' actress and icon of an age-less lifestyle, Jane Fonda (Kagan and Morse 1988, 165). Although Fonda had initially concentrated upon workouts for young mothers, her workout books and videos increasingly targeted middle-aged people who did not want to become old, using messages that resonated with the various empowerment ideals expressed by second wave feminism.

Kagan and Morse recognised the generational split between the old and the new 'fitness and exercise' regimes, expressed by the transition from collectivist masculine callisthenics to an individualised, commercial aesthetic crossing many of the old gender barriers. But, they argued, 'the cultural boundaries which had once limited women from organized forms of movement' were, in the 1980s, 'displaced to a struggle within the body itself' where the implicit enemy was 'the body itself as it ages' (Kagan and Morse 1988, 169). The incorporation of a cosmetic and medical aesthetic into the new exercise regimes created a new gendered conflict around being 'forever feminine' while staying 'forever functional'. Developments from the 1970s onwards had established a new approach to exercise and fitness, associated with jogging, aerobics and personalised workouts that enabled women to pursue the freedom from bodily restraint, the pleasure of the dance and the empowerment of the workout in a manner they had not previously been able to practice. These new 'practices of freedom', however, would soon create new internalised conflicts over the feasibility of bodily control and the power of the individual self to maintain such bodily definition. The demise of the 'revolutionary' 1960s seemed to usher in a sense of growing danger, a sense not so much of a new age emerging but of an age that was heading out of control. This furthered a new kind of body panic concerned not with the freedom of youth but with the constraints of age.

Ageing, Exercise and the Crisis of Masculinity

If women began to engage their bodies as a new site of agency and subjectivity in the period following the 1960s, by the late 1970s a new crisis of postmodern masculinity seemed imminent. Without the collective disciplines of work or war providing resolution, concerns over men's fitness merged with concerns over their mortality. Deaths while jogging became a topical issue of concern in the medical journals of the late 1970s and early 1980s. A masculine physique had become a symbol of masculinity, a masculinity that was valued not because of the work it could perform and the resources it could control, but by how 'fit' it looked. Men with bodies that epitomised the new, hegemonic masculinity and matched the cultural ideal – lean, muscular and youthful – now held the physical capital that was most valued (Coles 2009). As the embodied qualities of youth were viewed as 'essentially masculine', ageing and old age represent the negation of that ideal, threatening men as they aged with the obvious failure of their inability to match up to such representations. Once secure in, or unaffected by, their body image men were now subject to fears of personal devaluation (Whitehead 2002). There emerged what Watson has termed 'backward glancing' (2000, 96), when middle-aged men look back to their own younger selves in order to sustain their present self-identities.

This 'idealised image' of the young, fit body Watson sees as being retained by older men. This active yet 'dated' image 'attached to current masculine identity', he believes, helps explain men's reluctance to acknowledge bodily changes regarded as intrinsically negative. Bodily ageing requires men in effect to renegotiate their masculine identities. Just as the body is transformed through ageing, so notions of masculinity become influenced by age. Exercise offers one way for men to renegotiate their way through age while still expressing and retaining this hegemonic ideal. Male lifestyles of 'excess' have become recognised as being dangerous to health, prompting increasing reference to a contemporary 'crisis' afflicting men and masculinity. This crisis, whilst referred in generic terms to men of all ages and stages of life, is seen to be more applicable to men as they become older and as masculine identity can no longer be portrayed or performed through a visually youthful male body.

As the 1980s passed, so too did the concerns over death by jogging. The postwar baby boomer generation seemed more able to challenge the entrenched views and traditional expectations of aging and masculinity. Members of this demographic cohort embody elements of the postmodern 'ideal', individuals who can control their bodies through their lifestyle and consumer choices, who can 'appear to age successfully and thus defend themselves against ageism' (Calasanti and King 2007, 359). Critics of this view, of course, tend to see men and women equally, if differently, duped by the commercialisation of age resistance and gender: endlessly dancing, jogging and working out in a fruitless attempt to deny the universal truth of the body's decline, decay and death. Behind these criticisms is an articulation of ageing as a 'natural' process which men and women should and would accept as a revealed truth, if it was not for the interventions of a youth orientated, 'venal' mass consumerism (Vincent 2006, 2009).

Just as the commodification of exercise seems so far to have won the cultural war over exercise and fitness as desirable individual goals, so too has the individualistic ethic also triumphed in terms of the social virtue of individual health and fitness. Not only has exercise become an important dimension of social distinction that operates at all ages, it has also become an individualised public health imperative. Health promotion and the emergence of what Deborah Lupton (1995) has termed the 'regulated body' continually suggest that individual health is more than a personal concern but is a public duty that functions as a 'will to health'. This will to health must be demonstrated at all points and in nearly all conditions of life. While this development has been closely identified with the rise of neo-liberal modes of health policy it is also connected to the rise of citizenship as a form of Foucauldian governmentality (Higgs et al. 2009). Older people's engagement with the various technologies of the self that are designed to promote fitness is now set against the changing notions of what the norms are that are expected to be reached. In part this is an expansion of the polysemous nature of health and fitness in a consumer society that we will explore later, but it can also be seen as part of the collapse in the inter-relationship between normal ageing and the normativity of ageing in a world where diversity is not just tolerated but expected (Jones and Higgs 2010). This sets up its own normative expectations of what individuals could do or choose not to do. To use Mitchell Dean's distinction between the 'civilised' and the 'marginalised', we can see how a failure to engage with exercise and fitness throughout adult life can result in some individuals finding themselves transferred to a position of marginalisation (Dean 1995).

Bauman, Consumerism and Fitness

The idea of fitness as a phenomenon of postmodernity has been discussed extensively by Zygmunt Bauman. Going beyond a simple notion of fitness as an aspect of health, Bauman sees fitness as a defining feature of the somaticised consumer culture where the anxieties of a more contingent 'liquid modernity' are recreated and acted upon

(Bauman 2000). For Bauman the pursuit of fitness is much more than a peripheral aspect of people's lives; it acts he argues as the organising principle for a whole range of social actions. He situates his argument by pointing out that modern society has moved from being a 'society of producers' to a 'society of consumers'. This is not just an economic transformation, it is a thoroughgoing ontological transformation where each person's body becomes seen as the focus of individual action rather than being seen simply as a factor of production, reproduction or military might. He writes:

> The post-modern body is first and foremost a receiver of sensations, it imbibes and digests experiences; the capacity of being stimulated renders it an instrument of pleasure. That capacity is called fitness; obversely the 'state of unfitness' stands for langour, apathy, listlessness, dejection, a lackadaisical response to stimuli; for a shrinking or just 'below average' capacity for, and an interest in, new sensations and experiences. (Bauman 1995, 116)

The 'fitness' of the postmodern body is central to the practices of contemporary consumerism, setting up both discourses of 'engagement' and feelings of unease and dissatisfaction with that engagement. This benefits a consumer culture because these feelings of dissatisfaction provoke a constant need to attempt to reach ever higher ideals of fitness whatever level has previously been reached. In a significant passage Bauman writes:

> 'Fitness' is to a consumer in the society of consumers what 'health' was to the society of producers. It is a certificate of 'being in', of belonging, of inclusion, of the right of residence. 'Fitness' knows no upper limit; it is, in fact, defined by the absence of limit [...] However fit your body is – you could make it fitter. However fit it may be at the moment, there is always a vexing helping of 'unfitness' mixed in, coming to light or guessed at whenever you compare what you have experienced with the pleasures suggested by the rumours and sights of other people's joys which you have failed to experience thus far and can only imagine and dream of living through yourself. In the search for fitness, unlike in the case of health, there is no point at which you can say: now that I have reached it I may as well stop and hold onto and enjoy what I have. There is no 'norm' of fitness you can aim at and eventually attain. (Bauman 2005, 93)

Bauman's views echo Featherstone's (1991) notion of the 'performing self' who is driven by consumption and the moral imperative 'not to let one's self go' in an endless quest to enhance one's own health and marketability. Jones and Higgs (2010) have argued that this focus meshes closely with the cultural habitus of the third age through constantly rising expectations placed upon individuals to demonstrate their 'will to health' and their capacity to engage with all manner of techniques and regimes 'not to become old'. This moves the idea of health in later life away from the concerns of health and social policy and towards a further engagement with consumer markets. Ideas of 'healthy' or 'successful' ageing follow this same logic where the reflexive 'older' self is expected to act agentically through making the right choices for their present and future well-being in order to age without disease, dysfunction or indeed, any diminishment of adult selfhood (Rose 2001). The drive to demonstrate fitness at older ages furnishes a new normativity separating out those capable of maximising their participation in the culture of the third age from those whose identity is overshadowed by the discourses of a coming fourth age. Instead of an overarching 'natural' ageing accommodating all those deemed to be old, a fracturing of the various statuses and states of later life is encouraged by state and market alike. This helps ensure that 'consumers' can be separated from 'proxy consumers' in order to maximise both market penetration for those able to demonstrate a state of agentic 'agelessness' and market optimisation for those deemed to have lost that capacity.

Because of the role that a concentration on exercise and health in later life seems to have on the moral value of old age, some gerontologists have positively endorsed what they term an 'anti-anti-ageing' position which concentrates on the problems of challenging 'nature' (Vincent, Tulle and Bond 2008). Unlike past views of the unsuitability of exercise in later life or concerns with the risk it represented in achieving a good old age, the new critique of exercise as 'anti-ageing' demonstrates an ambivalence confounded by a general wish to promote an ideal of 'healthy ageing' as an individual and public virtue while descrying the promotion of a 'fit' body in later life as a signifier of fashion driven consumerism. The anti-ageing properties of exercise are criticised for creating the narrative fiction of 'a new older adult, strong, trainable with improved psychological and health status' (Tulle 2008, 344) which thus imagined, brings into contrast, oppresses even, those who in ageing unsuccessfully demonstrate their abjection before the masculine motif of the 'master athlete'. This conflict between the acceptance of 'natural' ageing and old age and those who see later life as having expanding possibilities for not performing 'age' or 'old', becomes a key line of fracture in understanding later life. Calasanti and Slevin (2001) posit this as a moral issue: individuals not only can, but should exert control over their ageing. However as we have seen, others see this differently. The narratives of the master athlete embody a desired extension of life not dominated by oldness replacing decline with an increasing 'performativity'.

The Master Athlete: Ageing with Strength and Endurance

The extension of physical exercise to mid-life in the late 1960s and to later life in the 1980s is also demonstrated by the increasing number of active older individuals who remain recreational or competitive athletes (Reaburn and Dascombe 2009). Once termed 'veterans', these individuals are now more commonly known as 'master athletes'. As such they occupy the medical more than the cosmetic element in contemporary fitness narratives, displaying their successful ageing through time spent running, rowing or jumping or through weights lifted and heights scaled. Master athletes have become a particular focus of interest to exercise physiologists who use them as models defining the 'true' narrative of decline, that should be evident 'despite' the powerful investment that such individuals have made in retaining the muscular power, strength and endurance of earlier adulthood (Bortz and Bortz 1996). Master athletes' performances, it is claimed, reveal the unmediated corporeality of ageing. As such master athletes both celebrate and define the ageing body, and have become a new presence in the field of sports medicine, turning it at the same time into a field of anti-ageing medicine (Tulle 2008; Phoenix and Smith 2011).

Master performances of cyclists (Brown, Ryan and Brown 2007), distance runners (Celie et al. 2010; Leyk, Erley and Bilzon 2007), rowers (Seiler, Spirduso and Martin 1998), sprinters (Hamilton 1993; Korhonen, Mero and Suominen 2003), swimmers (Donato et al. 2003; Weir et al. 2002) and weightlifters (Pearson et al. 2002) have all been studied in order to explore 'ageing and maximal performance' (Suominen 2011), 'expertise and aging' (Horton, Baker and Schorer 2008) as well as 'the struggle for maintenance' (Deakin, Baker and Horton 2004). While the growth in the number of such studies demonstrates the rise of master sports and the shifting normativities around age decline, they also reveal the complexity and indeterminacies in defining the corporeal limits to an 'ageless' performativity.

While some aspects of age-associated master athlete performance differences have been linked to measured changes in muscle mass, muscle fibre atrophy, maximal oxygen consumption and so forth, other aspects make salient 'embodied practice' and the impact of training technique and strategy. Even the 'sub-components' identified as physiological constraints to an ageless performance, such as muscle mass and atrophy are themselves subject to modification, since even experienced specialist master athletes appear able to improve their performance, for example, when additional practices such as strength and resistance training are added to their already existing training regimes (Cristea et al. 2008).

As practice improves, and as master athletes participate in more athletic events, the better their performances appear. Between the 1980s and the 2000s, for example, the number of women aged between 60 and 80, who completed the New York City Marathon, rose from 249 to 2469, while for men the numbers finishing rose from 2442 to 11, 463. The mean time to complete the marathon of both decreased significantly as did the gender gap, suggesting that male and female master runners 'have probably not yet reached their limits in marathon performance' (Lepers and Cattagni 2011). In another study involving the Nijmegen Seven Hills 15 km run, mean running time decreased over time along with a similar increase in rates of participation, suggesting that secular improvements in older adults' peak performance are common (Celie et al. 2010) and, more generally, that plasticity of performance remains at all stages of life (Suominen 2011). Complexity of function is compounded by complexity of the meaning-making associated with master athletic participation. Studies of the meaning attributed by individuals to their participation in master sports have found that it provides 'a strategy for fighting, monitoring, adapting to, avoiding and/or accepting the aging process' (Dionigi 2010, 138). Such a multiplicity of meanings suggest that the individual desire to be 'masterful' and to pursue an active, functional and fit lifestyle is as complex and multidimensional as any other consumerist passion, and involves considerations beyond those associated with the narrowly framed ethos of fitness, and so excoriated by the anti-anti-agers (Vincent 2009). A similar multiplicity of meanings applies to the embodied practices of fitness pursued by non-master athletes as much perhaps as it does to all forms of consumerist behaviour (Miller 2012, 184), not the least of which is the virtue associated with physical activity that is undertaken not out of the necessity of labour, but through the reflexive practices of freedom.

Ageing and the Exercise of Virtue

Ageless athletic activity is more than a deliberate tactic of seeking distinction and power through 'age resistance'. It is part of a broader social response to the changing balance between work and leisure, reflecting what Bauman has characterised as a shift from a society of producers to a society of consumers. As work has declined as a form of necessary physical labour, compensatory routines have emerged through a concomitant increase in physically active leisure. Unlike the work-dependent patterns of physical activity, associated with first modernity, active leisure can be more easily extended beyond the circumstances of working life. In a period when the end of work meant the end of labour, more often than not it lead to an inactive retirement – hence mid-twentieth-century retirement being framed as a tragedy of loss. By the late 1970s and early 1980s, the inactivity of retirement was beginning to be replaced by a new 'busy ethic' of leisure perfected in the USA (Ekerdt 1986). Formerly proscribed, exercise and activity in mid-life and in retirement began to be positively promoted. In 1972, less than half the Finnish population in their fifties were physically active in their leisure time; by 1992 that figure had risen to just over three-quarters (Borodulin et al. 2008). No longer expected to labour, older bodies were now exercised with more care, and within the context of active leisure. For those no longer working, later life seems to have become progressively more active, as the 'sportification' of society expands to include growing numbers of older men and women (Tischer, Hartman-Tews and Combrink 2011).

The full extent of this change can be seen in European comparisons of sporting activity conducted a half century or so apart. In one of the earliest reported studies, a 1953 Danish national survey of over 1000 adults found that only 9 per cent of those aged over 50 reported any active engagement with sport, with most reporting none or only a passive engagement as spectators (Andersen et al. 1956). In 2003, the German National Health Interview found that some 30 per cent of men and 22 per cent of women in their *seventies* reported participating in at least 2 hours of sporting activities per week, the most popular activities being cycling, gymnastics and swimming (Hinrichs et al. 2010). Recent Danish, Dutch and Swedish studies confirm this upward trend across the generations (Petersen et al. 2010; Agahi and Parker 2005; Cozijnsen et al. 2013). Unpublished data from the 2009 Sport England survey based upon some 100,000 interviewees aged 50 and above indicate that 35 per cent of men and 32 per cent of women had actively pursued one or other sporting or athletic activity in the previous month (authors' own calculations from data supplied by Sport England).

National surveys and reports of health and physical activity – conducted at all stages of life – still reflect gendered imbalances in the way in which men and women engage in sports and other deliberate physical activities. Individualised regimes of exercise, like walking, swimming, jogging and cycling are practiced more commonly by older

Figure 9.1. Finnish men and women's leisure time physically active 1971–2002 (data derived from Borodulin et al. 2007).

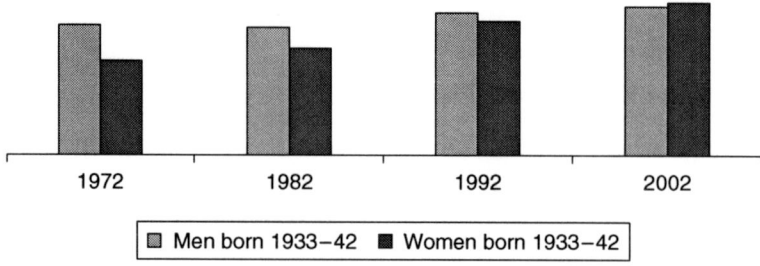

men, no doubt reflecting the historically different value placed on exercise by men compared with women (Vertinsky 1994). Gymnastic and aerobic exercises on the other hand are practiced more often in groups and by older women (Tischer, Hartman-Tews and Combrink 2011) although there is also evidence that overall gender differences in exercise and activity are declining (Borodulin et al. 2008).

Such investments in the body are pursued more through the market than the state. Commercial and semi-commercial organisations such as gyms, leisure centres and various not-for-profit social clubs provide the main venues. Commercial products and services, such as workout regimes on video or DVD, computer exercise games, such as the Nintendo Wii, cycling, rowing or other exercise machines, treadmills and other forms of fitness machinery provide much of the means. Some form of home trainer can be found in over 30 per cent of 'later life' German households (Gilleard and Higgs 2011c, 365). While pensioners clubs and other local authority settings still offer free fitness classes, such settings increasingly demand some form of payment. In contrast to the private gyms and leisure centres, the not-for-profit institutes/social clubs, the municipal day centres for the elderly and the regimes they provide resemble more the poor choices of the marginalised senior citizen, than expressing the later lifestyles of society's more successfully embodied citizen consumers.

Fitness as we have noted is more than the exercise of a consumerist 'interpellation'. If ageing is, at bottom, no more than the consequence of an inadequate genetic investment in the soma, as Kirkwood and others have implied (Kirkwood 2001; Kirkwood and Austad 2000), compensating for this lack of genetic investment by a refashioned lifestyle seems a logical response. Within the 'new ageing' paradigm, exercise and fitness-oriented practices can be seen as deliberate social and cultural investments in the soma not becoming old. The success of such investments in actively promoting health, functionality and longevity has empirical support (American College of Sports Medicine 2009; Leyk et al. 2010). Indeed some have gone so far as to argue that, with exercise, 'the effects of age on physiological functional capacity may be slowed, halted or even be reversed' (Leyk, Erey and Bilzon 2007, 7.4). Proponents of activity and exercise argue that 'lifestyle factors' have a greater impact upon adult endurance and strength than chronological age does, and there is evidence that continued participation in sports can modify the trajectory of declining performance traditionally attributed to 'age' (Young et al. 2007). But as with all embodied practices performed to resist the master narrative of decline, the virtues of successful exercise can also reinforce the vices of failure with the consequence of dividing rather than diversifying later life.

Conclusions

The pursuit of fitness in later life has become part of the new ageing ethic embodied in the ideals of successful or productive ageing. We have used the term exercise to cover what are in fact a wide variety of embodied practices ranging from body building to walking; marathon running to step and dance aerobics. What distinguishes the physical exercise regimes of first modernity from those of second modernity, we have argued, is their individualisation, their commercialisation and their integration into the broader 'lifestyles' of those no longer young. Jogging and aerobics, home trainers and DVD fitness exercises, computerised 'activity' games and the complex electronic devices used to monitor progress are able to target the individual consumer at all ages of adult life. This expanding keep fit industry vastly overshadows the old fashioned body building regimes of Eugen Sandow and the 'dynamic tension' methods promoted by Charles Atlas in the dying decades of first modernity.

This process of individualised fitness has also facilitated less exclusionary practices with respect to gender as well as age. Aerobics, jogging, marathons sports and workouts are as accessible to those in mid- and later life as to those still young and increasingly as much to women as to men. This is true not just for the more 'cosmetic' forms of fitness involved in workouts and aerobics but for those activities where master athletes compete. Over the last three decades, for example, older women have increased their participation in the New York City Marathon more than any other demographic group (Lepers and Cattogni 2011). Similar secular improvements in performance specifically of older participants have been noted in 'Ironman' race performances (Lepers et al. 2012). From another source, the numbers of disabled athletics have also grown in size and significance, transforming the image of the wheelchair user from that of the 'frail old lady' to that of the 'fit young man' (Pullin 2009). Wheelchair sports may still be dominated by young disabled people, but they have served to bridge a previously unbridgeable gap between sport and fitness and immobility and impairment.

As exercise oriented body work has moved from the realms of production to those of leisure and consumption, it is more easily incorporated into leisured later lifestyles. While the forms of physical activity undertaken by older bodies are still connected with the embodied identities of gender, race and disability, they are less connected to the productive processes of society and the needs for an army of labour. Age does not so much constrain as segment the market. Exercise in later life, as in earlier life, is still performed through gender. More older men than women engage in 'senior' or 'disability' sports, while more older women than men engage in aerobics and pursue workout regimes based upon DVDs and videos. Older men engage more often in the 'solitary' pursuits of walking, cycling and swimming, while older women engage more often in the socialised exercises of group walks, swim-aerobics and dance exercise. Racialised identities raise other issues we have not touched upon. Older African American men engage less often in physical activities, generally, and senior sports compared with older European Americans, perhaps because age and seniority remain structured through a predominantly 'white' lens (King et al. 2000; Trost et al. 2002). The slow demise of the 'white/black' binary within US society may be modifying this patterning. Part of the multiculturalism of the new ageing seems already to be broadening what constitutes 'activity' or 'exercise'. The adoption by many older non-Asian individuals of traditional 'Asian' technologies of self-care such as Tai Chi suggest future diversification may well take place in exercise oriented body work. Disability sports and athletics now dominated by younger people may also see further change as young disabled athletes continue playing sports into later life, performing roles other than those prescribed for the 'impaired' elderly, in effect creating new groups of master athletes. This is not to ignore the possibility that as participation in exercise and fitness becomes the new 'norm' for later life, issues of distinction might become issues of marginalisation, markers of a failure not to become old, by failing to remain self-constituting and agentic adults at all points in the life course (Higgs et al. 2009). Whatever the outcome, it is necessary to acknowledge the reality of the shift taking place toward 'exercising' the body in later life, irrespective of the consequences that follow. Adopting one of Foucault's later formulations, exercise and physical activity can be seen as part of the agonistic exploration of what human bodies can be and what they can become (Foucault 1982). And of course exercise can be a means of people having fun, simply enjoying being a body that performs without reference to age or gender, for at least some of the time (Tulle 2008).

Chapter 10

AGEING AND ASPIRATIONAL MEDICINE

In the last three chapters we have discussed how the various embodied practices promoting sexual activity, personal attractiveness and bodily fitness have become aligned with the new ageing. We turn now to the fourth of Francis Bacon's 'sciences for the good of the body', namely medicine and its recent re-orientation toward ageing through the aspirational science of corporeal betterment. Although prolongevity has been a longstanding interest of medicine, what is distinct about late modernity is the growth in 'rejuvenative' technologies that go well beyond the homilies and the herbaria of past eras. As Forth has pointed out 'what most clearly separates twentieth century bodily ideals from those of earlier periods is not the strong social emphasis that is placed on appearance and performance but the ever expanding technologies that allow one to alter one's body in hitherto unexpected ways' (Forth 2010, 145). In this chapter we will explore the emergence and expansion within medicine and surgery of a widening variety of techniques that offer individuals, not so much treatments for their disease, as choices over their appearance. One key element in this search for enhancement is delivering a choice over how much 'age' individuals wish to display. The application of medicine (including surgery) to this particular task of corporeal enhancement is what we refer to as 'rejuvenative medicine'.

Encultured by the consumerist belief that things can and should only 'get better' and that individuals have a lifelong right to health and well-being, an 'aspirational' medicine has emerged concerned less with disease than with building better bodies (Gilleard and Higgs 2000, 187). This aspect of medicine does not focus upon any particular organ, nor does it confine itself to any particular form of pathology or, indeed, ally itself with a particular technology or procedure. Aspirational medicine aims to deliver something other than treatment, something other than health promotion, namely somatic enhancement, whether that is in the form of improved physical performance, enhanced physical appearance or increased physical resilience. In some ways this is a return to medicine's 'classical' roots, for medicine has always claimed to serve two different ends: that of promoting and enhancing health and well-being, and that of curing or relieving disease. While the latter has led to considerable clinical specialisation over the last 200 years, the promotion of health has been continuing with less visible success for well over 2000 years as physicians have competed with priests and politicians as sources of public influence, mixing medical with moral advice that touches upon all aspects of life, work and leisure.

As discussed in the previous chapter, the goals of modern nation states to improve their (male) population's capacity to wage war and work well began to be replaced, in the period after the Second World War, by fears about the growing indolence of the population. Regular physical activity, fresh air and an appropriate diet with the supplementary consumption of various minerals and vitamins and not too much stress were promoted as desirable methods for living a long, healthy and productive life. Arguably, those postwar public health messages amounted to little more than re-vamped versions of Galen's health promoting six 'non-naturals', of healthy air, good diet, appropriate exercise, regular bowels, freedom from stress and adequate sleep (Jarcho 1970). Meanwhile, clinical medicine moved forward, slowly entering the field of positive health and the possibilities of corporeal enhancement. Aspirations for delivering better health – not primarily in the sense of curing people with cancer or cardiovascular disease, but of improving or enhancing individual health, fitness and beauty – were not confined to any one branch of medicine but emerged in many forms of 'hospital medicine'. Ophthalmic surgeons began to strive to make eyes keener for longer – even to eliminate ocular 'ageing' altogether. Orthopaedic surgeons learned to replace old joints with new improved ones from materials less subject to 'normal' corporeal wear and tear while witnessing steadily improving outcomes. Dermatologists began to seek ways of removing, renovating or refurbishing old skin while endocrinologists offered ways of reconditioning declining or defunct hormone systems. Even gynaecologists – albeit still only a minority – have shown themselves prepared to try extending the boundaries of 'reproductive age' by facilitating birth at later and later ages. It is no longer enough to inoculate the young against the diseases of youth and advise the not so young to practice healthy 'lifestyles'; for a small but growing minority of physicians and surgeons, the goal is to make bodies, old or young, better, fitter and more resilient.

First among equals in the sub-field of rejuvenative medicine has been plastic and reconstructive surgery. Once derided as a fairground for showmen, mountebanks and charlatans, plastic surgery has become one of the most eagerly pursued (and remunerated) specialisms in medicine and surgery (Sullivan 2001). For many plastic surgeons, health is beauty and beauty health. Within this framework, age is acknowledged as the common enemy and it is combated not through science fiction ideals built by imaginary medical nanotechnologists and avant-garde stem cell therapists, but through the millions of practical day to day tasks undertaken to improve bodies of various ages, shapes, sizes, ethnicities and genders. While plastic surgery is especially emblematic of aspirational medicine it is by no means the only field where aspirational medicine is practiced and where clinicians seek to help individuals 'age better' by 'not becoming old'. A host of medical and surgical specialties have now become implicated in rejuvenative medicine, whether directly or indirectly. Dental implants and cochlear implants, hip replacements and hormone replacements, hair transplants and organ transplants can all be subsumed as interventions designed to facilitate 'anti-ageing' (Giampapa, Fuente del Campo and Ramirez 2004) or 'ageing well' (Wollina and Payne 2010). Their differences are more a matter of emphasis.

In early modernity, poverty and lack were once considered the lot of people who looked, acted and were classified as 'old'. Their poverty was not just financial, but included poor teeth or a lack of teeth, poor eyesight or a lack of sight, poor hearing or a lack of hearing, poor mobility or a lack of mobility, and so on. The necessity of such diffuse impoverishment by ageing is now questioned, though somewhat less by geriatricians and other clinicians concerned with the 'care of the elderly' than by other clinical specialities responding less to collective needs than to individual desires.

In charting the development of plastic surgery's engagement with age and ageing, we want to illustrate how medicine has re-legitimated its role in enhancing or restoring beauty, fitness and health to those who feel neither. In the process, we also want to draw attention to the increasing intertwining that is taking place between medical and self-care practices, from the one off 'heroic' surgical interventions designed to permanently remove some aspect of the corporeality of age to the more every day, less intensive interventions designed to maintain or restore a smarter, fresher appearance to an ageing face or body. As surgery has become less intensive and as minimally invasive interventions have become more extensive the distinction between surgical, medical and cosmetic procedures has lessened. Just as 'invasive' and 'minimally invasive' surgical procedures have become more closely linked, so 'minimally invasive' procedures such as microdermabrasion, radiofrequency skin tightening, Botox injections and the use of dermal fillers have become more akin to routine 'non-medical' cosmetic practices, such as visits to hair salons, nail parlours, tanning and tattooing studios as well as to other forms of mediated self-care practiced in health spas, hotels, leisure centres and community centres.

Rejuvenation and Modernity

As with all forms of practice and knowledge directed at the good of men's and women's bodies, rejuvenation medicine has existed both in the form of medical interventions and as folk remedies well before the modern period. Gabriele Zerbi, for example, described several remedies for wrinkles in old men in 1489 as well as methods to prevent their hair going grey (Zerbi 1988). Most of these premodern recommendations concerned the use of potions and lotions and were little more than systematising folk practices or reiterating ancient material read in translation on the topic of *hygieina*. Few people would have read these manuals and fewer still would have followed their advice, a point that was made by Roger Bacon in his manual for *The Cure of Old Age* (1683). It was not until the early decades of the twentieth century that rejuvenative methods emerged as phenomena with mass appeal, as practiced by the new breed of 'beauty doctors'. Amongst the various techniques on offer, the beauty doctors promised to reveal new skin by peeling off the 'old', using acetic, carbolic (phenol) or salicylic acids (Peters 1991; Landau 2008; Sullivan 2001) or, more daringly, to 'plump out' ageing, thinning faces by injecting Vaseline or paraffin under the skin (Quinlan 1902). A few began to pioneer radical skin lifting procedures to remove crow's feet, bags below the eyes and facial lines. By the first decade of the twentieth century, the American surgeon, Charles Miller, was using surgery to remove bags from under the eyes and paraffin injections to remove wrinkles, while in Europe, Eugene Hollander and Erich Lexer had executed the first 'full' facelifts (Rogers

1976). The Paris-based plastic surgeon, Julien Bourguet, is credited with performing the first cosmetic blepharoplasty by removing pockets of perio-orbital fat from under the eyes of a middle-aged patient (Lam 2004). These three surgical techniques – forehead lifts, facelifts (rhytidectomy) and the removal of eye bags (blepharoplasty) – together with the two 'minimally invasive' procedures of skin peels and skin fillers, would continue, albeit in modified form, to provide the basic medical technology for removing or reducing the signs of facial ageing well into the twenty-first century.

These 'early' practitioners were an extremely varied group, ranging from the frankly charlatan, such as Howard Crum and Henry Julius Schireson to the seriously committed, like Miller and Malianak (Haiken 1997; Sullivan 2001). Though most of the rejuvenators were men, there were also women beauty doctors. Some, like the 'first wave' feminist and entrepreneurial soroptomist, Dr Suzanne Noel, were innovative pioneers in the art of rejuvenation. She developed the concept of the 'mini-lift' offering women the opportunity to attend her clinic in Paris regularly for repeated surgery to 'update' their appearance (Davis 1999). Other women were less committed and less scrupulous. Among the more notorious was the self-styled beauty doctor and 'naturopath', Dr Gertrude Steele, whose license to practice was eventually revoked after two of her 'face peel' patients died as a result of her ministrations (Pinkham 1926). Steele subsequently fled to Germany after which little seems to have been heard of her (Haiken 1997, 92).

Progress in medical rejuvenation proved slower than in the field of cosmetics and self-care. Thanks to the unscrupulous practices and showmanship of practitioners like Crum, Schireson and Steele, cosmetic surgery became an increasingly precarious profession. These early attempts at 'surgical rejuvenation' raised sufficient opposition within the popular media and importantly within institutional medicine to curtail any expansion of cosmetic medicine within the academy (Haiken 1997). In the eyes of the medical establishment, these early practitioners were nothing but 'ignorant, unscrupulous and uneducated "beauty doctor[s]"' (Oppenheimer 1920, 596). But though the development of *cosmetic* plastic surgery was halted, *reconstructive* plastic surgery advanced significantly. As Elizabeth Haiken has pointed out, the interwar years saw the emergence of 'a gendered spectrum' of practice 'with the reconstructive work men needed at one end and the cosmetic or aesthetic work women desired at the other' (Haiken 1997, 103). Since the prestige to gain entry into the ranks of institutionalised medicine was reserved for the 'heroic' reconstruction of war-damaged, male bodies, reconstructive surgery rose to prominence by denigrating the latter. As John Staige Davis, the author of the first comprehensive textbook on plastic surgery, made clear: 'plastic surgery [...] is absolutely distinct and separate from what is known as cosmetic or decorative surgery' (cited by Sullivan 2001, 56). The latter, he felt, had little place in plastic surgery proper while the former was amongst the foremost new branches of surgery. Suitably cast in such truths, in the 1940s, plastic surgery became a recognised medical specialty such that, when plastic surgery was added to the medical school curriculum, in the 1950s, 'few procedures other than reconstructive [surgery] were covered' (Sullivan 2001, 56).

According to Sullivan's account of the institutional emergence of cosmetic or aesthetic surgery, surgeons who performed cosmetic operations did so mostly by working 'surreptitiously', often using false diagnoses when operating and restricting any public acknowledgement of their work to 'acceptable' cosmetic procedures such as rhinoplasty (Sullivan 2001, 56). Most technical developments took place in reconstructive surgery as a result of war injuries, both those of the Second World War and the Korean War, aided significantly by the development of effective antibiotics. In contrast, the procedures developed by Hollander, Lexer, Miller and Noel for face-lifting, forehead lifting and eye bag removal remained largely unchanged. Not only were the techniques unchanged but they were often inadequately learned and poorly performed. Even finding cosmetic surgery work had become difficult and some US cosmetic surgeons had to devise alternative ways of making money by a 'round robin' scheme, 'accusing each other of shoddy work and testifying against each other [and then] settl[ing] out of court and collect[ing] expert witness fees' (Hait 1994, 26a).

The Postwar Rehabilitation of Cosmetic Surgery

In the 1960s cosmetic surgery resurfaced. It began with an article published in the 20 May 1960 issue of *Harper's Bazaar*, written by the PR team working on behalf of the American Society for Plastic and Reconstructive Surgery (ASPRS), a small group of surgeons who were growing increasingly anxious about the 'silent' threat to their financial hold over cosmetic surgery by other emerging groups of surgeons. The article outlined some of the costs and benefits of surgery and recommended that the magazine's readers stick to registered members of the ASPRS rather than risk going under the knife of ENT and other less 'specialised' surgeons. This was followed by a riposte from the ENT surgeons in an article published in *Mademoiselle* advising *its* readers to choose a surgeon qualified by the American Board of Otolaryngology. The war of the magazines had begun (Hait 1994, 57a). Shortly after this initial blaze of publicity, the cosmetic side of plastic surgery returned in the media with the introduction of silicone breast implants in 1962.

After the Second World War, liquid silicone had been employed by dermatologists as a safer approach to treating wrinkles than the earlier debacle of paraffin and Vaseline injections. Its apparent safety profile encouraged wider experimentation. In 1962, a silicone sac filled with liquid silicone was implanted into women's breasts by Texan surgeons, Thomas Cronin and Frank Gerow. Suddenly breast augmentation was in the news and despite a number of horror stories emerging at the time 'silicone breast augmentation [...] [became] one of the leading cosmetic operations of its day' (Haiken 1997, 257), as 'surgeons and women came to see breast augmentation – like other cosmetic surgical operations – as simply another form of self-improvement' (Haiken 1997, 281).

A 'new' generation of plastic surgeons had now graduated who started practicing after the Second World War. The number of trained plastic surgeons in America rose from 111 in 1940 to 225 in 1950, and by 1964 there were over 600 trained surgeons. During and immediately before the war, there were only 3 training programmes in plastic and reconstructive surgery in the USA, with 8 residency positions. By 1950 the number of programs had grown to 22 and by 1960, there were fifty programmes operating from nearly seventy hospitals with some 150 residency positions (Conway 1965). Among the 'new' generation of plastic surgeons the most politically active was Simon Fredricks. In 1967, he co-opted an older colleague, John Lewis, to become president of the newly founded American Society for Aesthetic Plastic Surgeons. A new legitimacy was conferred on cosmetic surgery and from this point onwards publications about cosmetic surgery began to occupy space not only in popular magazines, but in academic surgical journals.

Despite the lack of further significant developments, by the late 1960s aesthetic/cosmetic surgery had become an accepted part of legitimate medical practice. Perhaps more significantly, it was increasingly featured in fashion and beauty magazines like *Esquire, Harper's, Ladies Home Journal, McCall's* and *Vogue* – and in popular current affairs weeklies such as *Newsweek* and *Time Magazine* (Haiken 1997). The culture of youth that emerged during the long 1960s had transformed young people into the vanguard of a mass consumerist revolution. Until then, the economics of cosmetic surgery had restricted access largely if not exclusively to the elites – and to those popular celebrities who began entering the elite circles. By the 1960s, however, costs had been brought down and, as Elizabeth Haiken has documented, cosmetic surgery gained a growing popularity across the generations – with facelifts for the middle aged and breast augmentation for the young and the bold (Haiken 1997).

Cosmetic Surgery in Late Modernity: Domesticated and Democratised

As surgical face-lifting procedures continue to become easier and cheaper to perform, rejuvenative appearance management has become even more popular (Elliot 2008). Expertise in newer and less invasive surgical techniques has expanded. The number of physicians designating themselves plastic surgeons grew from 1970 to 1996 by over 250 per cent – more than double the overall increase in US doctors (Sullivan 2001). Procedures even less invasive than the 'mini-lifts' that were pioneered by Suzanne Noel were developed during this period so that a temporary rejuvenation of the face can be achieved almost as quickly and cheaply as a facial beauty makeover. Developments in laser technology and increasing experience in the use of Botox and a wide range of chemical fillers have led to a massive expansion in minimally invasive 'age reduction' procedures. Along with the expansion of techniques, anti-ageing surgical and minimally invasive procedures are now being performed by an increasing range of surgical and medical specialities, including dermatologists, family doctors, general physicians, general surgeons, ophthalmologists, ENT surgeons as well as general and specialist plastic surgeons (Housman et al. 2008). Many 'minimally invasive' techniques are provided in beauty salons, dental clinics, health clubs and 'well-being' centres. As well as expanding the number of techniques and sites where rejuvenation occurs there has also been an expansion in the number of countries offering such procedures. Developing countries can significantly undercut the costs charged in highly developed countries for dental implants, facelifts and hip replacements, leading to new forms of medical tourism that offer the dedicated tourist much more than a simple tan (Lunt and Carrera 2010).

Figure 10.1. Research on wrinkles: Ratio of papers on 'wrinkles' compared with those on 'acne', published in peer-reviewed dermatology journals, 1960–2009 (Web of Science, 2011).

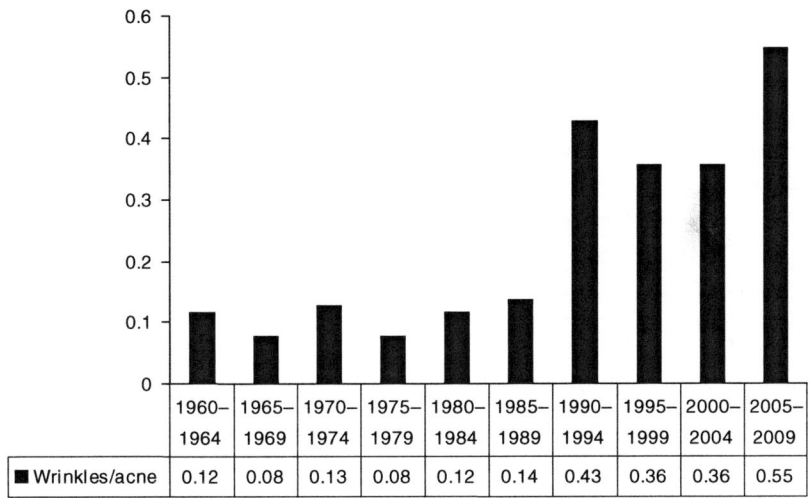

	1960–1964	1965–1969	1970–1974	1975–1979	1980–1984	1985–1989	1990–1994	1995–1999	2000–2004	2005–2009
■ Wrinkles/acne	0.12	0.08	0.13	0.08	0.12	0.14	0.43	0.36	0.36	0.55

Alongside this expansion of techniques, specialities and destinations have come more sophisticated approaches to measuring the morphology of age changes to the face and body in order to more clearly elucidate the mechanisms underlying corporeal agedness (Lemperle et al. 2001; Valet et al. 2009; Yaar 2006). Geriatrics and gerontology have pretty much given up on reporting developments in rejuvenation procedures – Brown's is the only article on facial rejuvenation ever published in the *Journal of Gerontology* and that was back in 1953 when the field was still young (Brown 1953). Other branches of medicine and surgery now dominate the field of rejuvenation. Increasingly the pharmaceutical industry has been involved, while new research centres are being set up and supported by the cosmetics and self-care industry. Wrinkles are an illustrative example. Prior to 1980, little research had been published on the topic of wrinkles which were treated generally as matters of little medical or scientific interest (Kligman 1976). With the development of synthetic analogues of Vitamin A as potential reducers of facial lines and wrinkles, a new interest emerged focusing upon the biological activity of trans retinoic acid on so-called 'photo aging'. This research provided one of the first pieces of 'medical' evidence for the effectiveness of such topical treatments in reducing the facial lines of 'exogenous' ageing (Kligman et al. 1986). The prospect of effective non-surgical anti-ageing products and procedures stimulated interest in what had hitherto been a dermatological backwater. Topical anti-aging products began to be promoted, for both cosmetic reasons and as a means of preventing disease in later life (Kafi et al. 2007), as a rising number of articles were published on the topic of 'wrinkles' in peer reviewed dermatology journals.

We have compared the number of articles with 'wrinkles' in their title or summary *as a ratio* to those on the classical dermatological topic of 'acne', in order to offset the general increase in papers published in dermatology journals. The results are illustrated in Figure 10.1 using data summed over five year periods from 1960–64 to 2005–09.

As the figure shows after 1990, 'wrinkles' took off as a topic of academic dermatological interest. During the same period, from 1990 to 2010, there has been an equal expansion in non-invasive methods of skin tightening and skin smoothing ranging from soft tissue fillers such as collagen and hyaluronic acid to laser resurfacing techniques, the use of intense ultra sound and of radiofrequency thermal energy (Fitzpatrick et al. 2003; Houk and Humphreys 2007; Shpall et al. 2004). Botox injections, developed for aesthetic use in the late 1980s, received approval for cosmetic use by the FDA in 1995. They have since become the most commonly applied antiageing surgical procedure (American Academy of Cosmetic Surgery 2010; American Society of Plastic Surgeons, 2010).

Traditional surgical methods of facial rejuvenation, however, remain the 'gold standard'. Yet, even in this area, surgeons have tried to keep pace with the low cost minimally invasive methods mentioned above by developing techniques for reducing the 'down-time' associated with undertaking surgery. Relatively less invasive methods of rejuvenative surgery have been developed, such as Tonnard's 'mini facelift', known as the Minimal Access Craniofacial Suspension lift (MACS-lift) (Tonnard et al. 2002), Wu's 'sutures only' or 'Woffles' lift (Wu 2004) and the Platysma SMAS plication or 'PSP' lift (Berry and Davies 2010). Claims for originating particular rejuvenation techniques are now hotly contested (van der Lei, Cromheecke and Hofer 2007; Clark 2006) in marked contrast to the secretive 'marketing' that characterised cosmetic surgery a half century ago. Unmentioned and virtually 'taboo' until the 1970s, rejuvenation has become a commonplace term in surgery.

This expansion into the academy of rejuvenative technologies has occurred across a number of fronts. Numerous graphs could be drawn demonstrating the rising number of papers published in peer reviewed academic journals about 'rhytidectomies', 'blepharoplasties', trials of minimally invasive procedures such as botulinum toxin type A (Botox), the relative effectiveness of hyaluronic acid gel fillers, comparative trials of skin resurfacing techniques or investigations of hair restoration techniques and comparative studies of treatments for hair graying. Outcome studies, rarely reported before the 1990s, are now common. Honigman and his colleagues (Honigman et al. 2004) found only one outcome study of facelifts published before 1990. Now meta-analytic reviews of individual outcome studies of invasive facelift procedures have been reported (Chang, Pusic and Rohrich 2011). Prospective and comparative outcome studies of minimally invasive procedures have multiplied (De Boulle et al. 2010; Fagien and Carruthers 2008; Hexsel et al. 2012; Rubino et al. 2005; Zager and Dyer 2005), and although indicators of 'customer satisfaction' still dominate the outcome literature (e.g. Friel et al. 2010; Hessler et al. 2009; Kosowski et al. 2009), less subjective measures based on 'age reduction' (Taub et al. 2010) and the 'objective' measurement of facial lines and wrinkling are beginning to replace them (Kafi et al. 2007; Rubino et al. 2005).

What is notable about the penetration of 'rejuvenation practices' into the academy is not only that these approaches are being routinely taught in medical schools but that they are also stimulating basic research. Where once the signs of ageing were deemed 'beneath notice by serious professionals' (Kligman, Zheng and Lavker 1985, 37) surgeons are now beginning 'to examine the process of aging not just from the point of view of effect and procedure but from the point of view of cause and effect' (Giampapa, del Campo and Ramirez 2004, 493). Just as the development of anti-ageing products and procedures has stimulated the growth of a scientific infrastructure within the beauty industry so developments in surgical practice have stimulated an interpretative, interrogatory and evaluative narrative supporting further research into these procedures and products.

As noted above, the increasing engagement with 'anti-ageing' procedures by different medical specialists has taken place alongside a similar growth in the number of non-medical self-care technicians, providing similar or related rejuvenative products and services. Dental surgeries, department stores, hairdressing salons, health food stores, nail parlours, pharmacies, fitness centres, health spas, generic 'therapy centres' and even supermarkets are competing to provide accessible outlets for a range of 'non-surgical' cosmeceutical and minimally invasive procedures, ranging from light rejuvenation to fillers and Botox injections. Several key features can be observed in the process. Firstly, there has been an expansion of techniques that either reduce the costs of invasive rejuvenation surgery or increase the longevity of their effects (Chang, Pusic and Rohrich 2011). Secondly, there has been an expansion in the number of minimally invasive rejuvenative techniques designed to achieve quick and relatively painless results (American Academy of Cosmetic Surgery 2010; American Society of Plastic Surgeons 2010). Thirdly the use of these latter technologies now encompasses a broad range of ages (American Academy of Cosmetic Surgery 2010; Housman et al. 2008). Infrastructural research on skin and facial ageing – notably, but not only, in relation to topical products designed to reduce wrinkles and facial lines – has grown commensurately (Holtkötter et al. 2005), while these new rejuvenative techniques have more thoroughly penetrated popular culture, most noticeably through the medium of television. Since the beginning of the twenty-first century, shows such as *The Swan* and *I Want a Famous Face* in the USA and *Ten Years Younger* in the UK have captivated TV audiences (Markey and Markey 2010; Petrie, Faasse and Fuhrmann 2008). Cosmetic rejuvenative surgery has become integrated into the market economy (Wong et al. 2010) as the aspirations of the market, of medicine and of the public have converged on the importance of maintaining an appearance of health fitness and beauty in the face of ageing. An old body has never been desirable; now it is beginning just to seem cheap.

Rejuvenation: New Practices of Freedom Versus the Disciplining of Docile Old Bodies?

Within the broad spectrum of self-care and body work practices that are oriented toward 'not becoming old', aspirational medicine represents one of the most challenging developments. Like sex, cosmetics and exercise, it too is oriented toward ideals of health, fitness and beauty that are increasingly contextualised within the binary of youth versus age. The binary that inflects these practices is at the same time

Figure 10.2. Anti-ageing procedures by age group, 1995–2003 (Housman et al. 2008, fig. 3).

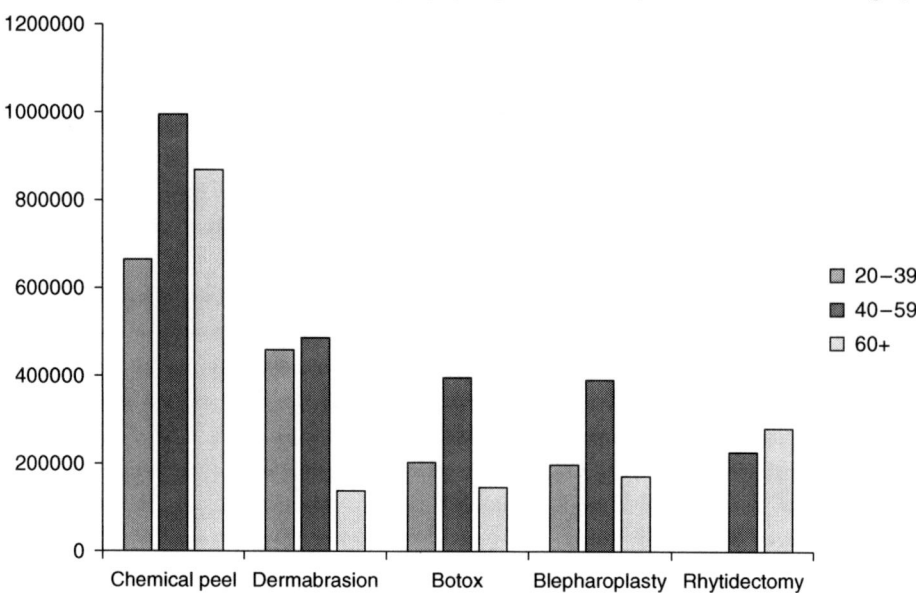

undermined by them. Just as sex, in becoming a practice actively extended into later life has confounded this binary, so too does rejuvenative surgery, and then some. By extending its remit from age to youth cosmetic surgery confounds the specificity of age and claims its practices are equally suited to all seasons. Figure 10.2 demonstrates how different 'rejuvenative' procedures are differentially taken up by different age groups, with only full on facelifts (rhytidectomies) confined exclusively to mid- and later life.

Equally important as the trend away from age boundaries in rejuvenation is the corresponding rejection of a singular ethnic ideal of beauty or attractiveness. Just as most surgeons do not believe (nor do they mean) that 'rejuvenation' means a restoration of youth, they also no longer rely upon a standard white European model of attractiveness. As differently gendered, racialised and aged clients seek to improve their appearance by something a little more invasive than a hairstyle or a makeover, so the 'outcome' criteria of cosmetic surgery have diversified (Harris 2004). This is not to say that the aim of achieving a better appearance has been abandoned, simply that the criteria of what is better have become more contingent. Unlike 'conventional' modern medicine, where the physician or surgeon treating a condition or illness rarely doubts what the desired outcome should be – for him or herself as much as for the patient – aspirational medicine entails a greater conditionality about outcomes and a greater engagement with the patient as a still desiring subject, whose own ideas of personal 'betterment' are married with what is professionally and technically feasible. This negotiation over appearances is clearly one of power, but it is a different kind of 'bio-power' than that exercised in traditional doctor-patient relationships, because the surgeon generally sees the criteria for his or her success in terms similar to those of the patient.

Cosmetic surgery, it has been claimed, is keen to seek 'not only a positive effect on the feature in question, but also a far-ranging enrichment of global well-being, sense of satisfaction and self-assurance' (Litner et al. 2008, 83). In doing so, it reflects and reinforces the desire for self-improvement and lifestyle enhancement that resonates within contemporary society (Elliot 2008). Responses and reactions to rejuvenative surgery make it evident that 'ageism' cuts both ways. Thus one study of people undergoing rejuvenative surgery found that the interviewees/patients:

> Linked several negative attributes to people with negative attitudes to cosmetic surgery, such as totalitarianism, fundamentalism, ugliness, feminism, malevolence, bitterness, peasantry, timidity, depression, ignorance, psychic instability, backwardness, and failure. In contrast, they linked positive attitudes to cosmetic surgery with tolerance, individualism, femininity, courage, carefulness, development, cosmopolitanism, happiness, joyfulness, realism, curiosity, education. (Kinnunen 2010, 261)

As Haiken has pointed out, plastic surgery first achieved acceptance when it emphasised its masculine virtues, restoring and making whole those whose bodies had been traumatised by war. War is a product of social relations, and the trauma inflicted by steel and shrapnel are not natural diseases. By treating bodily agedness as equally traumatic, plastic surgery has achieved a new kind of legitimation for its rejuvenative practices, whether as a rescuer of the victims of the war of age or as a saver of souls and a master designer of more fashionable lifestyles. Those who have had surgery are regarded differently by different people. Some evince the moral disgust once meted out when 'ordinary' women went out wearing makeup; others respond with a mix of anger and envy for those who seem to have refused to wait in line along with the rest taking their turn to grow old; while still others can acknowledge, with a glad or a grudging admiration, something of the transgression that has taken place.

Much righteous indignation is directed toward those whose post-operative rejuvenation is judged a failure. Even though chronological age does not seem to be an independent risk factor for post-operative complications (Becker and Castellano 2004; Martén et al. 2011), there is still a sense that older people undergoing cosmetic surgery deserve to see their wishes thwarted. It is notable how people who are considered not to show their age 'naturally' are applauded for their good fortune, good genes or good habits, while those who choose to make their own luck by carving out an equivalent distance between their chronological and corporeal age are excoriated for doing so. Some cultural commentators such as Anthony Elliot see the 'cosmetic surgery culture' as an embodiment of 'a pervasive addiction to the ethos of instant self-reinvention' (Elliot 2008, 145) which can only have social costs. Those who have gone through such procedures are seen as exhibiting an internalised ageism (Hurd-Clarke 2011, 137) in much the same way as African Americans who straighten their hair or who have their lips thinned are accused of demonstrating an internalised racism. Such practices of choice are still hard won and their boundaries endlessly policed. For those who want to enjoy their skin without reducing their lives to the conformity of a colour, being black can be treated as a form of self-care, or a lifestyle choice rather than an essentialised biological necessity. Practices of freedom are needed for such ideas to be realised. In the same way, those who have lived long may still wish to live well on their own terms and by their own standards. Choosing to age differently can be seen as an equally necessary part in the practices of freedom that constitute choosing not to become old, even though these choices are rarely exercised in unconstrained circumstances.

Those who choose to rejuvenate – whether via mini-lifts, Botox, fillers, laser skin peels or fractional radio frequency skin tightening procedures – create a place for themselves to be other than they once were. Through such choices, the possibility of individuals 'not becoming old' can be raised. To argue that such choices are the result of the 'alienation' of the market implies that all consumers are alienated by the appeals of goods and services that offer something other than meeting basic 'needs'. But in contemporary society 'being natural', like being 'authentic', exists as one potential choice among a variety of alternative constructions. As Elias noted, the possibility of choosing not to go 'natural' was once the basis for civilisation (Elias 1984). The possibility of not becoming old, of ageing by choice and not by necessity might be a late modern equivalent.

Aspirational medicine expresses the notion of autonomy, choice, self-expression and pleasure that, we have argued, distinguish third age cultures (Gilleard and Higgs 2000, 2011a). Its close links with the market, particularly the market for health, beauty and fitness aligns it with other services and practices that mediate self-care but which are excluded from the domain of 'health care'. The rise of quick, short-term rejuvenation techniques draws an ever thinner line between the practices of aspirational medicine and that of commercial cosmetics, perhaps nowhere better exemplified than in the practice of cosmetic tattooing in later life (Armstrong, Saunders and Roberts 2009). In the process, the divide between the vain and the virtuous narrows, between interventions lauded for helping us 'age well' (Wollina and Payne 2010) and those excoriated for being oriented to a self-centred 'anti-ageing' (Ring 2002).

Conclusion

However much the age-old currency of attractiveness loses its value with age, few people see a new beauty emerging from old age. That is not to say that there are no attractive older people; undoubtedly there are many. But generally that is despite rather than because of old age. For most people, ageing brings unwanted changes in appearance, not just in the number of lines and wrinkles but in many other small but significant ways, from excessive hair growth or hair loss, the various 'benign growths' of actinic keratoses or sebaceous hyperplasia, the appearance of brown spots or lentigoes on the skin, the thinning and loss of volume in the lips and cheeks, the dryness and skin pigmentation of rosacea and so on, and so on (Yaar 2006). Viewing these changes as 'the body doing what it naturally does' (Brooks 2010, 252) and doing nothing about them reinforces an emerging alienation between self and body that makes ageing a mask, hiding the authentic, ageless self beneath (Featherstone and Hepworth 1991). Caring for one's self through the body challenges such alienation, and in so doing, challenges our understanding of what ageing 'naturally' is. More than conventional medicine, aspirational medicine acts as a kind of mediator between self-care and contemporary culture. Instead of reinforcing the alienation of the body by objectifying it through illness, lack and need, aspirational medicine seeks to establish a new set of possibilities that allow for a more embodied subjectivity in later life, of ageing as one chooses.

As we have emphasised throughout this book, what is read from the body as age and what features and phenomena are privileged as 'signs of ageing' are not simply matters of common sense. Nor are the corporeal boundaries of age more likely to be revealed in human inertia. What matters more than categorising or delimiting that which constitutes 'true' or 'essential' bodily ageing is trying to change how age is realised through the body; to discover by what embodied practices and by what somatic discourses it is currently realised and the extent to which the techniques mediated by the care of the self can and do succeed in altering such realisations. As Kathy Davis has pointed out: 'cosmetic surgery [...] [can] provide an avenue towards becoming an embodied subject rather than [being] an objectified body' (Davis 1997, 114). It is, we should stress, but one avenue; there are many others, with lower risks of failure. However, it is an avenue that millions of people have chosen and many more millions follow with interest (Frederick, Lever and Peplau 2007). Rather than seeing it solely through the lens of gendered oppression, or the idealisation of whiteness, or the domination of the market over the moral economy of the life course, we have chosen to examine it through the prism and practices of 'self-care'. Doing so, we believe, helps move the debate about ageing from the binaries of young and old; of resisting or embracing age; of rejecting or accepting rejuvenation. Seeing rejuvenative procedures as yet another mediated form of caring for one's self, as both a vulnerable as well as a desiring body, may also contribute to thinking about ageing through the body differently.

Conclusions

AGEING, FOREVER EMBODIED

Our aim in writing this book has been to pursue a debate about the place of the body in ageing studies and, more broadly, in the social sciences. Central to this debate has been the contested framework by which the body is seen to mediate the relationship between the individual and society. While each individual is, or owns, his or her body, the meaning of that body and the meaning that confers on the self who owns the body is realised only and necessarily within social relations. This is the case, whether in the way that individual bodies are used to represent social identities, in the way that they express cultural distinctions, perform social functions or reproduce social positions and in the way that bodies are realised as distinct kinds of individuals, within the medium of our social imaginaries. In order to distinguish between two different ways of understanding the body and the body's relation to society, we have deployed the contrasting concepts of corporeality and embodiment. The corporeality of the body – its fleshy materiality and capacity to grow, generate and decay – serves as a contrast to the more thoroughly socialised concept of embodiment. It represents a materiality which, even if reproduced socially can never be socially produced. It starts each human being off as a human being whose history is located not so much in society as in its *species being*. Embodiment, conversely, represents the metaphorical 'imbrication' of the body within the particular social relations of its time, from its coming into being to its dissolution. But embodiment too has a history, distinct from the body's history as a species being, developed within the particular cultural history of a society and its institutions, and its customary way of narrating and practising embodiment. However realised, embodiment can never escape its historical location both in individual lives and in social relations, no more than the body's corporeality can ever escape its history as a member of a species.

We have focused upon embodiment not corporeality, for otherwise this would have been a book about biology. Within this explicitly social framework we have distinguished between two general forms of embodiment; those realised through embodied identities and those realised through embodied practices. Although the two are linked they can be considered conceptually distinct phenomena. Embodied identities refer to selective aspects of the corporeal appearance of the body or its corporeal functions that have come to define a distinct social position for the individual in society. Embodied practices on the other hand refer to those activities that orientate the body toward distinct social, cultural and personal identities and their associated lifestyles. Embodied practices may directly support and help realise a particular identity or they can indirectly express styles or ways of living that are either positively enhanced by those practices or that negate other alternative identities and lifestyles.

In second modernity, there has been a (re)turn to a more somatic society, where the 'body without organs' has acquired a new significance, as the world of work and labour power has become subordinated to the world of consumption and leisure. Released from its subservient role in relation to the forces of production and social reproduction, the body has taken on a role outside the sphere of paid and domestic labour, redefining old identities as well as realising new, alternative lifestyles. This 'somatic turn' has re-problematised the corporeality of the body and its relationship to both the self and society, particularly its role in signifying social identity. Several writers have argued that with the re-embodiment of identity in contemporary modernity, particularly when expressed through the various binary oppositions of male/female, black/white, heterosexual/homosexual or able-bodied/disabled, has come a new instability in the meanings of corporeality – in how the body is 'read'. The somatic turn in society has led to a pervasive questioning of the old binary framings of the body that had been stabilised (and rendered less visible) within the relations of production of classical modernity. As choice, autonomy, self-expression and pleasure emerged as motifs permeating the cultural ferment of the long 1960s, a new, critical interrogation of bodily identities began, challenging both their biological essentialism as well as their social fixity. This new 'discourse of choice' proved 'a powerful dissolvent of old verities' (Weeks 1995, 28) and has continued to extend its influence across a wider range of social issues and a wider expanse of the life course. The consequence has been to make the body a focal point of dissent in the cultural ordering of society and of the self in second modernity.

Ageing has emerged as a rather late addition in this process of cultural destabilisation. The new social movements were fashioned in the context of the youth sub-cultures of the 1960s. It was among the 'young' that the corporeal dualisms of first modernity, of gender, race, able-bodiedness and sexuality were first challenged. As the avant-garde of this period of generational schism, the cohorts within whom these youth sub-cultures were fashioned have become no longer young. Reared on a rejection of all that was old and 'out-dated', the corporeality of ageing can appear as a threat to the new forms of identity and lifestyle that emerged during this period, threatening a return of the oppression of the old, but in circumstances which cannot, however, be so easily externalised as the 'old other' of a past generation. Corporeal ageing has come to be seen as a different form of alienation, a potential disjunction between self and the world conferring on the body a hitherto unaddressed and unacknowledged dimension that threatens to close down the openness that those other earlier forms of embodiment seemed to promise.

The 'new ageing' can be seen, in part at least, as a response to this emerging predicament. The youthful desire for the body to remain a site of choice, autonomy, self-expression and pleasure has been extended to all portions of the adult life course. The increasing space that has opened up for this as a result of a more or less secure, more or less healthy, more or less leisure oriented later life has meant that the time, space and resources for practising 'age resistance' have grown. The first signs of this new style ageing were noted in the USA, perhaps as early as the mid-1970s, when Richard Calhoun first wrote about the emergence of a 'new' old age, (Calhoun 1978) one that was less marginalised, less restricted and less dependent than in the old days of old age. Since then, various paradigms of 'healthy', 'positive', 'productive' and/or 'successful' ageing have been outlined (Bass, Caro and Chen 1993; Butler, Oberlink and Schechter 1990; Rowe and Kahn 1997) leading to the fuller flowering of the idea that a new ageing has indeed begun (Gergen and Gergen 2000). This response we have formulated elsewhere as the emergence of a third age cultural field with its later lifestyles framed around 'not becoming old' (Gilleard and Higgs 2000, 2011a). The particular practices and narratives by which 'not becoming old' has become *embodied* have been the subject of this book. They are, we have argued, shaped in part by the forms of body work that have been deployed in fashioning the identities, narratives and performances of gender, race, sexuality and able-bodiedness and in the general enhancement of self through the practices of self-care. These practices, we suggest, can be seen as 'the practices of freedom' that Foucault referred to at the end of his life, in the sense that they are deliberately and reflexively performed as ways of disciplining the self to remain fit, healthy, open and attractive and, thereby, not old (Foucault 1994, 3).

Of course, such motives are not new, nor are most of the practices designed to realise them. Their origins predate modernity, consumerism and the market. They have been evidenced in late antiquity (Foucault 1988, 19) and no doubt can be found, like consumption itself, in all societies and at all times. In the seventeenth century they were characterised by Francis Bacon as 'human sciences' concerned with promoting 'the good of man's body' (Bacon 2002, 208). Bacon grouped these 'bodies of knowledge' into four distinct fields of inquiry and practice, medicine or the art of cure, cosmetics or the art of decoration, gymnastics or the art of activity and the art voluptuary or the 'sensuous' sciences. Marginalised by the changed emphasis upon machinery and manufacturing during the industrialising period, these individual desires and the disciplines concerned with the good of man's body re-emerged within the new context of a mass consumerist culture, new social movements and the policies of voice and choice. While the former promoted these practices to the desiring subject through aspirational advertising, market segmentation and a new sensibility born of the street, the latter has encouraged their 'individualised' take up as part of a 'bio-politics' aimed at re-balancing responsibility for the public good from the institutions of the state to the personalised agendas of individual citizen consumers.

Embodiment, Identity and Lifestyle

We set the scene for this debate by first contextualising the study of the body in the social sciences before exploring the relationship of the new sociologies of the body to the paradigm of the 'new ageing'. We then examined the embodiments of identity and lifestyle that arose in the generational rupture of the 'long 1960s' (Marwick 1998), focusing particularly on the 'postmodern' embodiment of gendered, racialised, disabled and sexualised identities, and their various 'agonistic' relations with ageing. Drawing upon Foucault's distinction between relations of power and relations of domination, we argued that the revisioning of the 'subaltern' positions associated with gender, race, disability and sexuality established the possibility of other ways of performing identity that celebrated difference rather than disputed equality (Foucault 1994). These approaches were represented, by their proponents at least, as a kind of 'liberation' from old ways of thinking about and interpreting bodily difference and in so doing they established new practices of freedom. Despite the emergence of these new practices, however, gender studies, ethnic and racial studies, gay and lesbian studies and disability studies have all experienced difficulties in engaging with, let alone coming to terms with, the destabilising influence of age and ageing. While there are signs that some of the new 'cultural studies' are beginning to develop some engagement with ageing – more than was the case when the fields of study emerged in the 1970s and 1980s – there is little evidence of any reciprocity of focus, in that ageing is rarely used as a lens by which to consider the contingencies that apply to the positioning of these otherwise embodied identities. Within ageing studies there is more evidence of an engagement with the concerns of cultural studies – and particularly issues of identity and embodiment than vice versa. It is no longer unusual, for example, to find studies of ageing in gay, lesbian and African American communities or to discover outlines for a feminist or queer gerontology, even if such developments are still limited compared with the more common structuralist examinations of the 'effects' of race, gender, sexuality 'on' ageing.

The racialisation of late life identities is clearly a more complex issue. Ageing remains predominantly a white topic. While the weight of the 'colour line' that has burdened American society throughout modernity began to shift through the destabilising effects of the civil rights and Black Power movements, the racialised structuring of modern American society still remains and resonates today. Although the new social movements fostered modifications, they failed to alter its salience in structuring American identity and lifestyle. In this sense, race still structures age more than age structures race. Theories of cumulative advantage/disadvantage, double jeopardy and weathering have helped stimulate research into the lifelong determinants of late life health and longevity in African American populations (Ferraro and Farmer 1996; Geronimus 2001; O'Rand 1996). But these structural analyses, and their inter-sectionality with other apparently enduring categories such as class, education or wealth, implicitly reinforce a narrative of 'docile bodies' which infers that ageing is fashioned or constructed by conditions external to the subject. The capacity of bodies to orientate themselves agentically to age, to still perform and celebrate age within the context of a racialised society and within a culture of oppression goes largely unrecognised (Shenk, Zablotsky and Croom 1998; Trotman 2002). Just as race can be reified as a hierarchical social category, so the ageing body can be reified by its representation as a 'health' or 'disability' status. Even when issues of agency are recognised – as in Dannefer's comment that 'an explanatory role for personal agency is also integral to a full account of the processes underlying trajectories of inequality' (Dannefer 2003, S333) – the overwhelming concern of such analyses remains with the 'effects' of race, gender or class as unambiguous structural influences, rather than as the polysemous forms of vulnerable embodiment and opportunity by which they can also be examined.

Considerations of vulnerability have been particularly central to the disability movement. By moving the focus from the vulnerabilities of disabled bodies to the insufficiencies of public spaces and social policies, the social model of disability enabled professionals, politicians and practitioners to rethink the place of the body both in gerontology and the social sciences. Instead of treating bodily functionality as the principle measure of individual worth or value, the disability movement and the theorising that accompanied it have sought to restore agency to the disabled body especially within the struggle by which people with bodily impairments achieve a place for themselves in the world from which they can fashion a distinctive lifestyle that is equal to and different from that of able bodied persons. But things are more complicated and the status of the body within disability studies is now more actively contested. There is a divide between those whose focus is upon how to challenge and resist the social institutions that oppress or limit the embodied agency of people with bodily impairments, and those whose focus is primarily upon the oppression and limitations that the body itself presents and the fluid understandings through which such oppression and alienation is experienced, enacted and understood. At the risk of oversimplification, the division lies between a focus upon structured social disadvantage and the validation of personal suffering. While the latter counters the risk of a politics of disembodiment by highlighting the everyday corporealities of disability, the former – i.e. the 'social model of disability' – provides a clearer strategy for locating the potential for collective betterment in society and its institutions; it points toward collective action instead of emphasising personal agonism.

While it may be superficial to suggest a 'both/and' position, what is important in the social model of disability is its representation of disability as a putative agentic 'restriction' that is modifiable in ways that can potentially benefit all age groups. The model also recognises the need for agency in making use of social cultural and technological resources without ignoring the suffering created by bodies with limits that neither the individual nor society can always get around. As we and others have pointed out, disability studies have tended to support a status model of disability, privileging those with lifelong stable and 'healthy' disabilities over those whose bodily identity is rendered unstable whether by age, by ill-health or by some underlying disease process (Wendell 2001). As a result both these approaches have eschewed thinking about ageing as a source of 'becoming' disabled, differently.

Unsurprisingly less resistant, ageing studies has also struggled to obtain a strong enough purchase in its engagement with disability whether as an identity or as exemplifying practices of freedom in the context of personal and social constraints. This reflects the history of both ageing and disability studies. Gerontology has long treated disability as an index of unsuccessful, premature or excess ageing rather than as a form of embodied identity and differential subjectivity. Within this structuralist tradition, the progressive elimination or reduction of disability within the older population remains a much contested good. Certainly, no gerontologist would ever celebrate rising levels of disability. At the same time the growing longevity of once young disabled people is a reason for rejoicing; rates of survival into later life of people with spinal cord injuries, for example, have increased by nearly 2000 per cent (Kemp 2005).

But while some writers and researchers have begun exploring the 'careers' of disabled people across the life course and their various negotiations with age, there has been less acknowledgement on both sides that 'disability' more often than not, is realised not in youth but in later life (Verbrugge and Yang 2002, 265). Ageing with a disability may add further limitations, but it also can bring the benefits of experience and maturity in forms and ways of resistance (Yorkston et al. 2010). Acquiring a disability in later life may also constrain the potential for a more active engagement with the new 'cultures of ageing', both because of corporeal limitations and because of the difficulties – on both sides – of engaging equally with the cultures of disability. The mutual suspicion that exists between some people in later life and some people with disabilities reflects, in part, their conflicting views of embodiment. The consequence is that their different practices of freedom can seem restrictive to both, making any alliance a risky and potentially costly business.

'Queering' these variously embodied representations of identity has been explored as an alternative avenue for examining the relationship between ageing, the body and society. By questioning the fixity and stability attached to gay and lesbian identities, queer theorists sought to expose the instability of all embodied identities, and their implicit or explicit binary oppositions. Their goal in 'queering' identity has been 'for the purpose of diminishing its force and releasing new possibilities for desire, identity and social organization' (Seidman 1998, 291). This critique has been extended by some queer theorists beyond issues of sexuality and identity to queer other binary oppositions, including those of gender, race and able-bodiedness and has been recently extended to considerations over the binary opposition between youth and age. Rather than being enslaved by youth or made subject to the tyranny of old age, the body can be approached as always more open than this, an inexorably polysemous vehicle that allows for the expression of multiple lifestyles that can be realised and modified at different times and in points in the lifecycle.

In the final section of the book, we moved from the embodiment of identity to a consideration of embodied practices and their orientation toward age and later life. Loosely following Bacon's categorisation of human sciences for the good of the body, we explored the significance of sexual practices, fashion and cosmetics, fitness and exercise as well as rejuvenative medical technologies as fields in which the body, identity, lifestyle and self-improvement may be reconstituted. Although all the practices we explored constitute products born of twentieth-century modernity, their modernity must be understood both in the context of premodern traditions of self-care and the practices of self-betterment in Foucault's technologies of self, as well as the transformation of a society whose mass has moved beyond the simple categorisations of caste and class. Ageing, old and new, we have argued, has long been implicated in these practices.

The corporeality of ageing was seen in Greek mythology as a condition inflicted upon humans to remind them that they are humans, not gods (Gilleard 2007). But at the same time, there was also within Greek culture a willingness to question the authority of the gods – or the powers of nature – in defining the features of humanity (Galen 1971). Premodern responses to the uncertainty surrounding old age varied. While the Greeks and Romans questioned it conceptually, the later medieval world sought empirical means of challenging age, through the use of magic, medicine and spirituality, as well as by pursuing the search for better health and greater comfort in old age (Gilleard 2013). The cyclical nature of life was overturned by the progress of modernity, and the rise of the new and the demise of the old fitted the modern model. Youth and progress were aligned to the good, while age was attached to decline and decay. Considerations of chronology overcame corporeality; old age was fashioned as the marginal end of the labouring life course, put to rest in a pauper's home. The new ageing challenged those old narratives of chronological decline and in making this challenge, like other 'rebel sells', the new ageing became more distinctly integrated into the consumerist lifestyles that define second modernity.

Despite the dominance of chronological age for the masses, it was first modernity that introduced the opportunities to 'not become old' through the cultivation of sex and the prolongation of an ageless, forever sexualised identity amongst key members of the new elite of the twentieth century. As class-divided society morphed into a mass consumer society, and a divided society became a diverse society, sex and gender had become important vectors of embodiment oriented toward ageing and not becoming old. This point has been neatly made by the title 'Forever Functional' in Marshall and Katz's paper on the marketing of the 'anti-impotence pill', Viagra (Marshall and Katz 2002). Equally caught up in the prolongation of an ageless, gendered identity, we turned from sex and sexual practices to self-care and the evolution of body work as beauty work in the cosmetics, clothing and fashion industries of the twentieth century.

As in other areas (and books), we have treated the 1960s as a watershed, when age and generation emerged as the dominant sources of distinction and market segmentation in the beauty and fashion industries. The subsequent transition of the 'sixties' generation out of their sub-culturally defined market segment, we have argued, saw the decline of market segmentation by age group. Since the 1980s, cosmetics have acquired a new lease of life through the development of 'anti-ageing' cosmetics. The appeal of these products has since extended above and below its original mid-life demographic. Around the same time, a new fashion for all ages came into existence as qualitative and quantitative market research attested to the continuing desire of older men and women to remain smart, fashionable and to want to look after themselves with and through their bodies. From such a standpoint, extending the body work associated with youthful identities to later life reflected the extension of the youthful values of choice, autonomy, self-expression and pleasure across the life course. The new ageing body also serves as a vehicle of the still desiring subject. For many gerontologists, such positive readings of the endless plasticity and fluidity that bodies possess risked creating a new binary opposition, between successfully and unsuccessfully ageing bodies. Set against this new binary, the ideology of 'the new ageing' can be criticised for failing to acknowledge – let alone accept – corporeal vulnerability and the part this discourse plays in creating new and equally oppressive binaries. Promoting self-expression and the individual practices of freedom, the new ageing can be seen as masking the hidden operations of a post-welfare state bio-politics, intent on ceding power to the market by transferring responsibility for the shape and fitness of one's body from the concerns of the collective to matters of individualised consumerist responsibility (Polivka 2011).

By denying the place of the corporeal in the shaping of the moral economy of the life course, critics have argued, a 'simulacrum' of agelessness has been created lacking any foundation either in our corporeality or our connections with our species being. Those who pursue such simulacra are criticised not just for their vanity or their capacity to be duped, but because by asserting their individualised desires they succeed only in oppressing and marginalising those whose docile bodies have failed to be other.

Set against such criticisms is the empirical evidence that bodies can become better and can do so at almost any age. Certainly bodies are not predestined to get worse once a particular age is reached. We have stressed these points in the chapters on fitness and on aspirational medicine. But perhaps more importantly, by excoriating those who pursue the 'vain' goals of fitness, health and beauty in later life, there is a failure to acknowledge that the pursuit of the goods of the body is not fixed within any corporeal hierarchy, be it constituted by age, gender, race, able-bodiedness or sexuality. Enabling an individual to be still 'minded' to cultivate his or her body irrespective of class, chronology or complexion may be as important as whether his or her body reaches a particular airbrushed standard of attractiveness or fitness. In being minded to bother about one's body, individuals can feel that their body still matters, that those embodied identities they have struggled with earlier in life still matter and that the corporeal limitations in exercising self-care can be, if not eliminated, at least attenuated by the care and social mediation of others. The inability to forever sustain beauty, fitness and health may be an inherent feature of our species being, but the desire to look good, to feel good and to be good need not be devalued because these goals can never be fully individually realised. Taking care of oneself by taking care of one's body is not obviously motivated by a wish to deprive others of such opportunities, nor is it motivated by a desire to render others weaker, sicker or uglier. The desire to live better longer cannot be opposed on the grounds that not all will succeed or because such goals can never be permanently realised. To use an oft quoted maxim from the playwright Samuel Beckett we must learn to fail, but we can also learn to fail better.

In conclusion, we have argued that the agency associated with embodiment, of performing and reforming the embodied identities of disability, gender, race and sexuality still continues in later life. The continuation into later life of the various narratives and practices associated with these identities contributes significantly to what the Gergens have termed 'the new ageing' (Gergen and Gergen, 2000). Resisting 'old age' is resisting old age's neutering of these identities, foreclosing the practices that sustain them. Staying 'black', staying 'gay', staying 'gendered' and staying 'disabled' in later life is not so much about clinging on to youth as it is about retaining the 'virtues' of these particular identities and their embodiment. The same can be said for the wider narratives and practices of a generation that has learned to privilege choice, autonomy, self-expression and pleasure. There is, of course, another side to such virtues. We would be remiss to ignore the extent to which these practices of freedom, these 'agonisms' can prove too onerous, too difficult or too painful. For some people, at some times, the costs of failing can be too great. The option of seeking a haven in the neutrality of an otherwise embodied old age can hardly then be denied.

REFERENCES

Abberley, Paul. 1987. 'The Concept of Oppression and the Development of a Social Theory of Disability'. *Disability, Handicap & Society* 2, no. 1: 5–19.
Acton, William. 1867. *The Functions and Disorders of the Reproductive Organs in Childhood, Youth, Adult Age and Advanced Life*. Philadelphia: Lindsay and Blakiston.
Agahi, Neda and Parker, Marti G. 2005. 'Are Today's Older People more Active than their Predecessors? Participation in Leisure-Time Activities in Sweden in 1992 and 2002'. *Ageing & Society* 25, no. 6: 925–41.
Ahmed, S. M. Faisal. 2006. 'Making Beautiful: Male Workers in Beauty Parlors'. *Men and Masculinities* 9: 168–85.
Alborn, Timothy L. 1999. 'Age and Empire in the Indian Census, 1871–1931'. *Journal of Interdisciplinary History* 30, no. 1: 61–89.
Albrecht, Gary L. and Verbrugge, Lois M. 2003. 'The Global Emergence of Disability'. In *The Handbook of Social Studies in Health & Medicine*, edited by Gary L. Albrecht, Ray Fitzpatrick and Susan C. Scrimshaw, 293–307. London: Sage Publications.
Allen, C. 1961. 'The Aging Homosexual'. In *The 'Third' Sex*, edited by I. Rubin, 91–5. New York: New Book Company.
Allyn, David. 2000. *Make Love Not War: The Sexual Revolution, an Unfettered History*. Boston: Little, Brown & Co.
American Academy of Cosmetic Surgery. 1996. '1996 National Statistics'. http://www.cosmeticsurgery.org/consumer/stats/1996national.html (accessed 18 March 1999).
———. 2000. 'Statistics of Cosmetic Surgery Procedures'. http://www.cosmeticsurgery.org/Media_Center/stats/2000statistics/00statsummary.html (accessed 29 June 2002).
———. 2006. '2005 AACS Procedural Statistics'. http://www.cosmeticsurgery.org/surgeons/2005_procedural_stats.pdf (accessed 12 May 2010).
———. 2007. '2002–2007 American Academy of Cosmetic Surgery (AACS) Procedural Census Age Facts'. http://www.cosmeticsurgery.org/media/FactSheet-Age.pdf (accessed 19 May 2010).
———. 2010. '2009 AACS Procedural Statistics'. http://www.cosmeticsurgery.org/media/2009_full_report.pdf (accessed 12 May 2010).
———. 2010. 'Society More Open than Ever about Cosmetic Surgery. Press Release, January 28th 2010'. http://www.cosmeticsurgery.org/media/pr_012810.pdf (accessed 20 April 2010).
American College of Sports Medicine. 2009. 'Position Stand: Exercise and Physical Activity for Older Adults'. *Medicine & Science in Sports & Exercise* 41, no. 7: 1510–30.
American Psychiatric Association. 2000. *Diagnostic and Statistical Manual of Mental Disorders*. 4th ed. Washington, American Psychiatric Association.
American Society of Plastic Surgeons. 2001. 'Report of the 2000 Statistics'. http://plasticsurgery.org/ (accessed 7 April 2010).
———. 2010. 'Report of the 2009 Statistics. National Clearing House of Plastic Surgery Statistics'. http://plasticsurgery.org/ (accessed 7 April 2010).
Anastadias, A. G., Davis, A. R., Ghafar, M. A., Burchardt, M. and Shabsigh, R. 2002. 'The Epidemiology and Definition of Female Sexual Disorders'. *World Journal of Urology* 20: 74–8.

Andersen, Helge, Bo-Jensen, Aage, Elkær-Hansen, N. and Sonne, A. 1956. 'Sports and Games in Denmark in the Light of Sociology'. *Acta Sociologica* 2, no. 1: 1–27.
Anderson, Michael. 1985. 'The Emergence of the Modern Lifecycle in Britain'. *Social History* 10, no. 1: 69–87.
Andrews, Molly. 1999. 'The Seduction of Agelessness'. *Ageing & Society* 19, no. 3: 301–18.
Appel, Jacob M. 2010. 'Sex Rights for the Disabled?' *Journal of Medical Ethics* 36: 152–4.
Arber, Sara and Ginn, Jay. 1993. 'Gender and Inequalities in Health in Later Life'. *Social Science & Medicine* 36, no. 1: 33–46.
Ardagh, John. 1973. *The New France: A Society in Transition, 1945–1973*. 2nd ed. Harmondsworth: Penguin Books.
Armstrong, Myrna L., Saunders, Jana C. and Roberts, Alden E. 2009. 'Older Women and Cosmetic Tattooing Experiences'. *Journal of Women & Aging* 21, no. 2: 186–97.
Åstrand, I., Åstrand, P. O. and Rodahl, K. 1959. 'Maximal Heart Rate during Work in Older Men'. *Journal of Applied Physiology* 14: 562–6.
August, Kristin J. and Sorkin, Dara H. 2010. 'Racial and Ethnic Disparities in Indicators of Physical Health Status: Do they Still Exist throughout Late Life?' *Journal of the American Geriatrics Society* 58: 2009–15.
Bacon, Francis. 2002. 'The Advancement of Learning, Book 2'. In *Francis Bacon: The Major Works* edited by Brian Vickers, 169–299. Oxford: Oxford University Press.
Bacon, Roger. 1683. *The Cure of Old Age and the Preservation of Youth*. Translated by R. Browne. London.
Bailey, Eric J. 2008. *Black America, Body Beautiful*. Westport: Prager Publishers.
Bajos, N., Bozon, M., Beltzer, N., Laborde, C., Andro, A., Ferrand, M., Goulet, V., Laporte, A., Le Van, C., Leridon, H., Levinson, S., Razafindratsima, N., Toulemon, L., Warszawski, J. and Wellings, K. 2010. 'Changes in Sexual Behaviours: From Secular Trends to Public Health Policies'. *AIDS* 24: 1185–91.
Bakhtin, Mikhail. 1981. *The Dialogic Imagination: Four Essays*. Translated by C. Emerson and M. Holquist. Austin: University of Texas Press.
Banks, James, Marmot, Michael, Oldfield, Zoe and Smith, James P. 2006. 'Disease and Disadvantage in the United States and in England'. *JAMA* 295, no. 17: 2037–45.
Barnes, Colin. 1991. *Disabled People in Britain and Discrimination: A Case for Anti-Discrimination Legislation*. London: C. Hurst & Co.
———. 1997. 'A Legacy of Oppression: A History of Disability in Western Culture'. In *Disability Studies: Past, Present and Future*, edited by Len Barton and Mike Oliver, 3–24. Leeds: Disability Press.
Barnes, Colin, Mercer, Geoff and Shakespeare, Tom. 1999. *Exploring Disability: A Sociological Introduction*. Cambridge: Polity Press.
Barry, A. J., Daly, J. W., Pruett, E. D. R., Steinmetz, J. R., Page H. F., Birkhead, N. C. and Rodahl, K. 1966. 'The Effects of Physical Conditioning on Older Individuals. I. Work Capacity, Circulatory-Respiratory Function and Electrocardiogram'. *Journal of Gerontology* 21: 182–91.
Bartky, Susan. 1988. 'Foucault, Femininity and the Modernization of Patriarchal Power'. In *Feminism and Foucault: Reflections on Resistance*, edited by I. Diamond and L. Quinby, 61–86. Boston: Northeastern University Press.
Bass, Scott A., Caro, Francis G. and Chen, Y. P., eds. 1993. *Achieving a Productive Aging Society*. Westport: Auburn House.
Basson, R., Leiblum, S., Brotto, L., Derogatis, L., Fourcroy, J., Fugl-Meyer, K., Graziottin, A., Heiman, J.R., Laan, E., Meston, C., Schover, L., van Lankveld, J. and Schultz, W. W. 2003. 'Definitions of Women's Sexual Dysfunction Reconsidered: Advocating Expansion and Revision'. *Journal of Psychosomatic Obstetrics and Gynecology* 24, no. 4: 221–7.
Basting, Anne Davis. 1998. *The Stages of Age: Performing Age in Contemporary American Culture*. Ann Arbor: University of Michigan Press.

Batchelder, Alan B. 1964. 'Decline in the Relative Income of Negro Men'. *The Quarterly Journal of Economics* 78, no. 4: 525–48.
Bauman, Zygmunt. 1995. *Life in Fragments*. London: Basil Blackwell.
———. 2000. *Liquid Modernity*. Cambridge: Polity Press.
———. 2005. *Liquid Life*. Cambridge: Polity Press.
Beck, Ulrich. 2007. 'Beyond Class and Nation: Reframing Social Inequalities in a Globalizing World'. *British Journal of Sociology* 58, no. 4: 679–705.
Beck, Ulrich and Beck-Gersheim, E. 2001. *Individualization*. London: Sage Publications.
Beck, Ulrich, Bonz, Wolfgang and Lau, Christoph. 2003. 'The Theory of Reflexive Modernisation: Problematic, Hypotheses and Research Programme'. *Theory, Culture & Society* 20, no. 2: 1–33.
Becker, Ferdinand F. and Castellano, Richard D. 2004. 'Safety of Face Lifts in the Older Patient'. *Archives of Facial Plastic Surgery* 6, no. 5: 311–14.
Beckman, Nils, Waern, Margda, Gustafson, Deborah and Skoog, Ingmar. 2008. 'Secular Trends in Self Reported Sexual Activity and Satisfaction in Swedish 70 year olds: Cross Sectional Survey of Four Populations, 1971–2001'. *BMJ* 337: a279.
Beeson, Diane. 1975. 'Women in Studies of Aging: A Critique and some Suggestions'. *Social Forces* 23, no. 1: 52–9.
Bell, Colin and Newby, Howard. 1971. *Community Studies*. London: George Allen & Unwin.
Bellah, Robert N., Madsen, Richard, Sullivan, William M., Swidler, Ann and Tipton, Steven M. 1996. *Habits of the Heart: Individualism and Commitment in American Life*. Berkeley: University of California Press.
Benjamin, Harry. 1945. 'Eugen Steinach, 1861-1944: A Life of Research'. *The Scientific Monthly* 61, no. 6: 427–42.
Bennett, Andy and Hodkinson, Paul. 2012. 'Introduction'. In *Ageing and Youth Culture*, edited by Andy Bennett and Paul Hodkinson, 1–8. London: Berg.
Bennett, Kate Mary. 1998. 'Gender and Longitudinal Changes in Physical Activities in Later Life'. *Age and Ageing* 27, S3: 24–8.
Bennett, Keith C. and Thompson, Norman L. 1980. 'Social and Psychological Functioning of the Ageing Male Homosexual'. *British Journal of Psychiatry* 137: 361–70.
Benson, John. 1997. *Prime Time: A History of the Middle Aged in Twentieth-Century Britain*. London: Longman.
Berger, Raymond M. 1984. 'Realities of Gay and Lesbian Aging'. *Social Work* 20, no. 1: 57–62.
Berlin, Ira. 2010. *The Making of African America: The Four Great Migrations*. New York: Penguin Books.
Berman, Marshall. 1982. *All That Is Solid Melts into Air: The Experience of Modernity*. London: Verso Books.
Bernal, Martin. 1987. *Black Athena: The Afroasiatic Roots of Classical Civilization*. New York: Rutgers University Press.
Bernauer, James. 1994. 'Michel Foucault's Ecstatic Thinking'. In *The Final Foucault*, edited by James Bernauer and David Rasmussen, 45–82. Harvard: MIT Press.
Berry, M. G. and Davies, D. 2010. 'Platysma-SMAS Plication Facelift'. *Journal of Plastic Reconstructive and Aesthetic Surgery* 63: 793–800.
Biggs, Simon. 1997. 'Choosing Not to be Old? Masks, Bodies and Identity Management in Later Life'. *Ageing & Society* 17, no. 4: 553–70.
———. 1999. *The Mature Imagination*. Buckingham: Open University Press.
Black, Dan, Gates, Gary, Sanders, Seth and Taylor, Lowell. 2000. 'Demographics of the Gay and Lesbian Population in the United States: Evidence from Available Systematic Data Sources'. *Demography* 37, no. 2: 139–54.
Black, Paula. 2004. *The Beauty Industry: Gender, Culture, Pleasure*. London: Routledge.
Blaikie, Andrew. 2002. 'The Secret World of Sub-Cultural Aging: What Unites and What Divides?' In *Cultural Gerontology*, edited by Lars Andersson, 95–110. Westport: Greenwood Publishing.

Blaikie, Andrew and Hepworth, Mike. 1997. 'Representations of Old Age in Painting and Photography'. In *Critical Approaches to Ageing and Later Life*, edited by Anne Jamison, Sarah Harper and Christina Victor, 102–17. Buckingham: Open University Press.

Blanker, M. H., Bosch J. L. H. R., Goenevekld, F. P. M. J., Bohnen A. M., Prins, A. and Thomas, S. 2001. 'Erectile and Ejaculatory Dysfunction in a Community Based Sample of Men 50–78 Years Old: Prevalence, Concern and Relation to Sexual Activity'. *Urology* 57: 763–8.

Blumer, Herbert. 1969. 'Fashion: From Class Differentiation to Social Selection'. *Sociological Quarterly* 10: 275–91.

Bois, Jean-Pierre. 1994. *Histoire de la vieillesse*. Paris: Presses Universitaires de France.

Boltanski, Luc and Chiapello, Eve. 2005. 'The New Spirit of Capitalism'. *International Journal of Politics, Culture, and Society* 18: 161–88.

Bordo, Susan. (1993) 2003. *Unbearable Weight: Feminism, Western Culture and the Body*. Tenth Anniversary Edition. Berkeley: University of California Press.

Borodulin, Katja, Laatikainen, Tiina, Juolevi, Anne and Jousilahti, Pekka. 2008. 'Thirty-Year Trends of Physical Activity in Relation to Age, Calendar Time and Birth Cohort in Finnish Adults'. *European Journal of Public Health* 18, no. 3: 339–44.

Borsay, Anne. 2002. 'History, Power and Identity'. In *Disability Studies Today*, edited by Colin Barnes, Mike Oliver and Len Barton, 98–119. Cambridge: Polity Press.

Bortz, W. M. IV and Bortz, W. M. II. 1996. 'How Fast Do we Age? Exercise Performance over Time as a Biomarker'. *Journals of Gerontology: Series A, Biological Sciences and Medical Sciences* 51a, no. 5: M223–5.

Boston Women's Health Book Collective (BWHC). (1973) 1984. *Our Bodies, Ourselves*. Harmondsworth: Penguin Books.

Boswell, John. 1991. 'Revolutions, Universals and Sexual Categories'. In *Hidden from History: Reclaiming the Gay and Lesbian Past*, edited by George Chauncey, Jr., Martin Duberman and Martha Vicinus, 17–36. London: Meridian Books.

Botto, Lori A., Petkau, A., John, Labrie, Fernand, and Basson, Rosemary. 2011. 'Predictors of Sexual Desire Disorders in Women'. *Journal of Sexual Medicine* 8: 742–53.

Botwinick, Jack and Shock, Nathaniel W. 1952. 'Age Differences in Performance Decrement with Continuous Work'. *Journals of Gerontology* 7, no. 1: 41–6.

Bourdieu, Pierre. 1977. *Outline of a Theory of Practice*. Cambridge: Cambridge University Press.

Bowerman, William J. and Harris, Waldo E., with Shea, James M. 1967. *Jogging*. New York: Grosset & Dunlap.

Boxer, Andrew M. 1997. 'Gay, Lesbian and Bisexual Aging into the Twenty-First Century: An Overview and Introduction'. *Journal of Gay, Lesbian and Bisexual Identity* 2: 187–97.

Brandon, Ruth. 2011. *Ugly Beauty: Helena Rubenstein, L'Oréal and the Blemished History of Looking Good*. New York: HarperCollins.

Braun, M., Wasmerr, G., Klotz, T., Reifenrath, B., Mathers, M. and Engelmann, U. 2000. 'Epidemiology of Erectile Dysfunction: Results of the Cologne Male Survey'. *International Journal of Impotence Research* 12: 305–11.

Brissett, Anthony E. and Naylor, Michelle C. 2010. 'The Aging African American Face'. *Facial Plastic Surgery* 26: 154–63.

British Association of Aesthetic Plastic Surgery. 2005. 'Plastic Surgery: It's Not Teens, It's their Grandparents'. http://www.baaps.org.uk/about-us/press-releases/131-plastic-surgery-its-not-teens-its-their-grandparents (accessed 12 June 2010).

———. 2008. 'Female Facelifts Reach Record Highs, Men Choose Nose Jobs'. http://www.baaps.org.uk/about-us/press-releases/280-over-32400-cosmetic-surgery-procedures-in-the-uk-in-2007 (accessed 12 June 2010).

Brooks, Abigail T. 2010. 'Aesthetic Anti-Ageing Surgery and Technology: Women's Friend or Foe?' *Sociology of Health & Illness* 32: 238–57.

Brown, A. M. 1953. 'Surgical Restorative Art for the Aging Face: Notes on the Artistic Anatomy of Aging'. *Journal of Gerontology* 8, no. 2: 173–84.

Brown, Maria T. 2009. 'LGBT Aging and Rhetorical Silence'. *Sexuality Research and Social Policy* 6, no. 4: 65–78.
Brown, Stephen J., Ryan, Helen J. and Brown, Julie A. 2007. 'Age-Associated Changes in VO2 and Power Output: A Cross-Sectional Study of Endurance Trained New Zealand Cyclists'. *Journal of Sports Science and Medicine* 6: 477–83.
Browne, Ruth C. 2006. 'Most Black Women Have a Regular Source of Hair Care – But Not Medical Care'. *Journal of the National Medical Association* 98, no. 10: 1652–3.
Budd, John W. and Guinnane, T. W. 1991. 'Intentional Age-Misrepresenting, Age Heaping and the 1908 Old Age Pensions Act in Ireland'. *Population Studies* 45, no. 1: 497–518.
Bureau of Economic Accounts. 2010. 'National Economic Accounts, National Income and Product Accounts Tables: Table 2.1. Personal Income and Its Disposition'. http://www.bea.gov/national/nipaweb/TableView.asp?SelectedTable=58&ViewSeries=NO&Java=no&Request3Place=N&3Place=N&FromView=YES&Freq=Year&FirstYear=1990&LastYear=2009&3Place=N&Update=Update&JavaBox=yes (accessed 29 May 2010).
Burgess, Ernest W. 1960. 'Aging in Western Culture'. In *Ageing in Western Societies*, edited by Ernest W. Burgess, 3–28. Chicago: University of Chicago Press.
Burkitt, Ian. 1999. *Bodies of Thought: Embodiment, Identity & Modernity*. London: Sage Publications.
Burrow, Roger. 1986. *The Ages of Man*. Oxford: Clarendon Press.
Butler, Amy C. 2005. 'Gender Differences in the Prevalence of Same Sex Sexual Partnering: 1988–2002'. *Social Forces* 84: 421–49.
Butler, Judith. 1986. 'Sex and Gender in Simone de Beauvoir's Second Sex'. *Yale French Studies* 72: 35–49.
———. 1988. 'Performative Acts and Gender Constitution: An Essay in Phenomenology and Feminist Theory'. *Theatre Journal* 40: 519–31.
———. 1990. *Gender Trouble: Feminism and the Subversion of Identity*. London: Routledge.
———. 1993. *Bodies that Matter: On the Discursive Limits of 'Sex'*. London: Routledge.
Butler, Robert N. and Lewis, Myrna I. 1976. *Sex After Sixty: A Guide for Men and Women for Their Later Years*. New York: HarperCollins.
Butler, Robert N., Oberlink, M. R. and Schechter, M. 1990. *The Promise of Productive Aging: From Biology to Social Policy*. New York: Springer Publishing.
Byrd, W. Michael and Clayton, Linda A. 2002. *An American Health Dilemma: Race, Medicine and Healthcare in the United States, 1900–2000*. New York: Routledge.
Caddick, Diana. 1986. 'Feminism and the Body'. *Arena* 74: 60–90.
Cahill, Spencer E. 1989. 'Fashioning Males and Females: Appearance Management and the Social Reproduction of Gender'. *Symbolic Interaction* 12, no. 2: 281–98.
Calasanti, Toni M. 1993. 'Introduction: A Socialist-Feminist Approach to Aging'. *Journal of Aging Studies* 7, no. 2: 117–31.
———. 2004. 'Feminist Gerontology and Old Men'. *Journals of Gerontology, Series B, Psychological Sciences and Social Sciences* 59, no. 6: S305–14.
Calasanti, Toni M. and King, Neil. 2007. '"Beware of the Estrogen Assault": Ideals of Old Manhood in Anti-Aging Advertisements'. *Journal of Aging Studies* 21: 357–68.
Calasanti, Toni, M. and Slevin, Katherine, F. 2001. *Gender, Social Inequalities and Aging*. Walnut Creek: AltaMira Press.
Calhoun, Richard B. 1978. *In Search of the New Old: Redefining Old Age in America, 1945–1970*. New York: Elsevier.
Campbell, Erin J. 2006. '"Unenduring Beauty": Gender and Old Age in Early Modern Art and Aesthetics'. In *Early Modern Europe: Cultural Representations*, edited by Erin J. Campbell, 153–68. Aldershot: Ashgate.
Campbell, Fiona Kumari. 2008. 'Exploring Internalized Ableism Using Critical Race Theory'. *Disability & Society* 23, no. 2: 151–62.
———. 2009. *Contours of Ableism: The Production of Disability and Ableness*. Basingstoke: Palgrave Macmillan.

Campbell, Jane and Oliver, Mike. 1996. *Disability Politics: Understanding our Past, Changing our Future*. London: Routledge.
Campos, Paul. 2004. *The Obesity Myth: Why America's Obsession with Weight is Hazardous to our Health*. New York: Penguin Books.
Carpenter, William. 1859. *Principles of Human Physiology: With their Chief Applications to Psychology, Pathology, Therapeutics, Hygiene and Forensic Medicine*. Philadelphia: Blanchard and Lea.
Carstens, Lisa. 2011. 'Unbecoming Women: Sex Reversal in the Scientific Discourse on Female Deviance in Britain, 1880–1920'. *Journal of the History of Sexuality* 20, no. 1: 62–94.
Celie, Floortje, Faes, Miriam, Hopman, Maeria, Stalenhoef, Anton F. H. and Olde-Rikkert, Marcel G. M. 2010. 'Running on Age in a 15-km Road Run: Minor Influence of Age on Performance'. *European Review of Aging and Physical Activity* 7, no. 1: 43–7.
Chambers, Jason. 2006. 'Equal in Every Way: African Americans, Consumption and Materialism from Reconstruction to the Civil Rights Movement'. *Advertising & Society Review* 7, no. 1, via http://muse.jhu.edu/journals/asr/v0007/7.1chambers.html (accessed 17 May 2011).
Chang, Suzie, Pusic, Andrwa and Rohrich, Rod J. 2011. 'A Systematic Review of Comparisons of Efficacy and Complication Rates among Face-Lift Techniques'. *Plastic and Reconstructive Surgery* 127, no. 1: 423–33.
Chapman, D. L. 1994. *Sandow the Magnificent: Eugen Sandow and the Beginnings of Body-Building*. Urbana: University of Illinois Press.
Cheah, Pheng. 1996. 'Mattering: Review of "Bodies that Matter: On the Discursive Limits of 'Sex'" by Judith Butler and Volatile Bodies: Toward a Corporeal Feminism by Elizabeth Grosz'. *Diacritics* 26, no. 1, 108–9.
Cheddie, Janice. 2002. 'The Politics of the First: The Emergence of the Black Model in the Civil Rights Era'. *Fashion Theory* 6, no. 1: 61–82.
Chu, Priscilla Lee, McFaland, Willi, Gibson, Steven, Weide, Darlene, Henne, Jeff, Miller, Paul, Partridge, Teddy and Schwartz, Sandra. 2003. 'Viagra Use in a Community-Recruited Sample of Men who have Sex with Men, San Francisco'. *JAIDS Journal of Acquired Immune Deficiency Syndromes* 33, no. 2: 191–3.
Cicero, Marcus Tullius. 1971. 'Cato the Elder on Old Age'. In *Cicero's Selected Works* translated by M Grant, 211–47. Harmondsworth: Penguin Books.
Clark, D. and Maddox, G. 1993. 'Race, Aging and Functional Health: Evidence of Selective Survival?' *Journal of Aging and Health* 5: 536–57.
Clark, R. 2006. 'Reply to Carruthers and Carruthers (letters)'. *Plastic and Reconstructive Surgery* 117: 1355.
Claussen, B. 1997. 'Rehabilitation Efforts Before and After Tightening Eligibility for Disability Benefits in Norway'. *International Journal of Rehabilitation Research* 20: 139–47.
Cliff, Tony. 1984. *Class Struggle and Women's Liberation: 1640 to Today*. London: Bookmarks.
Clutton-Brock, T. H. and Isvaran, K. 2007. 'Sex Differences in Ageing in Natural Populations of Vertebrates'. *Proceedings of the Royal Society B* 274: 3097–3104.
Cocks, H. G. 2006. 'Modernity and the Self in the History of Sexuality'. *The Historical Journal* 49, no. 4: 1211–27.
Cohen, Lizabeth. 2003. *A Consumers' Republic: The Politics of Mass Consumption in Post-War America*. New York: Alfred A. Knopf.
Coleman, Vernon. 1990. *Bodysense*. London: Sheldon Press.
Coles, Thomas. 2009. 'Negotiating the Field of Masculinity: The Production and Reproduction of Multiple Dominant Masculinities'. *Men and Masculinities* 12, no. 1:30–44.
Collins, William J. and Margo, Robert A. 2011. 'Race and Home Ownership from the Civil War to the Present'. *NBER Working Paper: 16665*. Cambridge: NBER.
Condorcet, Jean Antoin Nicolas de Caritat, Marquis. 1795. *Esquisse d'un tableau historique des progrès de l'esprit humain*. Paris.
Conway, Herbert. 1965. 'Distribution of Plastic Surgeons in the United States'. *Plastic and Reconstructive Surgery* 35, no. 2: 183–90.

Conway-Turner, Katherine. 1995. 'Inclusion of Black Studies in Gerontology Courses: Uncovering and Transcending Stereotypes'. *Journal of Black Studies* 25: 577–88.
Cook, Hera. 2007. 'Sexuality and Contraception in Modern England: Doing the History of Reproductive Sexuality'. *Journal of Social History* 40, no. 4: 915–32.
Cookson, M. S. and Nadig, P. W. 1993. 'Long-term Results with Vacuum Constriction Device'. *Journal of Urology* 149, no. 2: 290–94.
Cooper, Kenneth H. 1970. *New Aerobics*. New York: Bantam Press.
Cooper, Richard S. 1993. 'Health and the Social Status of Blacks in the United States'. *Annals of Epidemiology* 3, no. 2: 137–44.
Cooter, Roger. 1993. *Surgery and Society in Peace and War: Orthopaedics and the Organisation of Modern Medicine: 1880–1948*. Basingstoke: Macmillan.
Coupland Justine. 2007. 'Gendered Discourses on the "Problem" of Ageing: Consumerized Solutions'. *Discourse & Communication* 1, no. 1: 37–61.
Covey, Herbert C. 1989. 'Perceptions and Attitudes toward Sexuality of the Elderly during the Middle Ages'. *The Gerontologist* 29: 93–100.
Cozijnsen, Rabina, Stevens, Nan L. and van Tilburg, Theo G. 2013. 'The Trend in Sport Participation among Dutch Retirees, 1983–2007'. *Ageing & Society* online first. DOI: http://dx.doi.org/10.1017/S0144686X12000189.
Crane, Diana. 2000. *Fashion and its Social Agendas: Class, Gender and Identity in Clothing*. London: University of Chicago Press.
Crane, Diana and Bovone, Laura. 2006. 'Approaches to Material Culture: The Sociology of Fashion and Clothing. *Poetics* 34: 319–33.
Cravit, David. 2008. *The New Old*. Toronto: ECW Press.
Crimmins, Eileen. 2001. 'Mortality and Human Life Spans'. *Experimental Gerontology* 36, no. 2: 885–97.
Cristea, A., Korhonen, M. T., Häkkinen, K., Mero, A., Alen, M., Sipila, S., Viitasalo J. Y., Koljonen, J. T., Suominen, H. and Larsson, L. 2008. 'Effects of Combined Strength and Sprint Training on Regulation of Muscle Contraction at the Whole-Muscle and Single-Fibre Levels in Elite Master Sprinters'. *Acta Physiologica* 193: 275–89.
Crockett, R. J., Pruzinsky, T. and Persing, J. A. 2007. 'The Influence of Plastic Surgery "Reality TV" on Cosmetic Surgery Patient Expectations and Decision Making'. *Plastic and Reconstructive Surgery* 120: 316–23.
Crossley, Nick. 1995. 'Body Techniques, Agency and Intercorporeality: On Goffman's Relations in Public'. *Sociology* 29, no. 1: 133–49.
———. 2001. *The Social Body: Habit, Identity and Desire*. London: Sage Publications.
———. 2007. 'Researching Embodiment by way of Body Techniques'. *Sociological Review* 55: 80–94.
Cruikshank, Margaret. 2003. *Learning to be Old: Gender, Culture and Aging*. Lanham: Rowman & Littlefield.
———. 2008. 'Aging and Identity Politics'. *Journal of Aging Studies* 22, no. 2: 147–51.
Daly, Mary. 1978. *Gynaecology: The Metaethics of Radical Feminism*. Boston: Beacon Press.
Danneels, Erwin. 1996. 'Market Segmentation: Normative Model Versus Business Reality: An Exploratory Study of Apparel Retailing in Belgium'. *European Journal of Marketing* 30, no. 6: 36–51.
Dannefer, Dale W. 2003. 'Cumulative Advantage/Disadvantage and the Life Course: Cross-Fertilizing Age and Social Science Theory'. *Journals of Gerontology* 58B, no. 6: S327–37.
Darling, Rosalyn B. and Heckert, D. Alex. 2010. 'Orientations toward Disability: Differences over the Lifecourse'. *International Journal of Disability, Development and Education* 57, no. 2: 131–43.
Davis, Angela Y. 1982. *Women, Race & Class*. London: The Women's Press.
Davis, Fred. 1992. *Fashion, Culture and Identity*. Chicago: University of Chicago Press.
Davis, Kathy. 1997. '"My Body is my Art": Cosmetic Surgery as Feminist Utopia?' *European Journal of Women's Studies* 4, no. 1: 23–37.

———. 1999. 'Cosmetic Surgery in a Different Voice: The Case of Madame Noel'. *Women's Studies International Forum* 22, no. 5: 473–88.
Davis, Lennard J. 1995. *Enforcing Normalcy: Disability, Deafness and the Body*. London: Verso Books.
Dawson, Percy M. and Hellebrandt, Frances A. 1945. 'The Influence of Aging in Man upon his Capacity for Physical Work and upon his Cardio-Vascular Response to Exercise'. *American Journal of Physiology* 143, no. 3: 420–27.
Deakin, J., Baker, J. and Horton, S. 2004. 'The Struggle for Maintenance: Performance Loss in Elite Golfers across a 25 Year Period'. *Journal of Sport and Exercise Psychology* 26: S62.
Dean, Mitchell. 1995. 'Governing the Unemployed Self in an Active Society'. *Economy & Society* 24, no. 6: 559–83.
de Beauvoir, Simone. 1974. *The Second Sex*. Translated by H. M. Parshley. New York: Vintage Books.
———. 1977. *Old Age*. Translated by P. O'Brien. Harmondsworth: Penguin Books.
De Boulle, Koenraad, Fagien, Steven, Sommer, Boris and Glogau, Richard. 2010. 'Treating Glabellar Lines with Botulinum Toxin Type A-Hemagglutin Complex: A Review of the Science, the Clinical Data and Patient Satisfaction'. *Clinical Interventions in Aging* 5: 101–18.
de Rigal, Jean, Des Mazis, Isabelle, Diridollou, Stephane, Querleux, Bernard, Yang, Grace, Leroy, Frederice and Barbosa, Victoria. 2010. 'The Effect of Age on Skin Color and Color Heterogeneity in Four Ethnic Groups'. *Skin Research and Technology* 16: 168–78.
DeLamater, John and Moorman, Sara M. 2007. 'Sexual Behavior in Later Life'. *Journal of Aging and Health* 19: 921–45.
Deleuze, Gilles and Guattari, Félix. (1980) 2004. *A Thousand Plateaus*. London: Continuum Books.
Delinsky, S. S. 2005. 'Cosmetic Surgery: A Common and Accepted Form of Self-Improvement?' *Journal of Applied Social Psychology* 35, no. 1: 2012–28.
Dell'Ollio, Anselma. 1973. 'The Sexual Revolution Wasn't our War'. In *The First Ms. Reader*, edited by Francine Klagsburn, 124–31. New York: Warner Books.
Deutsch, F. M., Zalenski, C. M. and Clark, M. E. 1986. 'Is there a Double Standard of Aging?' *Journal of Applied Social Psychology* 16: 771–85.
Dionigi, Ryelee A. 2006. 'Competitive Sport as Leisure in Later Life: Negotiations, Discourse and Aging'. *Leisure Sciences* 28, no. 3: 181–96.
———. 2010. 'Masters Sport as a Strategy for Managing the Aging Process'. In *The Masters Athlete: Understanding the Role of Sport and Exercise in Optimizing Aging*, edited by Joseph Baker, Sean Horton and Patricia Weir, 137–56. Oxford: Routledge.
Dissel, Maria, Rotterdam, Sebastian, Altmeyer, Peter and Gambichler, Thilo. 2009. 'Indoor Tanning in North Rhine-Westphalia Germany: A Self-Reported Survey'. *Photodermatology, Photoimmunology & Photomedicine* 25, no. 2: 94–100.
Donato, A. J., Tench, K., Glueck, D. H., Seals D. R., Eskurza, I. and Tanaka, H. 2003. 'Declines in Physiological Functional Capacity with Age: A Longitudinal Study in Peak Swimming Performance'. *Journal of Applied Physiology* 94, no. 10: 764–9.
Dow, Grove S. 1922. *Society and Its Problems*. New York: Thomas Y. Cromwell.
Draelos, K. 2008. 'The Cosmeceutical Realm'. *Clinics in Dermatology* 26: 200–208.
Drasin, Harry, Beals, Kristin P., Elliott, Marc N., Lever, Janert, Klein, David J. and Schuster, Mark A. 2008. 'Age Cohort Differences in the Developmental Milestones of Gay Men'. *Journal of Homosexuality* 54, no. 4: 381–99.
Du Bois, W. E. Burghardt. 1928. 'Race Relations in the United States'. *Annals of the American Academy of Political and Social Science* 140: 6–10.
du Laurens, André. 1599. *A Discourse of the Preservation of the Sight; of Melancholike Diseases; of Rheumes; and of Old Age*. Translated by Richard Surphlet. London.
Dumenil, Laura. 1995. *The Modern Temper: American Culture and Society in the 1920s*. New York: Hill & Wang.

Dutta, S. 2008. 'Cosmetic Surgery Market: Current Trends. Frost & Sullivan Market Insight'. http://www.frost.com/prod/servlet/market-insight-top.pag?Src=RSS&docid=153913646 (accessed 19 June 2010).
Dyhouse, Carol. 2010. *Glamour: Women, History, Feminism*. London: Zed Books.
Ekerdt, David. 1986. '"The Busy Ethic": Moral Continuity between Work and Retirement'. *The Gerontologist* 26, no. 3: 239–44.
Elders, M. Jocelyn. 2010. 'Sex for Health and Pleasure throughout a Lifetime'. *Journal of Sexual Medicine* 7, no. s5: 248–9.
Elias, Norbert. 1978. 'The Civilising Process Revisited'. *Theory and Society* 5: 243–53.
———. 1984. *The Civilising Process*. Oxford: Basil Blackwell.
Elliot, Anthony. 2008. *Making the Cut: How Cosmetic Surgery is Transforming our Lives*. London: Reaktion Books.
Ellis, Anthony. 2009. *Old Age, Masculinity and Early Modern Drama: Comic Elders on the Italian and Shakespearean Stage*. Farnham: Ashgate.
Ellwood, Charles A. 1918. *Sociology and Modern Social Problems*. New York: American Book Company.
Elo, Irma T. 2001. 'New African American Life Tables from 1935–1940 to 1985–1990'. *Demography* 38: 97–114.
Entwhistle, Joanne. 2000. *The Fashioned Body: Fashion, Dress and Modern Social Theory*. Cambridge: Polity Press.
Erikson, Erik H. 1963. *Childhood and Society*. Harmondsworth: Penguin Books.
———. 1980. *The Lifecycle Completed*. New York: Norton.
Euromonitor International. 2011. 'A Look at Global Anti-Ageing Drivers and Hinderers'. http://www.in-cosmetics.com/page.cfm/Link=346 (accessed 3 June 2011).
Evans, J., Grimley, Williams T., Franklin, Beattie B., Lynn, Michel J. P. and Wilcock, Gordon K. 1992. *Oxford Textbook of Geriatric Medicine*. Oxford: Oxford University Press.
Ewing, Elizabeth. 2005. *History of 20th Century Fashion*. London: Batsford.
Fagien, Steven and Carruthers, Jean D. A. 2008. 'A Comprehensive Review of Patient-Reported Satisfaction with Botulinum Toxin Type A for Aesthetic Procedures'. *Plastic and Reconstructive Surgery* 122, no. 6: 1915–25.
Fairclough, Adam. 2001. *Better Day Coming: Blacks and Equality, 1890–2000*. New York: Penguin Books.
Falk, Pasi. 1985. 'Corporeality and its Fates in History'. *Acta Sociologica* 28 no. 2: 115–36.
Falkner, Thomas M. 1995. *The Poetics of Old Age in Greek Epic, Lyric and Tragedy*. Norman: University of Oklahoma Press.
Falkner, Thomas M. and De Luce, Judith D., eds. 1989. *Old Age in Greek and Latin Literature*. Albany: State University of New York Press.
Favor, J. Martin. 1999. *Authentic Blackness: The Folk in the New Negro Renaissance*. Durham: Duke University Press.
Featherstone, Mike. 1982. 'The Body in Consumer Culture'. *Theory, Culture & Society* 1, no. 2: 18–30.
———. 1991. 'The Body in Consumer Culture'. In *The Body, Social Process and Cultural Theory*, edited by Mike Featherstone, Mike Hepworth and Bryan S. Turner, 170–96. London: Sage Publications.
———. 2010. 'Body, Image and Affect in Consumer Culture'. *Body & Society* 16, no. 1: 193–221.
Featherstone, Mike and Hepworth, Mike. 1983. 'The Midlifestyle of George and Lynn: Notes on a Popular Strip'. *Theory, Culture & Society* 1, no. 3: 85–92.
———. 1991. 'The Mask of Ageing and the Postmodern Lifecourse'. In *The Body, Social Process and Cultural Theory*, edited by Mike Featherstone, Mike Hepworth and Bryan S. Turner, 371–89. London: Sage Publications.
Felstein, Ivor. 1974. *Sex in Later Life*. Harmondsworth: Penguin Books.
Ferraro, Kenneth F. 1987. 'Double Jeopardy to Health for Black Older Adults?' *Journal of Gerontology* 42: 528–33.

Ferraro, Kenneth F. and Farmer, Melissa M. 1996. 'Double Jeopardy Aging as Leveler or Persistent Health Inequality? A Longitudinal Analysis of White and Black Americans'. *Journal of Gerontology: Social Sciences* 51b, no. 6: S319–28.

Fillit, Howard M., Rockwood, Kenneth and Woodhouse, Ken, W. eds. 2010. *Brocklehurst's Textbook of Geriatric Medicine and Gerontology*. 7th ed. Philadelphia: Saunders.

Finkelstein, Victor. 1980. *Attitudes and Disabled People: Issues for Discussion*. New York: World Rehabilitation Fund.

Firestone, Shulamith. 1971. *The Dialectic of Sex*. New York: Bantam Books.

Fisher, Dennis G., Malow, Robert, Rosenberg, Rhonda, Reynolds, Grace L., Farrell, Nisha and Jaffe, Adi. 2006. 'Recreational Viagra Use and Sexual Risk among Drug Abusing Men'. *American Journal of Infectious Diseases* 2, no. 2: 107–14.

Fitzpatrick, R., Geronemus, R. and Goldberg, D. 2003. 'Multicenter Study of Noninvasive Radiofrequency for Periorbital Tissue Tightening'. *Lasers in Surgery and Medicine* 33: 232–42.

Forth, Christopher E. 2010. 'Beauty and Concepts of the Ideal'. In *Cultural History of the Human Body, Vol. 6: The Modern Age*, edited by Ivan Crozier, 127–46. Oxford: Berg Publishing.

Fox, Nick. 1999. 'Postmodern Reflections on Risks, Hazards and Life Choices'. In *Risk and Sociocultural Theory: New Directions and Perspectives*, edited by Deborah Lupton, 12–33. Cambridge: Cambridge University Press.

Fox, Ragan Cooper. 2007. 'Gay Grows Up: An Interpretive Study on Aging Metaphors and Queer Identity'. *Journal of Homosexuality* 52, nos. 3/4: 33–61.

Foucault, Michel. 1970. *Madness and Civilisation*. London: Tavistock Pubications.

———. 1975. *The Birth of the Clinic*. New York: Vintage Books.

———. 1979. *Discipline and Punish: The Birth of the Prison*. Harmondsworth: Penguin Books.

———. 1982. 'The Subject and Power'. In *Michel Foucault: Beyond Structuralism and Hermeneutics*, edited by Hubert L. Dreyfuss and Paul Rabinow, 208–26. Hemel Hempstead: Harvester Wheatsheaf.

———. 1988. 'Technologies of the Self'. In *Technologies of the Self: A Seminar with Michel Foucault*, edited by Luther H. Martin, Huck Gutman and Patrick H. Hutton, 16–49. London: Tavistock Publications.

———. 1990a. *The History of Sexuality: Volume 1, An Introduction*. London: Penguin Books.

———. 1990b. *The History of Sexuality: Volume 3, The Care of the Self*. London: Penguin Books.

———. 1992. *The History of Sexuality: Volume 2, The Use of Pleasure*. London: Penguin Books.

———. 1994. 'The Ethic of Care for the Self as a Practice of Freedom: An Interview with Michel Foucault'. In *The Final Foucault*, edited by James Bernauer and David Rasmussen, 1–20. Cambridge: MIT Press.

———. 2005. *The Hermeneutics of the Subject: Lectures at the Collège de France 1981–1982*. Houndsmills: Palgrave.

———. 2008. *The Birth of Bio-Politics: Lectures at the Collège de France 1978–1979*. Houndsmills: Palgrave.

Fraser, Nancy. 1989. *Unruly Practices: Power, Discourse and Gender in Contemporary Social Theory*. Cambridge: Polity Press.

———. 1995. 'From Redistribution to Recognition? Dilemmas of Justice in a "Post Socialist" Age'. *New Left Review* 212: 68–93.

Frazier, E. Franklin. 1947. 'Sociological Theory and Race Relations'. *American Sociological Review* 12, no. 3: 265–71.

Frederick, David A., Lever, Janet and Peplau, Letitia Anne. 2007. 'Interest in Cosmetic Surgery and Body Image: Views of Men and Women across the Lifespan'. *Plastic and Reconstructive Surgery* 120, no. 5: 1407–15.

Fredriksen-Goldsen, Karen I. and Muraco, Anna. 2010. 'Aging and Sexual Orientation: A 25-Year Review of the Literature'. *Research on Aging* 32, no. 3: 372–413.

Friedan, Betty. 1963. *The Feminine Mystique*. New York: HarperCollins.

———. 1993. *The Fountain of Age*. London: Vintage Books.

Friel, Michael T., Shaw, Richard E., Trovato, Matthew J. and Owsley, John Q. 2010. 'The Measure of Face-Lift Patient Satisfaction: The Owsley Facelift Satisfaction Survey with a Long Term Follow-Up Study'. *Plastic and Reconstructive Surgery* 126, no. 1: 245–57.

Friend, R. 1990. 'Older Lesbian and Gay People: A Theory of Successful Aging'. *Journal of Homosexuality* 20, nos. 3/4: 99–118.

Fullmer, Elise M., Shenk, Dena and Eastland, Lynette J. 1999. 'Negating Identity: A Feminist Analysis of the Social Invisibility of Older Lesbians'. *Journal of Women & Aging* 11, nos. 2/3: 131–48.

Furlow, W. L., Goldwasser, B. and Gundian, J. C. 1988. 'Implantation of Model AMS 700 Penile Prosthesis: Long Term Results'. *Journal of Urology* 139, no. 4: 741.

Furman, Frida Kerner. 1997. *Facing the Mirror: Older Women and Beauty Shop Culture*. New York: Routledge.

Gagnon, John, H. and Simon, William. 1973. *Sexual Conduct: The Social Sources of Human Sexuality*. Chicago: Aldine.

Galen, Claudius. 1997. 'To Thrasyboulos: Is Healthiness a Part of Medicine or of Gymnastics?' In *Galen's Selected Works*, translated and edited by Peter N. Singer, 53–99. Oxford: Oxford University Press.

Gallop, Jane. 1988. *Thinking through the Body*. New York: Columbia University Press.

Garland-Thomson, Rosemarie. 2002. 'Integrating Disability, Transforming Feminist Theory'. *NWSA Journal* 14, no. 3: 1–32.

Gates, Henry L. 1988. 'The Trope of the New Negro and the Reconstruction of the Image of the Black'. *Representations* 24: 129–55.

Gergen, Kenneth J. and Gergen, Mary M. 2000. 'The New Aging: Self Construction and Social Values'. In *The Evolution of the Aging Self: The Societal Impact on the Aging Process*, edited by Richard W. Schaie and Jo Hendricks, 281–306. New York: Springer.

Geronimus, Arlene T. 2001. 'Understanding and Eliminating Racial Inequalities in Women's Health in the United States: The Role of the Weathering Conceptual Framework'. *Journal of the American Women's Medical Association* 56: 133–6.

Geronimus, Arline T., Bound, John, Waidmann, Timothy A., Colen, Cynthia G. and Steffick, Dianne. 2001. 'Inequality in Life Expectancy Functional Status and Active Life Expectancy across Selected Black and White Populations in the United States'. *Demography* 38: 227–51.

Geronimus, Arline T., Bound, John, Waidmann, Timothy A., Hillemeier, Marianne M. and Burns, Patricia B. 1996. 'Excess Mortality among Blacks and Whites in the United States'. *New England Journal of Medicine* 335, no. 21: 1552–8.

Geronimus, Arline T., Hicken, Margaret T., Pearson, Jay A., Seashols, Sarah J., Brown, Kelly L. and Cruz, Tracey Dawson. 2010. 'Do US Black Women Experience Stress-Related Accelerated Biological Aging? A Novel Theory and First Population Based Test of Black-White Differences in Telomere Length'. *Human Nature: An Interdisciplinary Biosocial Perspective* 21, no. 1: 19–38.

Giampapa, V. C., Fuente del Campo, A. and Ramirez, O. M. 2004. 'Anti-Aging Medicine and the Aesthetic Surgeon: A New Perspective for our Specialty'. *Aesthetic Plastic Surgery* 27: 493–501.

Gibson, Rose C. 1994. 'The Age-by-Race Gap in Health and Mortality in the Older Population: A Social Science Research Agenda'. *The Gerontologist* 34: 454–62.

Giddens, Anthony. 1991. *Modernity and Self-Identity: Self and Society in the Late Modern Age*. Cambridge: Polity Press.

———. 1992 *The Transformation of Intimacy: Sexuality, Love and Eroticism in Modern Societies*. Cambridge: Polity Press.

Gilbert, Charles. 1967. 'When Does a Man in the Renaissance Grow Old?' *Studies in the Renaissance* 14: 7–32.

Gilleard, Chris. 2002. 'Aging and Old Age in Medieval Society and the Transition to Modernity'. *Journal of Aging and Identity* 7, no. 1: 25–41.

———. 2007. 'Old Age in Ancient Greece: Narratives of Desire, Narratives of Disgust'. *Journal of Aging Studies* 21, no. 2: 81–92.

———. 2013. 'Renaissance Treatises on "Successful Ageing"'. *Ageing & Society* 33, no. 2: 189–215.

Gilleard, Chris and Higgs, Paul. 1998. 'Ageing and the Limiting Conditions of the Body'. *Sociological Research Online* 3, no. 4, http://www.socresonline.org.uk/3/4/4.html.

———. 2000. *Cultures of Ageing: Self, Citizen and the Body*. London: Prentice Hall.

———. 2009. 'The Power of Silver: Ageing and Identity Politics'. *Journal of Aging and Social Policy* 21: 277–95.

———. 2010. 'Aging without Agency: Theorizing the Fourth Age'. *Aging & Mental Health* 14, no. 2: 121–8.

———. 2011a. 'The Third Age as a Cultural Field'. In *Gerontology in the Era of the Third Age*, edited by Dawn Carr and Kathrin Komp, 33–50. New York: Springer.

———. 2011b. 'Frailty, Disability and Old Age: A Re-Appraisal'. *Health: An Interdisciplinary Journal for the Social Study of Health, Illness and Medicine* 15, no. 5: 475–90.

———. 2011c. 'Consumption and Aging'. In *Handbook of Sociology of Aging*, edited by Richard Setterson and Jacqueline L. Angel, 361–75. New York: Springer.

Gilroy, Paul. 2000. *Between Camps: Nations, Cultures and the Allure of Race*. London: Allen Lane.

Gimlin, Debra. 2002. *Body Work: Beauty and Self-Image in American Culture*. Berkeley: University of California Press.

———. 2007. 'What is "Body Work"? A Review of the Literature'. *Sociology Compass* 1, no. 1: 353–70.

Ginn, Jay and Arber, Sara. 1995. '"Only Connect": Gender Relations and Ageing'. In *Connecting Gender & Ageing: A Sociological Approach*, edited by Sara Arber and Jay Ginn, 1–14. Buckingham: Open University Press.

Glassner, Barry. 1989. 'Fitness and the Postmodern Self'. *Journal of Health and Social Behavior* 30, no. 6: 180–91.

Gleeson, Brian J. 1997. 'Disability Studies: A Historical Materialist View'. *Disability & Society* 12, no. 2: 179–202.

Goffman, Erving. 1970. *Stigma: Notes on the Management of Spoiled Identity*. Harmondsworth: Penguin Books.

———. 1971. *The Presentation of Self in Everyday Life*. Harmondsworth: Penguin Books.

Goldsberry, Ellen, Shim, Soyeon, and Reich, Naomi. 1996. 'Women 55 years and Older: Part I. Current Body Measurements as Contrasted to the PS 42-70 Data'. *Clothing and Textile Research Journal* 14, no. 2: 108–20.

———. 1996. 'Women 55 years and Older: Part II. Overall Satisfaction and Dissatisfaction with the Fit of Ready-to-Wear'. *Clothing and Textile Research Journal* 14, no. 2: 121–32.

Goldstein, Sidney. 1968. 'The Aged Segment of the Market, 1950 and 1960'. *Journal of Marketing* 32, no. 1: 62–8.

———. 1971. 'Negro-White Differentials in Consumer Patterns of the Aged 1960–1961'. *The Gerontologist* 11, no. 3: 242–9.

Goodson, Patricia. 2010. 'Sexual Activity in Middle to Later Life'. *BMJ* 340: 544–5.

Gosselink, Carol A., Cox, Deborah L., McClure, Sarissa J and De Jong, Mary L. G. 2008. 'Ravishing or Ravaged: Women's Relationships with Women in the Context of Aging and Western Beauty Culture'. *International Journal of Aging and Human Development* 66, no. 4: 307–27.

Gott, Merryn. 2004. *Sexuality, Sexual Health and Ageing*. Buckingham: Open University Press.

Gott, Merryn and Hinchliff, Sharron. 2003. 'How Important is Sex in Later Life? The Views of Older People'. *Social Science & Medicine* 56: 1617–28.

Graham, Jean Ann and Kligman, Albert M. 1984 'Cosmetic Therapy for the Elderly'. *Journal of the Society of Cosmetic Chemists* 35, no. 3: 133–45.

———. 1985. 'Physical Attractiveness, Cosmetic Use and Self-Perception in the Elderly'. *International Journal of Cosmetic Science* 7, no. 2: 85–97.

Grahame, Rodney. 2002. 'The Decline of Rehabilitation Services and its Impact on Disability Benefits'. *Journal of the Royal Society of Medicine* 95: 114–17.
Gray, Caroline. 2009. 'Narratives of Disability and the Movement from Deficiency to Difference'. *Cultural Sociology* 3: 317–32.
Gray, Heather and Dressel, Paula. 1985. 'Alternative Interpretations of Aging among Gay Males'. *The Gerontologist* 25, no. 1: 83–7.
Gray, S. L., Hanlon, J. T., Fillenbaum, G. G.,Wall, W. E. Jr. and Bales, C. 1996. 'Predictors of Nutritional Supplement Use by the Elderly'. *Pharmacotherapy* 16, no. 4: 715–20.
Greer, Germaine. 1991. *The Change: Women, Aging and the Menopause*. Harmondsworth: Penguin Books.
Grenier, Amanda. 2007. 'Constructions of Frailty in the English Language: Care Practice and the Lived Experience'. *Ageing & Society* 27, no. 3: 425–45.
Grimes, Pearl E. and Shabazz, Dwana. 2009. 'A Four Month Randomized Double Blind Evaluation of the Efficacy of Botulinum Toxin Type A for the Treatment of Glabear Lines in Women with Skin Types V and VI'. *Dermatological Surgery* 35: 429–36.
Grossman, A. H., D'Augelli, A. R. and O'Conell, T. S. 2001. 'Being Lesbian, Gay, Bisexual and 60 or Older in North America'. *Journal of Gay & Lesbian Social Services* 13, no. 1: 23–40.
Grosz, Elizabeth. 1994. *Volatile Bodies: Toward a Corporeal Feminism*. Bloomington: Indiana University Press.
Gruman, Gerald J. 2003. *A History of Ideas about the Prolongation of Life*. New York: Springer Publishing.
Guild, Warren. 1971. 'Fitness Forever'. *Vogue*, May: 172.
Gullette, Margaret M. 1997. *Declining to Decline: Cultural Combat and the Politics of the Midlife*. Charlottesville: University Press of Virginia.
———. 2004. *Aged by Culture*. Chicago: University of Chicago Press.
Gunn D. A., Rexbye H., Griffiths C. E. M., Murray P. G., Fereday, A., Catt, S. D., Tomlin, C. C., Strongitham, B. H., Perrett, D. I., Catt, M., Mayes, A. E., Messenger, A. G., Green, M. R., van der Ouderaa, F., Vaupel, J. W. and Christensen, K. 2008. 'Why Some Women Look Young for their Age'. *PLoS ONE* 4, no. 12: e8021, DOI: 10.1371/journal.pone.0008021.
Gutton, Jean-Pierre. 1988. *Naissance du vieillard: Essai sur l'histoire des rapports entre les vieillards et la société en France*. Aubier: Collection Historique.
Hacker, Jacob S. 2002. *The Divided Welfare State*. Cambridge: Cambridge University Press.
Haeck, Phillip C. and Hait, Pam. 2006. 'Into the Twenty First Century: The History of the American Society of Plastic and Reconstructive Surgeons from 1995 to 2006'. *Plastic and Reconstructive Surgery* Suppl. 5: 2S–31S.
Hahn, Harlan. 1985. 'Towards a Politics of Disability: Definition, Disciplines and Politics'. *The Social Science Journal* 22, no. 4: 87–105.
———. 1988. 'The Politics of Physical Differences: Disability and Discrimination'. *Journal of Social Issues* 44: 39–43.
———. 1994. 'The Minority Group Model of Disability: Implications for Medical Sociology'. In *Research in the Sociology of Health Care: Volume 11*, edited by R. Wetz and J. J. Kronenfeld, 3–240. Greenwich: JAI press.
———. 2002. 'Academic Debates and Political Advocacy: The US Disability Movement'. In *Disability Studies Today*, edited by Colin Barnes, Mike Oliver and Len Barton, 162–89. Cambridge: Polity Press.
Haiken, Elizabeth. 1997. *Venus Envy: A History of Cosmetic Surgery*. Baltimore: John Hopkins University Press.
———. 2000. 'Virtual Virility or Does Medicine Make the Man?' *Men and Masculinities* 2, no. 4: 388–409.
Hait, Pam. 1994. 'A History of the American Society of Plastic and Reconstructive Surgery'. *Plastic and Reconstructive Surgery* 94, no. 4, Suppl. 4: 1–109.
Hakim, Christine. 2011. *Honey Money: The Power of Erotic Capital*. London: Allen Lane.

Hall, Stuart. 1990. 'Cultural Identity and Diaspora'. In *Identity: Community, Culture, Difference*, edited by James Rutherford, 222–37. London: Lawrence and Wishart.

———. 1996. 'New Ethnicities'. In *Stuart Hall: Critical Dialogues in Cultural Studies*, edited by David Morley and Kuan-Hsing Chen, 442–51. London: Routledge.

Halliwell, Emma and Dittmar, Helga. 2003. 'A Qualitative Investigation of Women's and Men's Body Image Concerns and their Attitudes towards Aging'. *Sex Roles* 49, nos. 11/12: 675–84.

Halperin, David M. 2000. 'How to Do the History of Male Homosexuality'. *GLQ: A Journal of Lesbian and Gay Studies* 6, no. 1: 87–123.

———. 1995. *Saint Foucault: Towards a Gay Hagiography*. Oxford: Oxford University Press.

Hamilton, N. 1993. 'Change in Sprint Stride Kinematics with Age in Master's Athletes'. *Journal of Applied Biomechanics* 9, no. 1: 15–26.

Hansen, Joseph, Reed, Evelyn and Waters, Mary-Alice. 1986. *Cosmetics, Fashions, and the Exploitation of Women*. London: Pathfinder Press.

Haraway, Donna J. 1997. *Modest_Witness@Second_Millenium. FemaleMan©_Meets_OncoMouse™: Feminism and Technoscience*. London: Routledge.

Harris, M. B. 1994. 'Growing Old Gracefully: Age Concealment and Gender'. *Journal of Gerontology: Psychological Sciences* 49: 149–58.

Harris, Monte O. 2004. 'The Aging Face in Patients of Color: Minimally Invasive Surgical Facial Rejuvenation – A Targeted Approach'. *Dermatologic Therapy* 17, no. 2: 206–11.

Harris, W. E., Bowerman, W., McFadden, R. B. and Kerns, T. A. 1967. 'Jogging: An Adult Exercise Program'. *JAMA* 201, no. 10: 759–61.

Harrison, Jo. 1983. 'Women and Ageing: Experience and Implications'. *Ageing & Society* 3, no. 2: 209–35.

———. 1999. 'A Lavender Pink Grey Power: Gay and Lesbian Gerontology in Australia'. *Australasian Journal of Aging* 18: 32–7.

Harry, J. and DeVall, W. 1978. 'Age and Sexual Culture among Homosexually Oriented Males'. *Archives of Sexual Behavior* 7, no. 3: 199–209.

Hartmann, Uwe, Philippsohn, Susanne, Heiser, Kristina and Ruffer-Hesse, Claudia. 2004. 'Low Sexual Desire in Midlife and Older Women: Personality Factors, Psychosocial Development, Present Sexuality'. *Menopause: The Journal of the North American Menopause Society* 11, no. 6: 726–40.

Haslop, Craig, Hill, Helene and Schmidt, Ruth A. 1998. 'The Gay Lifestyle: Spaces for a Subculture of Consumption'. *Marketing Intelligence and Planning* 16, no. 5: 318–26.

Havighurst, Robert J. 1961. 'Successful Aging'. *The Gerontologist* 1, no. 1: 4–7.

Hawton, Keith, Catalan, Jose and Fagg, J. 1992. 'Sex Therapy for Erectile Dysfunction: Characteristics of Couples, Treatment Outcome and Prognostic Factors'. *Archives of Sexual Behavior* 21, no. 2: 161–75.

Hawton, Keith, Catalan, Jose, Martin, Philip and Fagg, J. 1986. 'Long Term Outcome of Sex Therapy'. *Behaviour Research and Therapy* 24, no. 6: 665–75.

Haycock, David Boyd. 2008. *Mortal Coil: A Short History of Living Longer*. New Haven: Yale University Press.

Hayes, Richard and Dennerstein, Lorraine 2005. 'The Impact of Aging on Sexual Function and Sexual Dysfunction in Women: A Review of Population-Based Studies'. *Journal of Sexual Medicine* 2: 317–30.

Hayes, Richard, Dennerstein, Lorraine, Bennett, Catherine M., Koochaki, Pastrica E., Leiblum, Sandra R. and Graziottin, Alessandra. 2007. 'Relationship Between Hypoactive Sexual Desire Disorder and Aging'. *Fertility and Sterility* 87, no. 1: 107–12.

Hayflick, Leonard. 2000. 'The Future of Ageing'. *Nature* 408: 267–9.

Heaphy, Brian, Yip, Andrew K. T. and Thompson, Debbie. 2004. 'Ageing in a Non-Heterosexist Context'. *Ageing & Society* 24: 881–902.

Hearn, H. L. 1971. 'Career and Leisure Patterns of Middle Aged Urban Blacks'. *The Gerontologist* 11, no. 4: 21–6.

REFERENCES

Heath, Kay. 2009. *Aging by the Book: The Emergence of Midlife in Victorian Britain*. New York: State University of New York Press.

Heath, Joseph and Potter, Andrew. 2005. *The Rebel Sell: How the Counterculture Became Consumer Culture*. Chichester: Capstone Publishing.

Heckman, C. J., Coups, E. J. and Manne, S. L. 2008. 'Prevalence and Correlates of Indoor Tanning among US Adults'. *Journal of the American Academy of Dermatology* 58: 769–80.

Heiman, Julia R. 2002. 'Psychologic Treatments for Female Sexual Dysfunction: Are they Effective and Do we Need Them?' *Archives of Sexual Behavior* 31, no. 5: 445–50.

Heiss, Sarah N. 2011. 'Locating the Bodies of Women and Disability in Definitions of Beauty: An Analysis of Dove's Campaign for Real Beauty'. *Disability Studies Quarterly* 31, no. 1, http://www.dsq-sds.org/article/view/1367/1497 (accessed 19 April 2013).

Hendricks, Jon. 2005. 'Moral Economy and Ageing'. In *The Cambridge Handbook of Age and Ageing*, edited in Malcolm L. Johnson, 510–17. Cambridge: Cambridge University Press.

Hennessy, C. H. 1989. 'Culture in the Use, Care and Control of the Aging Body'. *Journal of Aging Studies* 3: 39–54.

Henss, R. 1991. 'Perceiving Age and Attractiveness in Facial Photographs'. *Journal of Applied Social Psychology* 21: 933–46.

Hepworth, Mike and Featherstone, Mike. 1982. *Surviving Middle Age*. Oxford: Basil Blackwell.

Herbenick, Debby, Reece, Michael, Sanders, Stephanie A., Dodge, Brian, Ghassemi, Annahita and Fortenberry, J. Dennis. 2009. 'Prevalence and Characteristics of Vibrator Use by Women in the United States: Results from a Nationally Representative Study'. *Journal of Sexual Medicine* 6:1857–66.

Herbenick, Debby, Reece, Michael, Schick, Vanessa, Sanders, Stephanie A., Dodge, Brian and Fortenberry, J. Dennis. 2010. 'Sexual Behaviors, Relationships and Perceived Health Status among Adult Women in the United States: Results from a National Probability Sample'. *Journal of Sexual Medicine* 7, Suppl. 5: 277–90.

Herdt, Gilbert, Beeler, Jeff and Rawls, Todd W. 1997. 'Life Course Diversity among Older Lesbians and Gay Men: A Study in Chicago'. *International Journal of Sexuality and Gender Studies* 2, nos. 3/4: 231–46.

Herlihy, David and Klapisch-Zuber, Christiane. 1985. *Tuscans and their Families: A Study of the Florentine Catasto of 1427*. New Haven: Yale University Press.

Herzberg, Arlene J. and Dinehart, Scott, M. 1989. 'Chronologic Aging in Black Skin'. *The American Journal of Dermatopathology* 11: 319–28.

Hexsel, Doris, Brum, Cristiano, do Prado, Débora Zechmeister, Soirefmann, Mariana, Rotta, Francisco Telechea, Dal'Forno, Taciana and Rodrigues, Ticiana C. 2012. 'Field Effect of Two Commercial Preparations of Botulinum Toxin Type A: A Prospective, Double-Blind, Randomized Clinical Trial'. *Journal of the American Academy of Dermatology* 67, no. 2: 226–9.

Heyman, Dorothy K. 1970. 'Does a Wife Retire?' *The Gerontologist* 10, no. 2: 54–6.

Higgs, Edward. 1983. 'Leisure and the State: The History of Popular Culture as Reflected in the Public Records'. *History Workshop* 15, no. 1: 141–50.

Higgs, Paul. 2012. 'Consuming Bodies: Zygmunt Bauman on the Difference between Fitness and Health'. In *Contemporary Theorists for Medical Sociology*, edited by Graham Scambler, 20–32. London: Routledge.

Higgs, Paul, Leontowitsch, Miranda, Stevenson, Fiona and Jones, Ian. 2009. 'Not Just Old and Sick: The Will to Health in Later Life'. *Ageing & Society* 29, no. 5: 687–707.

Higgs, Paul and Jones, Ian R. 2009. *Medical Sociology and Old Age: Towards a Sociology of Health in Later Life*. London: Routledge.

Higgs, Paul and McGowan, Fiona. 2012. 'Ageing, Embodiment and the Negotiation of the Third and Fourth Ages'. In *Aging Men: Masculinities and Modern Medicine*, edited by Antje Kampf, Barbara Marshall and Alan Petersen, 21–34. London: Taylor and Francis.

Hill, Amelia. 2008. 'Cosmetics Firms Tempt Men over 50'. *The Observer*, 27 April.

Hinrichs, Timo, Trampisch, Ulrike, Burghaus, Ina, Endres, Heinz G., Klaaßen-Mielke, Renate, Moschny, Anna and Platen, Petra. 2010. 'Correlates of Sport Participation among Community-Dwelling Elderly People in Germany: A Cross-Sectional Study'. *European Review of Aging and Physical Activity* 7, no. 2: 105–15.

Hirschl, Thomas A. and Rank, Mark R. 2010. 'Homeownership across the American Life Course: Estimating the Racial Divide'. *Race and Social Problems* 2: 125–36.

Hirshbein, Laura Davidow. 2000. 'The Glandular Solution: Sex, Masculinity, and Aging in the 1920s'. *Journal of the History of Sexuality* 9, no. 3: 277–304.

Hofferth, Sandra L., Kahn, Joan R. and Baldwin, Wendy. 1987. 'Premarital Sexual Activity among U.S. Teenage Women over the Past Three Decades'. *Family Planning Perspectives* 19, no. 2: 46–53.

Hoffman, Martin. 1968. *The Gay World*. New York: Bantam Books.

Holly, Elisabeth, Lele, Chitra and Bracchi, Paige. 1998. 'Hair-Color Products and Risk for Non-Hodgkin's Lymphoma: A Population-Based Study in the San Francisco Bay Area'. *American Journal of Public Health* 88, no. 12: 1767–73.

Holmlund, Maria, Hagman, Anne and Polsa, Pia. 2011. 'An Exploration of How Mature Women Buy Clothing: Empirical Insights and a Model'. *Journal of Fashion Marketing and Management* 15, no. 1: 108–122.

Holtkötter, Olaf, Schotmann, K., Hofheinz, H., Obrisch, R. R. and Petersohn, D. 2005. 'Unveiling the Molecular Basis of Intrinsic Skin Aging'. *International Journal of Cosmetic Science* 27, no. 4: 263–9.

Honigman, Roberta, Phillips, Katharine and Castle, David J. 2004. 'A Review of Psychosocial Outcomes for Patients Seeking Cosmetic Surgery'. *Plastic and Reconstructive Surgery* 113, no. 4: 1229–37.

Horton, Sean, Baker, Joseph and Schorer, Jorg. 2008. 'Expertise and Aging: Maintaining Skills through the Lifespan'. *European Reviews in Aging and Physical Activity*, DOI: 10.1007/s11556-008-0034-5.

Houk, L. D. and Humphreys, T. 2007. 'Masers to Magic Bullets: An Updated History of Lasers in Dermatology'. *Clinics in Dermatology* 25: 434–42.

Housman, T. S., Hancox, J. G., Mir, M. R., Camacho, F., Fleischer, A. B., Feldman, S. R. and Williford, P. M. 2008. 'What Specialties Perform the Most Common Outpatient Cosmetic Procedures in the United States?' *Dermatological Surgery* 34: 1–8.

Howson, Alexandra and Inglis, David. 2001. 'The Body in Sociology: Tensions Inside and Outside Sociological Thought'. *Sociological Review* 49, no. 3: 297–317.

Hughes, Bill. 1995. 'What Can a Foucauldian Analysis Contribute to Disability Theory?' In *Foucault and the Government of Disability*, edited by Shelley Tremain 78–92. Michigan: University of Michigan Press.

———. 2009. 'Wounded/Monstrous/Abject: A Critique of the Disabled Body in the Sociological Imaginary'. *Disability & Society* 24: 399–410.

Hughes, Bill and Paterson, Kevin. 1997. 'The Social Model of Disability and the Disappearing Body: Towards a Sociology of Impairment'. *Disability & Society* 12: 325–340.

Hughes, Mark. 2006. 'Queer Ageing'. *Gay and Lesbian Issues and Psychology Review* 2, no. 2: 54–9.

Hurd-Clarke, Laura. 2011. *Facing Age: Women Growing Older in Anti-Aging Culture*. Lanham: Rowman & Littlefield.

Hurd-Clarke, Laura and Griffin, M. 2007a. 'The Body Natural and the Body Unnatural: Beauty Work and Aging'. *Journal of Aging Studies* 21, no. 3: 187–201.

———. 2007b. 'Becoming and Being Gendered through the Body: Older Women, Bodies and Body Image'. *Ageing & Society* 27, no. 5: 701–18.

Hurd-Clarke, Laura and Griffin, M. 2008. 'Visible and Invisible Ageing: Beauty Work as a Response to Ageism'. *Ageing & Society* 28, no. 5: 653–74.

Hurd-Clarke, Laura, Repta, R. and Griffin, M. 2007. 'Non-Surgical Cosmetic Procedures: Older Women's Perceptions and Experiences'. *Journal of Women & Aging* 19, nos. 3/4: 69–87.

Ibrahim, T., Bloch, B., Esler, C. N., Abrams, K. R. and Harper, W. M. 2010. 'Temporal Trends in Primary Total Hip and Knee Arthroplasty Surgery: Results from a UK Regional Joint Register, 1991–2004'. *Annals of the Royal College of Surgeons (England)* 92, no. 6: 231–5.

Iezzoni, Lisa I. and Freedman, Vicki A. 2008. 'Turning the Disability Tide: The Importance of Definitions'. *JAMA* 299, no. 3: 332–4.

International Cosmetic News. 2006. Vol. 88, 1 June.

Irigaray, Luce. 1985. *This Sex Which is Not One*. Ithaca: Cornell University Press.

Jagger, Elizabeth. 2005. 'Is Thirty the New Sixty? Dating, Age and Gender in a Postmodern Consumer Society'. *Sociology* 39, no. 1: 89–106.

Jarcho, S. 1970. 'Galen's Six Non-Naturals: A Bibliographic Note and Translation'. *Bulletin of the History of Medicine* 44: 372–7.

Jarow, Jonathan P., Nana-Sinkam, Patrick, Sabbagh, Mohsen and Eskew, Andrew. 1996. 'Outcome Analysis of Goal Directed Therapy for Impotence'. *Journal of Urology* 155, no. 5: 1609–12.

Jenß, Heike. 2004. 'Dressed in History: Retro Styles and the Construction of Authenticity in Youth Culture'. *Fashion Theory* 8, no. 4: 387–404.

Johnson, Roberta Ann. 1999. 'Mobilizing the Disabled'. In *Waves of Protest: Social Movements Since the 1960s*, edited by Joe Freeman and Victoria Johnson, 25–46. New York: Rowman & Littlefield.

Jones, Geoffrey. 2010. *Beauty Imagined: A History of the Global Beauty Industry*. Oxford: Oxford University Press.

———. 2008. 'Blonde and Blue-Eyed? Globalizing Beauty, c.1945–c.1980'. *Economic History Review* 61, no. 1: 125–54.

Jones, Ian Rees and Higgs, Paul. 2010. 'The Natural, the Normal and the Normative: Contested Terrains in Ageing and Old Age'. *Social Science & Medicine* 71, no. 8: 1513–19.

Jones, Meredith. 2004. 'Mutton Cut Up as Lamb: Mothers, Daughters and Cosmetic Surgery'. *Continuum: Journal of Media & Cultural Studies* 18, no. 4: 525–39.

Jonson, Hakan and Larsson, Anika Taghizadeh. 2009. 'The Exclusion of Older People in Disability Activism and Policies – A Case of Inadvertent Ageism?' *Journal of Aging Studies* 23: 69–77.

Jordanova, Ludmilla. 1989. *Sexual Visions: Images of Gender in Science and Medicine between the Eighteenth and Twentieth Centuries*. London: Harvester Wheatsheaf.

Jorm, Anthony F., Dear, K. B. G., Rodgers, B. and Christensen, H. 2003. 'Cohort Difference in Sexual Orientation: Results from a Large Age-Stratified Population Sample'. *Gerontology* 49, no. 6: 392–5.

Joung, Hyun-Mee and Miller, Nancy J. 2006 'Factors of Dress Affecting Self-Esteem in Older Females'. *Journal of Fashion Marketing and Management* 10, no. 4: 466–78.

Juvin, Hervé. 2010. *The Coming of the Body*. London: Verso Books.

Kadri, N., McHichi, Alami K. H., McHakra, Tahiri. S. 2002. 'Sexual Dysfunction in Women: Population Based Epidemiological Study'. *Archives of Women's Mental Health* 5: 59–63.

Kafi, R., Kwak, H. S. R., Schumacher, W. E., Cho, S., Hanft, V. N., Hamilton, T. A., King, A. L., Neal, J. D., Varani, J., Fisher, G. J., Voorhees, J. J. and Kang, S. 2007. 'Improvement of Naturally Aged Skin with Vitamin A (Retinol)'. *Archives of Dermatology* 143, no. 5: 606–12.

Kagan, Elizabeth and Morse, Margaret. 1988. 'The Body Electronic: Aerobic Exercise on Video: Women's Search for Empowerment and Self-Transformation'. *TDR* 32, no. 4: 164–80.

Kaiser, Daniel H. and Engel, Peyton. 1993. 'Time- and Age-Awareness in Early Modern Russia'. *Comparative Studies in Society and History* 35, no. 4: 824–39.

Karo, Margherita. 1967. 'The Cosmetics/Toiletries Industry'. *Financial Analysts Journal* 23, no. 3: 27–32.

Katz, Stephen. 2000. 'Busy Bodies: Activity, Aging, and the Management of Everyday Life'. *Journal of Aging Studies* 14, no. 2: 135–52.

Katz, Stephen, Ford A. B., Moskowitz R. W., Jackson, B. A. and Jaffe, M. W. 1963. 'Studies of Illness in the Aged: The Index of ADL: A Standardized Measure of Biomedical and Psychosocial Function'. *JAMA* 185: 914–19.

Katz, Stephen and Marshall, Barbara L. 2003. 'New Sex for Old: Lifestyle, Consumerism and the Ethics of Aging Well'. *Journal of Aging Studies* 17, no. 1: 3–16.

Keenan, Brigid. 1977. *The Women We Wanted to Look Like*. London: Macmillan.

Kelly, J. 1977. 'The Aging Homosexual: Myth and Reality'. *The Gerontologist* 17: 328–32.

Kemp, Brian J. 2005. 'Aging with Disability: What the Rehabilitation Professional and the Consumer Need to Know'. *Physical Medicine & Rehabilitation Clinics of North America* 16, no. 1: 1–18.

Kennedy, J. 2005. 'Herb and Supplement Use in the US Adult Population'. *Clinical Therapeutics* 27: 1847–58.

Kent, Donald P. 1971. 'The Negro Aged'. *The Gerontologist* 11: 48–51.

Kerscher, Martina and Buntrock, Heik. 2011. 'Update on Cosmeceuticals'. *JDDG: Journal der Deutschen Dermatologischen Gesellschaft* 9, no. 4: 314–28.

Khan, Parisa Islam and Tabassum, Ayesha. 2012. 'Beautification for Males in Dhaka: Exploring the Customer Groups, Services and Selection of Service Providers'. *World Review of Business Research* 2, no. 4: 71–85.

Kim, H., Kim, N., Jung, S., Mun, J., Kim, J., Kim, B., Lee, J. and Jung, H. 2009. 'Improvement in Skin Wrinkles from the Use of Photostable Retinyl Retinoate: A Randomized Controlled Trial'. *British Journal of Dermatology* 162: 497–502.

Kimmel, D. C. 1979. 'Adult Development and Aging: A Gay Perspective'. *Journal of Social Issues* 34, no. 3: 113–30.

———. 1980. 'Life History Interviews of Aging Gay Men'. *International Journal of Aging and Human Development* 10: 239–48.

King, Abby C., Castro, Cynthia, Wilcox, Sara, Eyler, Amy A., Sallis, James F. and Brownson, Ross C. 2000. 'Personal and Environmental Factors Associated with Physical Inactivity among Different Racial-Ethnic Groups of US Middle-Aged and Older Aged Adults'. *Health Psychology* 19, no. 4: 354–64.

Kinnunen, Taina. 2010. '"A Second Youth": Pursuing Happiness and Respectability through Cosmetic Surgery in Finland'. *Sociology of Health & Illness* 32: 258–71.

Kinsey, Alfred C., Pomeroy, Wardell B. and Martin, Clyde E. 1948. *Sexual Behavior in the Human Male*. New York: W. B. Saunders.

Kinsey, Alfred E. Pomeroy, Wardell, B., Martin, Clyde E. and Gebhardt, Paul. 1953. *Sexual Behavior in the Human Female*. New York: W. B. Saunders.

Kirkwood, Tom. 2001. *The End of Age*. London: Profile Books.

Kirkwood, Tom and Austed, Steven N. 2000. 'Why Do We Age?' *Nature* 408: 233–8.

Kleg, Milton and Yamamoto, Kaoru. 1998. 'As the World Turns: Ethno-Racial Distances after 70 Years'. *The Social Science Journal* 35, no. 2: 183–90.

Kligman, Albert M. 1976. 'Perspectives and Problems in Cutaneous Gerontology'. *Journal of Investigative Dermatology* 73: 39–46.

———. 1993 'Why Cosmeceuticals? The Role of Non Prescription Topical Treatment Products'. *Cosmetics & Toiletries* 108, no. 8: 37–8.

Kligman, Albert, M. and Graham, J. A. 1989. 'The Psychology of Appearance in the Elderly'. *Clinics in Geriatric Medicine* 5, no. 1: 213–22.

Kligman, Albert M., Grove, G. R., Hirose, R. and Leyden, J. J. 1986. 'Topical Tretinoin for Photoaged Skin'. *Journal of the American Academy of Dermatology* 15: 836–59.

Kligman, Albert M., Zheng, P. and Lavker, R. M. 1985. 'The Anatomy and Pathogenesis of Wrinkles'. *British Journal of Dermatology* 113: 37–42.

Kline, Chrysee. 1975. 'The Socialization Process of Women: Implications for a Theory of Successful Aging'. *The Gerontologist* 15, no. 6: 486–92.

Kohli, Martin. 1986. 'The World We Forgot: A Historical Review of the Life Course'. In *Later Life: The Social Psychology of Ageing*, edited by Victor W. Marshall, 271–303. Beverly Hills: Sage Publications.

———. 2007. 'The Institutionalization of the Life Course: Looking Back to Look Ahead'. *Research in Human Development* 4, nos. 3/4: 253–71.

Korhonen, Marko T., Mero, Antti and Suominen, Harri. 2003. 'Age-Related Differences in 100-m Sprint Performance in Male and Female Master Runners'. *Medicine & Science in Sports & Exercise* 35, no. 8: 1419–28.

Kosowski, T. R., McCarthy, C., Reavey, P. L, Scott, A. M., Wilkins, E. G., Cano, S. J., Klassen, A. F., Carr, N., Cordeiro, P. G. and Pusic, A. L. 2009. 'A Systematic Review of Patient Reported Outcome Measures after Facial Cosmetic Surgery and/or Nonsurgical Facial Rejuvenation'. *Plastic and Reconstructive Surgery* 123, no. 6: 1819–27.

Kramarow, Ellen, Lubitz, James, Lentzner, Harold and Gorina, Yelena. 2007. 'Trends in the Health of Older Americans, 1970–2005'. *Health Affairs* 26, no. 5: 1417–25.

Krekula, Clary. 2007. 'The Intersection of Age and Gender: Reworking Gender Theory and Social Gerontology'. *Current Sociology* 55, no. 2: 155–71.

Kurt, U., Özkardes, S. H., Altuğ, U., Germiyanoğlu, C., Gurdal, M. and Erol, D. 1994. 'The Efficacy of Anti-Serotinergic Agents in the Treatment of Erectile Dysfunction'. *Journal of Urology* 152: 407–9.

Kwan, Samantha and Trautner, Mary N. 2009. 'Beauty Work: Individual and Institutional Rewards, the Reproduction of Gender and Questions of Agency'. *Sociology Compass* 3, no. 1: 49–71.

Lam, S. M. 2004. 'Julien Bourguet: Father of Cervical Rhytidectomy'. *Archives of Facial Plastic Surgery* 6: 137.

Landau, M. 2008. 'Chemical Peels'. *Clinics in Dermatology* 26: 200–208.

Laqueur, Thomas, W. 1990. *Making Sex: Body and Gender from the Greeks to Freud*. Cambridge: Harvard University Press.

Lasch, Christopher. 1979. *The Culture of Narcissism*. New York: W. W. Norton & Co.

Laslett, Peter. 1989. *A Fresh Map of Life: The Emergence of the Third Age*. London: Weidenfeld & Nicolson.

Latimer, Joanna. 2009. 'Introduction'. *Un/Knowing Bodies*, edited by Joanna Latimer and Michael Schillmeier, 1–22. London: Wiley-Blackwell.

Laumann, Edward O., Paik, Anthony, Glasser, Dae B., Kang, Jeong-Han, Wang, Tianfu, Levinson, Bernard, Moreira, Edson D., Nicolosi, Alfredo and Gingell, Clive. 2006. 'A Cross National Study of Subjective Sexual Well-Being Among Older Women and Men: Findings from the Global Study of Sexual Attitudes and Behaviors'. *Archives of Sexual Behavior* 35, no. 2: 145–61.

Laumann, Edward O., Paik, Anthony and Rosen, R. C. 1999. 'Sexual Dysfunction in the United States: Prevalence and Predictors'. *JAMA* 281: 537–44.

Lawton, M. Powell and Brody, Elaine M. 1969. 'Assessment of Older People: Self-Maintaining and Instrumental Activities of Daily Living'. *The Gerontologist* 9, no. 3: 179–86.

Lefebvre, Henri. 2002. *Critique of Everyday Life: Volume II*. London: Verso Books.

Leiblum, Sandra R., Koochaki, Patricia E., Rodenberg, Cynthia A., Barton, Ian P. and Rosen Raymond C. 2006. 'Hypoactive Sexual Desire Disorder in Postmenopausal Women: US Results from the Women's International Study of Health and Sexuality (WISHeS)'. *Maturitas* 13: 46–56.

Lemperle, Gottfried, Holmes, Ralph E., Cohen, Steven R. and Lemperle, Stefan M. 2001. 'A Classification of Facial Wrinkles'. *Plastic and Reconstructive Surgery* 108: 1735–50.

Leontowitsch, Miranda, Higgs, Paul, Stevenson, Fiona and Jones, Ian R. 2010. 'Taking Care of Yourself in Later Life: A Qualitative Study into the Use of Non-Prescription Medicines by People Aged 60+'. *Health (London)* 14, no. 2: 213–31.

Lepers, Romuald and Cattagni, Thomas. 2012. 'Do Older Athletes Reach Limits in their Performance during Marathon Running?' *Age* 34, no. 3: 773–81.

Lepers, Romuald, Rüst, Christoph A., Stapley and Knechtle, Beat. 2012. 'Relative Improvements in Endurance Performance with Age: Evidence from 25 Years of Hawaii Ironman Racing'. *Age*, DOI: 10.1007/s11357-012-9392-z.

Levy, Judith A. 1988. 'Intersections of Gender and Aging'. *The Sociological Quarterly* 29, no. 4: 479–86.

Leyk, Dieter, Erley, Oliver and Bilzon, James. 2007. 'Effects of Age on Operational Physical Performance'. In NATO report, *Intrinsic and Extrinsic Factors Affecting Operational Physical Performance*, Section 7.2: 7.2–7.5.

Leyk, Dieter, Rüther, Thomas, Wunderlich, Max, Sievart, Alexander, Eβfeld, Dieter, Witzki, Alexander, Erley, Oliver, Kuchmeister, Gerd, Piekarski, Claus and Löllgen, Herbert. 2010. 'Physical Performance in Middle Age and Old Age'. *Deutsches Ärzteblatt International* 107, no. 4: 809–16.

Lindau, Stacy Tesler and Gavrilova, Natalia. 2010. 'Sex, Health and Years of Sexually Active Life Gained Due to Good Health: Evidence from Two US Population-Based Cross Sectional Surveys of Ageing'. *BMJ* 340: c810s.

Linton, Simi. 1998. *Claiming Disability: Knowledge and Identity*. New York: New York University Press.

Lipovetsky, Gilles. 2002. *The Empire of Fashion: Dressing Modern Democracy*. Princeton: Princeton University Press.

Litner, J. A., Rotenberg, B. W., Dennis, M. and Adamson, P. A. 2008. 'Impact of Cosmetic Facial Surgery on Satisfaction with Appearance and Quality of Life'. *Archives of Facial Plastic Surgery* 10: 79–84.

Livingston, James. 1998. 'Modern Subjectivity and Consumer Culture'. *Getting and Spending: European and American Consumer Societies in the Twentieth Century*, edited by Susan Strasser, Charles McGovern and Matthias Judt, 413–30. Cambridge: Cambridge University Press.

L'Oréal. 2010. *The L'Oréal UK Men's Grooming Report 2010*. March 2010.

Loughman, Celeste. 1980. 'Eros and the Elderly: A Literary View'. *The Gerontologist* 20, no. 2: 182–7.

Luciano, Lynne. 2001. *Looking Good: Male Body Image in Modern America*. New York: Hill & Wang.

Lunt, Neil and Carrera, Percivil. 2010. 'Medical Tourism: Assessing the Evidence on Treatment Abroad'. *Maturitas* 66: 27–32.

Lupton, Deborah. 1995. *The Imperative of Health: Public Health and the Regulated Body*. London: Sage Publications.

Macdonald, Barbara. 1989. 'Outside Sisterhood: Ageism in Women's Studies'. *Women's Studies Quarterly* 17, nos. 1/2: 6–11.

Macfarlane, Andrew. 1977. 'History, Anthropology and the Study of Communities'. *Social History* 5, no. 5: 631–52.

Macinko, J. and Elo, I. T. 2009. 'Black-White Differences in Avoidable Mortality in the USA, 1980–2005'. *Journal of Epidemiology and Community Health* 63: 715–21.

Mahoney, F. I. and Barthel, D. 1965. 'Functional Evaluation: The Barthel Index'. *Maryland State Medical Journal* 14, no. 1: 56–61.

Mairs, Nancy. 1989. *Remembering the Bone House: An Erotics of Place and Space*. New York: Harper and Row.

Malik, Kenan. 1996. *The Meaning of Race*. London: Macmillan.

Manton, Kenneth G. 1988. 'A Longitudinal Study of Functional Change and Mortality in the United States'. *Journal of Gerontology* 43: S153–S161.

Manton, Kenneth G. and Gu, S. 2001. 'Changes in the Prevalence of Chronic Disability in the United States Black and Non-Black Population above Age 65 from 1982 to 1999'. *Proceedings of the National Academy of Sciences* 98: 6354–9.

Manton, Kenneth G., Patrick, C. H. and Johnson, W. K. 1987. 'Health Differentials between Blacks and Whites: Recent Trends in Mortality and Morbidity'. *Milbank Memorial Fund Quarterly* 65, S1: 129–99.

Marable, Manning. 1995. *Beyond Black and White*. London: Verso Books.

Marcuse, Herbert. 1969. 'Repressive Tolerance'. In *A Critique of Pure Tolerance*, edited by R. P. Wolff, Barrington Moore Jr. and Herbert Marcuse, 95–137. Boston: Beacon Opress.

Marinac, Jacqueline S., Buchinger, Colleen L., Godfrey, Lincoln A., Wooten, James M., Sun, Xchao and Willsie, Sandra K. 2007. 'Herbal Products and Dietary Supplements: A Survey of Use Attitudes and Knowledge among Older Adults'. *Journal of the American Osteopaths Association* 107, no. 1: 13–23.

Markey, C. N. and Markey, P. M. 2010. 'A Correlational and Experimental Examination of Reality Television Viewing and Interest in Cosmetic Surgery'. *Body Image* 7: 165–71.

Marshall, Barbara L. 1994. *Engendering Modernity: Feminism, Social Theory and Social Change*. Cambridge: Polity Press.

———. 2007. 'Climacteric Redux? (Re)Medicalizing the Male Menopause'. *Men and Masculinities* 9: 509–29.

———. 2009. 'Rejuvenation's Return: Anti-Aging and Re-Masculinization in Biomedical Discourse on the "Aging Male"'. *Medicine Studies* 1, no. 3: 249–65.

———. 2011. 'The Graying of "Sexual Health": A Critical Research Agenda'. *Canadian Review of Sociology* 48, no. 4: 390–413.

Marshall, Barbara L. and Katz, Stephen. 2002. 'Forever Functional: Sexual Fitness and the Ageing Male Body'. *Body & Society* 8, no. 4: 43–70.

Martén, Esteban, Langevin, Claude-Jean, Kaswan, Sumesh and Zins, James E. 2011. 'The Safety of Rhytidectomy in the Elderly'. *Plastic and Reconstructive Surgery* 127: 2455–63.

Martin, Claude R. 1976. 'A Transgenerational Comparison: The Elderly Fashion Consumer'. *Advances in Consumer Research* 3: 453–6.

Marwick, Arthur. 1998. *The Sixties*. Oxford: Oxford University Press.

Maseres, Francis. 1792. *A Proposal for Establishing Life-Annuities in Parishes for the Industrious Poor*. London.

Mauss, Marcel. 1973. 'Techniques of the Body'. *Economy & Society* 2: 70–88.

McCall, L. 2005. 'The Complexity of Intersectionality'. *Journal of Women in Culture and Society* 30, no. 3: 1771–1800.

McCruer, Robert. 2006. *Crip Theory: Cultural Signs of Queerness and Disability*. New York: New York University Press.

———. 2010. 'Disability Nationalism in Crip Times'. *Journal of Literary & Cultural Disability Studies* 4, no. 2: 163–78.

McDougall, Andrew. 2012. 'Big Opportunity in Men's Skin Care'. http://www.comsteicsdesign.com/content/view/print/612103 (accessed 12 March 2012).

McMullin, Julie. 1995. 'Theorizing Age and Gender Relations'. In *Connecting Gender & Ageing: A Sociological Approach*, edited by Sara Arber and Jay Ginn, 30–41. Buckingham: Open University Press.

McNay, Lois. 1992. *Foucault & Feminism*. Cambridge: Polity Press.

Mellor, Philip A. and Shilling, Chris. 1997. *Re-Forming the Body: Religion, Community and Modernity*. London: Sage Publications.

Merleau-Ponty, Maurice. 1962. *The Phenomenology of Perception*. London: Routledge.

———. 1968. *The Visible and the Invisible*. Evanston: Northwestern University Press.

Mendes, Valerie and de la Haye, Amy. 1999. *20th Century Fashion*. London: Thames & Hudson.

Michelon, L. C. 1954. 'The New Leisure Class'. *American Journal of Sociology* 59: 371–8.

Milam, Lorenzo W. 1983. *The Cripple Liberation Front Marching Band Blues*. Los Angeles: Mho & Mho Works.

Millard, Peter and Higgs, Paul. 1989. 'Geriatric Medicine beyond the Hospital'. *Age and Ageing* 18, no. 1: 1–3.

Miller, Daniel. 2012. *Consumption and its Consequences*. Cambridge: Polity Press.
Miller, Laura. 2003. 'Male Beauty Work in Japan'. In *Men and Masculinites in Contemporary Japan*, edited by James E. Robertson and Nobue Suzuko, 37–58. London: Routledge.
Millett, Kate. 1972. *Sexual Politics*. London: Abacus.
Minkler, Meredith and Cole, Thomas A. 1991. 'Political and Moral Economy: Not such Strange Bedfellows'. In *Critical Perspectives on Aging: The Political and Moral Economy of Growing Old*, edited by Meredith Minkler and Carol L. Estes, 37–50. Amityville: Baywood Publishing.
Minkler, Meredith and Fadem, Pamela. 2002. '"Successful Ageing": A Disability Perspective'. *Journal of Disability Policy Studies* 12, no. 4: 229–35.
Minkler, Meredith and Stone, Robyn L. 1983. 'The Feminization of Poverty and Older Women'. *The Gerontologist* 25, no. 4: 351–7.
Minnigerode, F. A. 1976. 'Age-Status Labeling in Homosexual Men'. *Journal of Homosexuality* 1, no. 3: 273–6.
Minois, George. 1989. *History of Old Age*. Cambridge: Polity Press.
Mitchell, David T. and Snyder, Sharon L. 2003. 'The Eugenic Atlantic: Race, Disability and the Making of an International Eugenic Science, 1800–1945'. *Disability & Society* 18: 843–64.
———. 2010. 'Disability as Multitude: Re-Working Non-Productive Labor Power'. *Journal of Literary & Cultural Disability Studies* 4, no. 2: 179–93.
Mitchell, Juliet. 1971. *Woman's Estate*. Harmondsworth: Penguin Books.
Montagna, William and Carlisle, Kay. 1991. 'The Architecture of Black and White Facial Skin'. *Journal of the American Academy of Dermatology* 24: 929–37.
Morley, John E. 2004. 'The Aging Man and Woman: Are the Differences Important?' *JMHG* 1, nos. 2/3: 224–6.
Morrison, Toni. 1974. 'Rediscovering Black History'. *The New York Times Magazine*, 11 August.
Morrell, Carolyn, M. 2003. 'Empowerment and Long-Living Women: Return to the Rejected Body'. *Journal of Aging Studies* 17, no. 2: 69–85.
Morrow-Howell, Nancy, Hinterlong, James and Sherraden, Michael. 2001. *Productive Aging: Concepts and Challenges*. Baltimore: John Hopkins University Press.
Moser, Ingunn. 2005. 'On Becoming Disabled and Articulating Alternatives'. *Cultural Studies* 19, no. 6: 667–700.
Muise, Amy and Desmarais, Serge. 2010. 'Women's Perceptions of and Use of "Anti-Aging" Products'. *Sex Roles* 63: 126–37.
Mumel, Damijan and Prodnik, Jadranka. 2005. 'Grey Consumers Are all the Same, they Even Dress the Same: Myth or Reality?' *Journal of Fashion Marketing and Management* 9, no. 4: 434–49.
Muraco, Anna, LeBlanc, Allen J. and Russell, Stephen T. 2008. 'Conceptualizations of Family by Older Gay Men'. *Journal of Gay & Lesbian Social Services* 20, nos. 1/2: 69–90.
Murray, John M., McDonald, Ann M. and Law, Matthew G. 2009. 'Rapidly Ageing HIV Epidemic among Men who Have Sex with Men in Australia'. *Sexual Health* 6: 83–6.
Mutchler, Jan E. and Burr, Jeffrey A. 2011. 'Race, Ethnicity and Aging'. In *Handbook of Sociology of Ageing*, edited by Richard A. Settersen and Jacqueline L. Angel, 83–101. New York: Springer.
Naidoo, Serena, Anderson, Stephanie, Mills, Joanna, Parsons, Stephanie, Breeden, Stephanie, Bevan, Emma, Edwards, Camilla and Otter, Simon. 2011. '"I Could Cry, the Amount of Shoes I Can't Get Into": A Qualitative Exploration of the Factors that Influence Retail Footwear Selection in Women with Rheumatoid Arthritis'. *Journal of Foot and Ankle Research* 4, no. 21.
Namaste, Ki. 1994. 'The Politics of Inside/Out: Queer Theory, Post Structuralism and a Sociological Approach to Sexuality'. *Sociological Theory* 12, no. 2: 220–31.
National Urban League. 1964. *Double jeopardy: The Older Negro in America*. New York: NUL.
Neal, Mark Anthony. 2002. *Soul Babies: Black Popular Culture and the Post-Soul Aesthetic*. New York: Routledge.

Nealon, Jeffery. 2008. *Foucault Beyond Foucault: Power and its Intensifications since 1984*. Stanford: Stanford University Press.
Neugarten, Bernice. 1974. 'Age Groups in American Society and the Rise of the Young-Old'. *The Annals of the American Academy of Political and Social Science* 415, no. 1: 187–98.
Newman, Andrew Adam. 2010. 'Men's Cosmetics Becoming a Bull Market'. *The New York Times*, 1 September. http://nytimes.com/2010/09/02/fashion/02skin.html?pagewanted=all (accessed 21 April 2011).
Newman, Katherine S. 2003. *A Different Shade of Gray: Midlife and Beyond in the Inner City*. New York: The New Press.
Nicolosi, Alfredo, Moreira, Edson D., Shirai, M., Bin Mohd Tambi, M. I. and Glasser, Dale B. 2003. 'Epidemiology of Erectile Dysfunction in Four Countries: Cross National Study of the Prevalence and Correlates of Erectile Dysfunction'. *Urology* 61: 201–6.
Nkengne, A., Bertin, C., Stamatas, G., Giron, A., Rossi, A., Issacher, N. and Fertil, B. 2008. 'Influence of Facial Skin Attributes on the Perceived Age of Caucasian Women'. *Journal of the European Academy of Dermatology and Venereology* 22: 982–91.
Norman, Alison. 1985. *Triple Jeopardy: Growing Old in a Second Homeland*. London: Centre for Policy on Ageing.
North, Joseph E. 1963. 'The Cosmetics and Toiletries Industry'. *Financial Analysts Journal* 19, 1: 39–50.
O'Connor, Kaori. 2008. 'The Body and the Brand: How Lycra Shaped America'. In *Producing Fashion: Commerce, Culture and Consumers*, edited by Regina Lee Blaszcyk, 207–27. Philadelphia: University of Pennsylvania Press.
Ó Gradá, Cormac. 2002. '"The Greatest Blessing of them All": The Old Age Pension in Ireland'. *Past and Present* 175: 124–61.
O'Rand, Angela M. 1996. 'The Precious and the Precocious: Understanding Cumulative Disadvantage and Cumulative Advantage over the Life Course'. *The Gerontologist* 36: 230–38.
Öberg, Peter and Tornstam, Lars. 2001. 'Youthfulness and Fitness – Identity Ideals for all Ages?' *Journal of Aging and Identity* 6, no. 1: 15–29.
Odunze, Millicent, Reid, Russell R., Yu, Maurice B. S. and Few, Julius W. 2006. 'Periorbital Rejuvenation and the African American Patient: A Survey Approach'. *Plastic and Reconstructive Surgery* 118, no. 4: 1011–18.
Ogbar, Jeffrey O. G. 2004 *Black Power: Radical Politics and African American Identity*. Baltimore: John Hopkins University Press.
Oldman, Christine. 2002. 'Later Life and the Social Mode of Disability: A Comfortable Partnership?' *Ageing & Society* 22, no. 6: 791–806.
Oliver, Michael. 1990. *The Politics of Disablement*. London: Macmillan Education.
Oliver, Michael. 1995. *Understanding Disability: From Theory to Practice*. Basingstoke: Palgrave.
Oliveria, Susan A., Christos, Paul J., Halpern, Allan C., Fine, Judith A., Barnhill, Raymond L. and Berwick, Marianne. 1999. 'Evaluation of Factors Associated with Skin Self-Examination'. *Cancer Epidemiology, Biomarkers & Prevention* 8, no. 7: 971–8.
Ongiri, Amy Abugo. 2010 *Spectacular Blackness: The Cultural Politics of the Black Power Movement and the Search for a Black Aesthetic*. Charlottesville: University of Virginia Press.
Oppenheimer, S. 1920. 'A Condemnatory Note on the Use of Paraffin in Cosmetic Rhinoplasty'. *The Laryngoscope* 30: 595–6.
Orel, Nancy A. and Fruhauf, Christine A. 2006. 'Lesbian and Bisexual Grandmothers' Perceptions of the Grandparent-Grandchild Relationship'. *Journal of GLBT Family Studies* 2, no. 1: 43–70.
Oriel, J. 2005. 'Sexual Pleasure as a Human Right: Harmful or Helpful to Women in the Context of HIV/AIDS'. *Women's Studies International Forum* 28, no. 8: 392–404.
Oudshoorn, Nelly 1994. *Beyond the Natural Body: An Archaeology of Sex Hormones*. London: Routledge.

Paine, Thomas. (1792) 1958. *The Rights of Man*. London: J. M. Dent & Sons.
Paleotti, Gabriele. 1506. *De Bono Senectutis*, Antwerp.
Palma, Diego Dalla. 2008. 'Looking Younger: Cosmetics and Clothing to Look More Vibrant'. *Clinics in Dermatology* 26, no. 6: 648–51.
Peacock, J. R. 2000. 'Gay Male Adult Development: Some Stage Issues of an Older Cohort'. *Journal of Homosexuality* 40, no. 1: 13–29.
Pearson, Stephen J., Young, Archie, Macaluso, Andrea, Devito, Giuseppe, Nimmo, Myra A., Cobbold, Matthew and Harridge, Stephen D. 2002. 'Muscle Function in Elite Master Weightlifters'. *Medicine & Science in Sports & Exercise* 34, no. 7: 1199–1206.
Peiss, Kathy. 1996. 'Making Up, Making Over: Cosmetics, Consumer Culture and Women's Identity'. In *The Sex of Things: Gender and Consumption in Historical Perspective*, edited by Victoria de Grazia and Ellen Furlough, 311–36. Berkeley: University of California Press.
———. 1998. *Hope in a Jar: The Making of America's Beauty Industry*. New York: Metropolitan Books.
Peters, Walter. 1991. 'The Chemical Peel'. *Annals of Plastic Surgery* 26: 564–71.
Petersen, Christina Bjørk, Thygesen, Lau Caspar, Helge, Jørn Wulff, Grønbæk, Morten and Tolstrup, Janne Schurmann. 2010. 'Time Trends in Physical Activity in Leisure Time in the Danish Population from 1987 to 2005'. *Scandinavian Journal of Public Health* 38, no. 2: 121–8.
Petigny, Alan. 2004. 'Illegitimacy, Postwar Psychology and the Reperiodization of the Sexual Revolution'. *Journal of Social History* 38, no. 1: 63–79.
Petrie, K. J., Faasse, K. E. and Fuhrmann, S. A. 2008. 'Influence of Television on Demand for Cosmetic Surgery'. *Medical Journal of Australia* 189, no. 5: 244–5.
Pfeiffer, Eric, Verwoerdt, Adriaan and Wang, Hsioh-Shan. 1968. 'Sexual Behavior in Aged Men and Women: Observations on 254 Community Volunteers'. *Archives of General Psychiatry* 19: 753–8.
———. 1969. 'The Natural History of Sexual Behavior in a Biologically Advantaged Group of Aged Individuals'. *Journal of Gerontology* 24: 193–8.
Phillipson, Chris. 1982. *Capitalism and the Construction of Old Age*. London: Macmillan Press.
Phoenix, Cassandra and Smith, Brett. 2011. 'Telling a (Good?) Counterstory of Aging: Natural Bodybuilding Meets the Narrative of Decline'. *Journals of Gerontology, Series B: Psychological and Social Sciences* 66, no. 5: 628–39.
Pickard, Susan. 2010. 'The Role of Governmentality in the Establishment, Maintenance and Demise of Professional Jurisdictions: The Case of Geriatric Medicine'. *Sociology of Health & Illness* 32, no. 7: 1–15.
———. 2011. 'Health, Illness and Normality: The Case of Old Age'. *BioSocieties* 6: 323–41.
Pinkham, Charles B. 1926. 'News Items from the Californian Board of Medical Examiners'. *California and Western Medicine* 25, no. 4: 531.
Pitts, Victoria. 2003. *In the Flesh: The Cultural Politics of Body Modification*. New York: Palgrave Macmillan.
Plann, Susan. 2006. *A Silent Minority: Deaf Education in Spain, 1550–1835*. Berkeley: University of California Press.
Pliner, Patricia, Chaiken, Shelly and Flett, Gordon L. 1990. 'Gender Differences in Concern with Body Weight and Physical Appearance over the Life Span'. *Personality and Social Psychology Bulletin* 16, no. 2: 263–73.
Pohl, Joanna M. and Boyd, Carol J. 1993. 'Ageism within Feminism'. *Journal of Nursing Scholarship* 25, no. 3: 199–205.
Polivka, Larry. 2011. 'Neoliberalism and the Postmodern Culture of Aging'. *Journal of Applied Gerontology* 48, no. 5: 564–72.
Pope, M. 1997. 'Sexual Issues for Older Lesbians and Gays'. *Topics in Geriatric Rehabilitation* 12: 53–60.
Prins, J., Blanker, M. H., Bohnen, A. M., Thomas, S. and Bosch, J. L. 2002. 'Prevalence of Erectile Dysfunction: A Systematic Review of Population-Based Studies'. *International Journal of Impotence Research* 14: 422–32.

Prus, Steven G., Tfaily, Rania and Lin, Zhiqiu. 2010. 'Comparing Racial and Immigrant Health Status and Health Care Access in Later Life in Canada and the United States'. *Canadian Journal on Aging* 29, no. 3: 383–95.

Pullin, Graham. 2009. *Design meets Disability*. Harvard: The Massachusetts Institute of Technology Press.

Putnam, Michelle. 2002. 'Linking Aging Theory and Disability Models: Increasing the Potential to Explore Aging with Physical Impairment'. *The Gerontologist* 42, no. 6: 799–806.

Quinlan, F. J. 1902. 'Paraffin Injections for Nasal and other Facial Deformities, with Exhibition of a New Instrument'. *The Laryngoscope* 12: 604–8.

Ray, Ruth E. 2004. 'Toward the Croning of Feminist Gerontology'. *Journal of Aging Studies* 18, no. 2: 109–21.

Reaburn, Peter and Dascombe, Ben. 2009. 'Anaerobic Performance in Masters Athletes'. *European Review of Aging and Physical Activity* 6, no. 1: 39–53.

Reece, Michael, Herbenick, Debby, Schick, Vanessa, Sanders, Stephanie A., Dodge, Brian and Fortenberry J. Dennis. 2010. 'Sexual Behaviors, Relationships and Perceived Health Status among Adult Men in the United States: Results from a National Probability Sample'. *Journal of Sexual Medicine* 7, Suppl. 5: 291–304.

Reel, Justine J., SooHoo, Sonya, Franklin Summerhays, Julia and Gill, Diane L. 2008. 'Age before Beauty: An Exploration of Body Image in African-American and Caucasian Adult Women'. *Journal of Gender Studies* 17, no. 4: 321–30.

Reid, K., Surridge, D. H., Morales, A., Condra, M., Harris, C., Owen, J. and Fenemore, J. 1987. 'Double-Blind Trial of Yohimbine in Treatment of Psychogenic Impotence'. *Lancet* 2: 421–3.

Reisenwitz, Timothy and Iyer, Rajesh. 2007. 'A Comparison of Younger and Older Baby Boomers: Investigating the Viability of Cohort Segmentation'. *Journal of Consumer Marketing* 24, no. 4: 202–13.

Reveille-Parise, J. H. 1854. *Traité de la vieillesse hygiénique, médical et philosophique*. Paris: J. B. Baillière.

Reynolds, Fred D. and Wells, William D. 1977. *Consumer Behavior*. New York: McGraw-Hill.

Richters, J., Grulich, A. E., de Visser, R. O., Smith, A. M. and Rissel, C. E. 2003. 'Sexual Difficulties in a Representative Sample of Adults'. *Australia New Zealand Journal of Public Health* 27: 164–70.

Ring, Anne L. 2002. 'Using "Anti-Ageing" to Market Cosmetic Surgery: Just Good Business or Another Wrinkle on the Face of Medical Practice?' *MJA* 176: 597–9.

Ringel, E. W. 1998. 'The Morality of Cosmetic Surgery for Aging'. *Archives of Dermatology* 134: 427–31.

Ritzer, George. 1996. *The McDonaldization of Society*. Thousand Oaks: Pine Forge Press.

Roberts, Celia. 2007. *Messengers of Sex: Hormones, Biomedicine and Feminism*. Cambridge: Cambridge University Press.

Robinson, Lucy. 2006. 'Three Revolutionary Years: The Impact of the Counter-Culture on the Development of the Gay Liberation Movement in Britain'. *Cultural and Social History* 3: 445–71.

Rodgers, Daniel T. 2011. *The Age of Fracture*. Boston: Harvard University Press.

Roebuck, Janet. 1979. 'When Does "Old Age" Begin? The Evolution of the English Definition'. *Journal of Social History* 12, no. 3: 416–28.

Roets, Griet and Braidotti, Rosi. 2012. 'Nomadology and Subjectivity: Deleuze, Guattari and Critical Disability Studies'. In *Disability and Social Theory: New Developments and Directions*, edited by Dan Goodley, Bill Hughes and Lennard Davis. Basingstoke: Palgrave Macmillan.

Rogers, Blair O. 1976. 'The Development of Aesthetic Plastic Surgery: A History'. *Aesthetic Plastic Surgery* 1: 3–24.

Romanelli, F. and Smith, K. M. 2004. 'Recreational Use of Sidenafil by HIV-Positive and -Negative Homosexual/Bisexual Males'. *Annals of Pharmacotherapy* 38, no. 6: 1024–30.

Rooks, Noliwe M. 1996. *Hair Raising: Beauty, Culture and African American Women*. New Brunswick: Rutgers University Press.

———. 2004. *Ladies' Pages: African American Women's Magazines and the Culture that Made Them*. New Brunswick: Rutgers University Press.

Rose, Nicholas. 2001. 'The Politics of Life Itself'. *Theory, Culture & Society* 18, no. 6: 1–30.

Rosen, Ruth. 2000. *The World Split Open: How the Modern Women's Movement Changed America*. New York: Viking.

Ross, Edward A. 1921. *Principles of Sociology*. New York: The Century Co.

Rothman, Sheila M. and Rothman, David J. 2004. *The Pursuit of Perfection: The Promise and Perils of Medical Enhancement*. New York: Vintage Books.

Rowbotham, Sheila. 2011. *Dreamers of a New Day*. London: Verso Books.

Rowe, James W. and Kahn, Robert L. 1987. 'Human Ageing: Usual and Successful'. *Science* 237: 143–9.

———. 1997. 'Successful Aging'. *The Gerontologist* 37, no. 4: 433–40.

Rowntree, Seebohm. 1902. *Poverty: A Study of Town Life*. London: Macmillan.

Rubino, Corrado, Farace, Francesco, Dessy, Luca A., Sanna, Marco P.G. and Mazzarello, Vittorio. 2005. 'A Prospective Study of Anti-Aging Topical Therapies Using a Quantitative Method of Assessment'. *Plastic and Reconstructive Surgery* 115: 1156–62.

Russell, Cherry. 1987. 'Ageing as a Feminist Issue'. *Women's Studies International Forum* 10, no. 2: 125–32.

———. 2007. 'What Do Older Women and Men Want? Gender Differences in the "Lived Experience" of Ageing'. *Current Sociology* 55, no. 2: 173–92.

Sakamoto, Arthur, Wu, Huei-Hsia and Tzeng, Jessie M.. 2000. 'The Declining Significance of Race among American Men during the Latter Half of the Twentieth Century'. *Demography* 37, no. 1: 41–51.

Sandberg, Linn. 2008. 'The Old, the Ugly and the Queer: Thinking Old Age in Relation to Queer Theory'. *Graduate Journal of Social Science* 5, no. 2: 117–39.

Sandoval, Daniel A., Rank, Mark R. and Hirschl, Thomas A. 2009. 'The Increasing Risk of Poverty across the American Life Course'. *Demography* 46, no. 4: 717–37.

Sassatelli, Roberta. 2007. *Consumer Culture: History, Theory and Politics*. London: Sage Publications.

Sawicki, Jana. 1988. 'Feminism and the Power of Discourse'. In *After Foucault: Humanistic Knowledge, Postmodern Challenges*, edited by J. Arac, 161–78. New Brunswick: Rutgers University Press.

Scherrer, Kristin S. 2009. 'Images of Sexuality and Aging in Gerontological Literature'. *Sexuality Research and Social Policy* 6, no. 4: 5–12.

Schofield, Nancy A. and LaBat, Karen L. 2005. 'Exploring the Relationships of Grading, Sizing and Anthropomorphic Data'. *Clothing and Textiles Research Journal* 23, no. 1: 13–27.

Schonfield, David. 1967. 'Geronting: Reflections on Successful Aging'. *The Gerontologist* 7, no. 4: 270–4.

Schope, Robert D. 2005. 'Who's Afraid of Growing Old?' *Journal of Gerontological Social Work* 45: 23–39.

Schwaiger, E. 2009. 'Performing Youth: Ageing, Ambiguity and Bodily Integrity'. *Social Identities* 15, no. 2: 273–84.

Schweik, Susan M. 2009. *The Ugly Laws: Disability in Public*. New York: New York University Press.

Scotch, Richard K. 1989. 'Politics and Policy in the History of the Disability Rights Movement'. *The Milbank Quarterly* 67, Suppl. 2: 380–400.

Scott, Joan W. 1986. 'Gender: A Useful Category of Historical Analysis'. *The American History Review* 91, no. 5: 1053–75.

Searle, G. 1971. *The Quest for National Efficiency: A Study in British Politics and Political Thought, 1899–1914*. London: Blackwell Publishers.

Sears, James T. 2008. 'Introduction: Queering Later Life'. *Journal of Gay & Lesbian Social Services* 20, no. 1: 1–4.
Seidman, Steven. 1997. *Difference Troubles: Queering Social Theory and Sexual Politics*. Cambridge: Cambridge University Press.
———. 1998. *Contested Knowledge: Social Theory in the Postmodern Era*. 2nd ed. London: Blackwell Publishers.
Seiler, K. S., Spirduso, W. W. and Martin, J. C. 1998. 'Gender Differences in Rowing Performance and Power with Aging'. *Medicine & Science in Sports & Exercise* 30, no. 1: 121–7.
Serri, Riccarda. 2008. 'Combating Aging Skin: Part II'. *Clinics in Dermatology* 26, no. 6: 589.
Seymour, Richard G. 2008. *Gay Men Getting Older: An Interpretive Study*. PhD diss., University of Sheffield.
Shakespeare, Tom. 1993. 'Disabled People's Self-Organisation: A New Social Movement?' *Disability, Handicap & Society* 8, no. 3: 249–64.
Shanas, Ethel, Townsend, Peter, Wedderburn, Dorothy, Friis, Henning, Milhoj, Poul and Stehouwer, Jan. 1968. *Old People in Three Industrial Societies*. London: Tavistock Press.
Sheehy, Gail. 1977. *Passages: Predictable Crises of Adult Life*. London: Corgi.
———. 1982. *Pathfinders: How to Achieve Happiness by Conquering Life's Crises*. London: Sidgwick and Jackson.
Shenk, Dena, Zablotsky, Diane and Croom, Mary Beth. 1998. 'Thriving Older African American Women: Aging after Jim Crow'. *Journal of Women & Aging* 10, no. 1: 75–95.
Sherkat, Darren E., Kilbourne, Cain, Van A., Hull, Pamela C., Levine, Robert S. and Husaini, Baqar A. 2007. 'The Impact of Health Service Use on Racial Differences in Mortality among the Elderly'. *Research on Aging* 29, no. 3: 207–24.
Shildrick, Margrit. 2005. 'The Disabled Body, Genealogy and Undecidability'. *Cultural Studies* 19: 755–70.
———. 2009. *Dangerous Discourses of Disability, Subjectivity and Sexuality*. London: Palgrave Macmillan.
Shilling, Chris. 1993. *The Body and Social Theory*. London: Sage Publications.
Shpall, Rebecca, Beddingfield, Fredrick C., Watson, Deborah and Lask, Gary P. 2004. 'Microdermabrasion: A Review'. *Facial Plastic Surgery* 20: 47–50.
Shuey, Kim M. and Willson, Andrea E. 2008. 'Cumulative Disadvantage and Black-White Disparities in Life Course Health Trajectories'. *Research on Aging* 30: 200–25.
Siebers, Tobin. 2001. 'Disability in Theory: From Social Constructionism to the New Realism of the Body'. *American Literary History* 13: 737–54.
Sigal, R. K., Weston, G. W., Poindexter, B. D. and Austin, H. W. 2000. 'Rejuvenating the Aged Face'. *Perspectives in Plastic Surgery* 14, no. 2: 1–36.
Silver, C. B. 2003. 'Gendered Identities in Old Age: Toward (De)Gendering?' *Journal of Aging Studies* 17, no. 4: 379–97.
Silverstein, Michael J. and Fiske, Neil. 2003. 'Luxury for the Masses'. *Harvard Business Review* 81, no. 4: 48–57.
Simmel, Georg. 1957. 'Fashion'. *American Journal of Sociology* 62: 541–58.
Simons, J. S and Carey, M. P. 2001. 'Prevalence of Sexual Dysfunctions: Results from a Decade of Research'. *Archives of Sexual Behavior* 30: 177–219.
Slater, Don and Tonkiss, Frank. 2001. *Market Society: Markets and Modern Social Theory*. Cambridge: Polity Press.
Slevin, Katherine F. and Linneman, Thomas. 2010. 'Old Gay Men's Bodies and Masculinities'. *Men and Masculinities* 12, no. 4: 483–507.
Smaje, Chris. 2000. *Natural Hierarchies: The Historical Sociology of Race and Caste*. Malden: Blackwell Publishers.
Smith, Dennis. 2001. *Norbert Elias & Modern Social Theory*. London: Sage Publications.
Solomon, Felicia M., Linnan, Laura M., Wasilewski, Yvonne, Lee, Ann Marie, Katz, Mira L. and Yang, Jingzhen. 2004. 'Observational Study in Ten Beauty Salons: Results Informing

Development of the North Carolina BEAUTY and Health Project'. *Health Education and Behavior* 31, no. 6: 790–807.

Soriano, Rainier P., Fernandez, Helen M., Cassel, Christine K. and Leipzig, Rosanne M. 2007. *Fundamentals of Geriatric Medicine: A Case-Based Approach*. New York: Springer.

Souiden, Nizar and Diagne, Mariam. 2009. 'Canadian and French Men's Consumption of Cosmetics: A Comparison of their Attitudes and Motivations'. *Journal of Consumer Culture* 26, no. 2: 97–109.

Snyder, J. E. 2011. 'Trend Analysis of Medical Publications about LGBT Persons: 1950–2007'. *Journal of Homosexuality* 58, no. 2: 164–88.

Snyder, Sharon L. and Mitchell, David T. 2001. 'Re-Engaging the Body: Disability Studies and the Resistance to Embodiment'. *Public Culture* 13, no. 3: 367–89.

———. 2006. *Cultural Locations of Disability*. Chicago: University of Chicago Press.

Sohm, Philip. 2007. *The Artist Grows Old: The Aging of Art and Artists in Italy, 1500–1800*. New Haven: Yale University Press.

Spector-Mersel, Gabriela. 2006. 'Never-Aging Stories: Western Hegemonic Masculinity Scripts'. *Journal of Gender Studies* 15, no. 1: 67–82.

Steinach, Eugen and Löbel, Josef. 1940. *Sex and Life: Forty Years of Biological and Medical Experiments*. London: Faber and Faber.

Steincrohn, Peter. 1942. *You Don't Have to Exercise: Rest Begins at Forty*. New York: Doubleday, Doran and Company.

Stern, Marc. 2008. 'The Fitness Movement and the Fitness Center Industry, 1960–2000'. *Business and Economic History Online* 6: 1–26. http://www.thebhc.org/publications/BEHonline/2008/stern.pdf (accessed 12 March 2012).

Strehler, Bernard. 1962. *Time, Cells and Aging*. New York: Academic Press.

Stiker, Henri-Jacques. 1999. *A History of Disability*. Ann Arbor: University of Michigan Press.

Struhkamp, Rita. 2005. 'Wordless Pain'. *Cultural Studies* 19, no. 6: 701–18.

Sturm-O'Brien, Angela K., Brissett, Annette E. A. and Brissett, Anthony E. 2010. 'Ethnic Trends in Facial Plastic Surgery'. *Facial and Plastic Surgery* 26: 69–74.

Sullivan, Deborah A. 2001. *Cosmetic Surgery: The Cutting Edge of Commercial Medicine in America*. London: Rutgers University Press.

Suominen, Harri. 2011. 'Ageing and Maximal Physical Performance'. *European Review of Aging and Physical Activity* 8, no. 1: 37–42.

Swearingen, S. G. and Klausner, J. D. 2005. 'Sildenafil Use, Risky Behavior and Risk for Sexually Transmitted Diseases, Including HIV Infection'. *American Journal of Medicine* 118, no. 6: 571–7.

Sydie, R. A. 2004. 'Sex and the Sociological Fathers'. In *Engendering the Social: Feminist Encounters with Sociological Theory*, edited by Barbara L. Marshall and Anne Witz, 36–53. Maidenhead: Open University Press.

Taub, Amy Forman, Sarnoff, Deborah, Gold, Michael and Jacob, Carolyn. 2010. 'Effect of Multisyringe Hyaluronic Acid Facial Rejuvenation on Perceived Age'. *Dermatologic Surgery* 36: 322–8.

Taylor, Miles G. 2008. 'Timing, Accumulation and the Black/White Disability Gap in Later Life: A Test of Weathering'. *Research on Aging* 30: 226–50.

Taylor, Paul C. 2007. 'Post-Black, Old Black'. *African American Review* 41, no. 4: 625–40.

Taylor, Paul C., Wang, Wendy, Parker, Kim, Passel, Jeffrey S., Patten, Eileen and Motel, Seth. 2012. *The Rise of Intermarriage*. Washington: Pew Research Centre.

Taylor, Susan C. 2002. 'Skin of Color: Biology, Structure, Function and Implications for Dermatologic Disease'. *Journal of the American Academy of Dermatology* 46: S41–62.

Teasley, Martell and Ikard, David. 2010. 'Barack Obama and the Politics of Race: The Myth of Postracism in America'. *Journal of Black Studies* 40, no. 3: 411–25.

Theoharides, Theoharis C. 1971. 'Galen on Marasmus'. *Journal of the History of Medicine and Allied Sciences* 26, no. 4: 369–90.

Thomas, Carol. 2004. 'How is Disability Understood? An Examination of Sociological Approaches'. *Disability & Society* 19, no. 6: 569–83.

———. 2007. *Sociologies of Disability and Illness. Contested Ideas in Disability Studies and Medical Sociology*. Basingstoke: Palgrave.

Thomson, A. P. 1949. 'Problems of Ageing and Chronic Sickness'. *BMJ* 2: 300–305.

Thompson, E. H. 2000. 'Older Men as Invisible Men in Contemporary Society'. In *Older Men's Lives*, edited by E. H. Thompson, 1–21. Thousand Oaks: Sage Publications.

Tiggemann, Marika and Kenyon, Sarah J. 1998. 'The Hairlessness Norm: The Removal of Body Hair in Women'. *Sex Roles* 39, nos. 11/12: 873–85.

Tischer, Ulrike, Hartmann-Tews, Ilse and Combrink, Claudia. 2011. 'Sport Participation of the Elderly – the Role of Gender, Age and Social Class'. *European Review of Aging and Physical Activity* 8, no. 1: 83–91.

Titmuss, Richard M. 1976. *Essays on the Welfare State*. 3rd ed. London: Allen & Unwin.

Tonnard, Patrick, Verpaele, Alexis, Monstrey, Stan, Van Landuyt, Koen, Blondeel, Philippe, Hamdi, Moustapha and Matton, Guido. 2002. 'Minimal Access Cranial Suspension Lift: A Modified S-Lift'. *Plastic and Reconstructive Surgery* 109, no. 6: 2074–86.

Tornstam, Lars. 1996. 'Gerotranscendence: A Theory about Maturing into Old Age'. *Journal of Aging and Identity* 1, no. 1: 37–50.

Townsend, Peter. 1963. *The Family Life of Old People*. Harmondsworth: Penguin Books.

———. 1973a. *The Social Minority*. London: Allen Lane Press.

———. 1973b. 'Elderly People with Disabilities'. In *Disability in Britain*, edited by Alan Walker and Peter Townsend, 52–72. Oxford: Martin Robertson.

Tremain, Shelley. 1995. 'Foucault, Governmentality and Critical Disability Theory'. In *Foucault and the Government of Disability*, edited by Shelley Tremain, 1–24. Ann Arbor: University of Michigan Press.

———. 2002. 'On the Subject of Impairment'. In *Disability/Postmodernity: Embodying Disability Theory*, edited by Mairian Corker and Tom Shakespeare, 32–47. London: Continuum.

Trost, Stewart G., Owen, Neville, Bauman, Adrian E., Salis, James F. and Brown, Wendy. 2002. 'Correlates of Adults' Participation in Physical Activity: Review and Update'. *Medicine & Science in Sports & Exercise* 34, no. 12: 1996–2001.

Trotman, Frances K. 2002. 'Historical, Economic and Political Contexts of Aging in African America'. *Journal of Women & Aging* 14, 3: 121–38.

Tsunokai, Glenn T. and McGrath, Allison R. 2011. 'Baby Boomers and Beyond: Crossing Racial Boundaries in Search of Love'. *Journal of Aging Studies* 25, no. 3: 285–94.

Tulle-Winton, Emmanuelle. 1999. 'Growing Old and Resistance: Towards a New Cultural Economy of Old Age?' *Ageing & Society* 19, no. 3: 281–99.

Tulle, Emmanuelle. 2008. 'Acting your Age? Sports Science and the Ageing Body'. *Journal of Aging Studies* 22, no. 6: 340–47.

Turner, Bryan S. 1984. *The Body and Society*. Oxford: Basil Blackwell.

———. 1991. 'Recent Developments in the Theory of the Body'. In *The Body: Social Process and Cultural Theory*, edited by Mike Featherstone, Mike Hepworth and Bryan S. Turner, 1–35. London: Sage Publications.

———. 1996. *The Body & Society: Explorations in Social Theory*. 2nd ed. London: Sage Publications.

Turner, Charles F., Danella, Rose D. and Rogers, Susan M. 1995. 'Sexual Behavior in the United States, 1930–1990: Trends and Methodological Problems'. *Sexually Transmitted Diseases* 22, no. 3: 173–90.

Twigg, Julia. 2004. 'The Body, Gender and Age: Feminist Insights in Social Gerontology'. *Journal of Aging Studies* 18, no. 1: 59–73.

———. 2007. 'Clothing, Age and the Body: A Critical Review'. *Ageing & Society* 27: 285–305.

———. 2012. 'Adjusting the Cut: Fashion, the Body and Age on the UK High Street'. *Ageing & Society*, DOI: 10.1017/S0144686X11000754.
Twigg, Julia and Atkin, Karl. 2000. 'Carework as a Form of Bodywork'. *Ageing & Society* 20: 389–411.
Valet, F., Ezzedine, K., Malvy, D., Mary, J. Y. and Guinot, C. 2009. 'Assessing the Reliability of Four Severity Scales Depicting Skin Ageing Features'. *British Journal of Dermatology* 161: 153–8.
Valocchi, Steve. 1999. 'Riding the Crest of a Protest Wave: Collective Action Frames in the Gay Liberation Movement, 1969–1973'. *Mobilization: An International Journal* 4, no. 1: 59–73.
van den Hoonaard, Deborah. 2007. 'Aging and Masculinity: A Topic whose Time has Come'. *Journal of Aging Studies* 21: 277–80.
van Hilvoorde, Ivo. 2008. 'Fitness: The Early (Dutch) Roots of a Modern Industry'. *The International Journal of the History of Sport* 25, no. 10: 1306–25.
van der Lei, B., Cromheecke, M. and Hofer, S. O. 2007. 'Mini Face Lift with Suspension Sutures: Historical Analysis of Development and Morphic Resonance'. *Plastic and Reconstructive Surgery* 119: 2317–18.
Vares, Tina. 2009. 'Reading the "Sexy Oldie": Gender, Age(ing) and Embodiment'. *Sexualities* 12, no. 4: 503–24.
Veblen, Thornstein. 1953. *The Theory of the Leisure Class*. New York: New American Library.
Verbrugge, Lois M. 1986. 'From Sneezes to Adieux: Stages of Health for American Men and Women'. *Social Science & Medicine* 22: 1196–1212.
Verbrugge, Lois M. and Yang, Li-shou. 2002. 'Aging with Disability and Disability with Aging'. *Journal of Disability Policy Studies* 12, no. 4: 253–67.
Vertinsky, Patricia. 1987. 'Exercise, Physical Capability and the Eternally Wounded Woman in Late Nineteenth Century North America'. *Journal of Sport History* 14, no. 1: 7–27.
———. 1991. 'Old Age, Gender and Physical Activity: The Biomedicalization of Aging'. *Journal of Sport History* 18, no. 1: 64–80.
Vincent, John. 2006. 'Ageing Contested: Anti-Ageing Science and the Cultural Construction of Old Age'. *Sociology* 40, no. 4: 681–98.
———. 2009. 'Ageing, Anti-Ageing and Anti-Anti-Ageing: Who are the Progressives in the Debate on Human Biological Ageing'. *Medicine Studies* 1, no. 3: 197–208.
Vincent, John, Tulle, Emmanuelle and Bond, John. 2008. 'The Anti-Aging Enterprise: Science, Knowledge, Expertise, Rhetoric and Values'. *Journal of Aging Studies* 22, no. 4: 291–4.
Vinken, Barbara. 2005. *Fashion Zeitgeist: Trends and Cycles in the Fashion System*. Oxford: Berg.
Vogel, Lise. 1995. *Woman Questions: Essays for a Materialist Feminism*. London: Pluto Press.
Voronoff, Serge. 1925. *Rejuvenation by Grafting*. Translated by Fred F. Imianitoff. London: George Allen & Unwin.
Wahler, Jim and Gabbay, Sarah G. 1997. 'Gay Male Aging: A Review of the Literature'. *Journal of Gay & Lesbian Social Services* 6, no. 3: 1–20.
Walsemann, Katrina M., Geronimus, Arline T. and Gee, Gilbert C. 2008. 'Accumulating Disadvantage over the Life Course: Evidence from a Longitudinal Study Investigating the Relationship between Educational Advantage in Youth and Health in Middle Age'. *Research on Ageing* 30: 169–80.
Ward, Richard and Holland, Caroline. 2011. '"If I Look Old, I Will be Treated Old": Hair and Later-Life Image Dilemmas'. *Ageing & Society* 31, no. 2: 288–307.
Ward, Russell, A. 1984. 'The Marginality and Salience of Being Old: When is Age Relevant?' *The Gerontologist* 24, no. 3: 227–32.
Warrel, David A., Cox, Timothy M. and Firth, John D., eds. 2010. *Oxford Textbook of Geriatric Medicine*. Oxford: Oxford University Press.
Warren, Marjorie A. 1943. 'Care of the Chronic Sick: A Case for Treating the Chronic Sick in Blocks in a General Hospital'. *BMJ* 2: 822–3.
Watkins, Elizabeth Siegel. 2008. 'Medicine, Masculinity, and the Disappearance of Male Menopause in the 1950s'. *Social History of Medicine* 21, no. 2: 329–44.

REFERENCES

Watson, J. 2000. *Male Bodies: Health, Culture and Identity*. Buckingham: Open University Press.
Weber, Max. 1976. *The Protestant Ethic and the Spirit of Capitalism*. London: George Allen & Unwin.
Weeks, Jeffrey. 1985. *Sex, Politics & Society: The Regulation of Sexuality since 1800*. London: Longman.
———. 1995. *Invented Moralities: Sexual Values in an Age of Uncertainty*. Cambridge: Polity Press.
Weinberg, M. S. 1969. 'The Aging Male Homosexual'. *Medical Aspects of Human Sexuality* 3, no. 12: 66–72.
Weir, P. L., Kerr, T., Hodges, N. J., McKay, S. M. and Starkes, J. L. 2002. 'Master Swimmers: How Are they Different from Younger Elite Swimmers? An Examination of Practice and Performance Patterns'. *Journal of Aging and Physical Activity* 10 no. 1: 41–63.
Weiss, Jonathan S., Ellis, Charles N., Headington, John T., Tincoff, Tom, Hamilton Ted A. and Voorhees, John J. 1988a. 'Topical Tretinoin for Photoaged Skin: A Double Blind Vehicle Controlled Study'. *JAMA* 259: 527–32.
Weiss, Jonathan S., Ellis, Charles N., Headington, John T. and Voorhees, John J. 1988b. 'Topical Tretinoin in the Treatment of Aging Skin'. *Journal of the American Academy of Dermatology* 19, no. 1: 169–75.
Weiss, Sarah. 2000. '"The Outcome of that Discontent": Oscar Michieux Motion Pictures and the Race for Dignity'. *The Concord Review* 11, no. 1: 1–32.
Wells, William D. and Gubar, George. 1966. 'Life Cycle Concept in Marketing Research'. *Journal of Marketing Research* 3, no. 4: 355–63.
Wendell, Susan. 2001. 'Unhealthy Disabled: Treating Chronic Illnesses as Disabilities'. *Hypatia* 16, no. 4: 17–33.
Wentzell, Emily. 2011a. 'Generational Differences in Mexican Men's Ideas of Age-Appropriate Sex and Viagra Use'. *Men and Masculinities* 14, no. 4: 392–407.
———. 2011b. 'Marketing Silence, Public Health Stigma and the Discourse of Risky Gay Viagra Use in the US'. *Body & Society* 17, no. 4: 105–25.
West, Cornel. 1990. 'The New Cultural Politics of Difference'. *October* 53: 93–109.
West, David J. 1967. *Homosexuality*. Harmondsworth: Penguin Books.
West, Suzanne L., D'Aloisio, Aimee, Agans, Robert P., Kalsbeek, William D., Borisov, Natalie N. and Thorp, John, M. 2008. 'Prevalence of Low Sexual Desire and Hypoactive Sexual Desire Disorder in a Nationally Representative Sample of US Women'. *Archives of Internal Medicine* 168, no. 13: 1441–9.
White, Lynn K. 1988. 'Gender Differences in Awareness of Aging among Married Adults Ages 20 to 60'. *The Sociological Quarterly* 29, no. 4: 487–502.
Whitehead, S. M. 2002. *Men and Masculinities*. Cambridge: Polity Press.
Wiersma, Elaine and Chesser, Stephanie. 2011. 'Masculinity, Ageing Bodies, and Leisure'. *Annals of Leisure Research* 14, no. 2/3: 242–59.
Wilkerson, Abby. 2002. 'Disability, Sex Radicalism and Political Agency'. *NWSA Journal* 14, no. 3: 33–57.
Willett, Julie A. 2000. *Permanent Waves: The Making of the American Beauty Shop*. New York: New York University Press.
Wilson, Elisabeth. 2003. *Adorned in Dreams: Fashion and Modernity*. New Brunswick: Rutgers University Press.
Wilson, Robert A. 1966a. *Feminine Forever*. New York: M. Evans.
———. 1966b. 'A Key to Staying Young' *Look*, 11 January: 66–73.
Wilson, Robert A. and Wilson, Thelma. 1963. 'The Fate of Nontreated Post-Menopausal Woman: A Plea for the Maintenance of Adequate Estrogen from Puberty to the Grave'. *Journal of the American Geriatrics Society* 11: 347–61.
Wilson, Thomas C. 1996. 'Cohort and Prejudice: Whites' Attitudes towards Blacks, Hispanics, Jews, and Asians'. *The Public Opinion Quarterly* 60, no. 2: 253–74.
Wilson, William Julius. 1980. *The Declining Significance of Race: Blacks and Changing American Institutions*. 2nd ed. Chicago: University of Chicago Press.

———. 2009. *More Than Just Race.* New York: W. W. Norton.
Witz, Anne and Marshall, Barbara, L. 2004. 'The Masculinity of the Social: Towards a Politics of Interrogation'. In *Engendering the Social: Feminist Encounters with Sociological Theory*, edited by Barbara Marshall and Anne Witz, 19–34. Maidenhead: Open University Press.
Wolf, Naomi. 1990. *The Beauty Myth: How Images of Beauty are Used Against Women.* London: Vintage Books.
Wollina, Uwe and Payne, Christopher R. 2010. 'Aging Well – The Role of Minimally Invasive Aesthetic Dermatological Procedures in Women over 65'. *Journal of Cosmetic Dermatology* 9, no. 1: 50–58.
Woloski-Wruble, Anna C., Oliel, Yulia, Leefsma, Miriam and Hochner-Celnikier, Drorith. 2010. 'Sexual Activities, Sexual and Life Satisfaction and Successful Aging in Women'. *Journal of Sexual Medicine* 7, no. 7: 2401–10.
Wong, Wendy W., Davis, Drew G., Son, A. K., Camp, Matthew C. and Gupta, Subhas C. 2010. 'Canary in a Coal Mine: Does the Plastic Surgery Market Predict the American Economy?' *Plastic and Reconstructive Surgery* 126: 657–66.
Woods, Robert. 2000. *The Demography of Victorian England and Wales.* Cambridge: Cambridge University Press.
Woodward, Kathleen. 1991. *Aging and its Discontents: Freud and other Fictions'.* Bloomington: Indiana University Press.
Wouters, Caz. 2007. *Informalization: Manners and Emotion since 1890.* Los Angeles: Sage Publications.
Wu, W. T. 2004. 'Barbed Sutures in Facial Rejuvenation'. *Aesthetic Surgery Journal* 24: 582–7.
Yaar, Mina. 2006. 'Clinical and Histological Features of Intrinsic Versus Extrinsic Skin Aging'. In *Skin Aging*, edited by Barbara Gilchrist and Jean Krutman, 9–22. Berlin: Springer Verlag.
Yang, Yang and Lee, Linda, C. 2009. 'Sex and Race Disparities in Health: Cohort Variations in Life Course Patterns'. *Social Forces* 87: 2093–2124.
Yorkston, Kathryn M., McMullan, Kara A., Molton, Ivan and Jensen, Mark P. 2010. 'Pathways of Change Experienced by People Aging with Disability: A Focus Group Study'. *Disability and Rehabilitation* 32, no. 10: 1697–1704.
Young, Bradley W., Weir, Patricia L., Starkes, Janet L. and Medic, Nikola. 2007. 'Does Lifelong Training Temper Age-Related Decline in Sport Performance? Interpreting Differences Between Cross-Sectional and Longitudinal Data'. *Experimental Aging Research* 34, no. 1: 27–48.
Zager, Warren H. and Dyer, Wallace K. 2005. 'Minimal Incision Facelift'. *Facial Plastic Surgery* 21, no. 1: 21–7.
Zames Fleischer, Doris, and Zames, Frieda. 2001. *The Disability Rights Movement: From Charity to Confrontation.* Philadelphia: Temple University Press.
Zerbi, Gabriele. 1988. *Gerontocomia: On the Care of the Aged.* Edited and translated by L. R. Lind. Philadelphia: American Philosophical Association.

INDEX

1920s 12, 38, 55, 106, 126
1940s 29, 59, 82, 127, 128, 132, 148
1950s 26–28, 39, 41, 44, 48, 60, 107, 127, 128, 135, 148
    early 59
    late 27, 106
    mid- 26
1960s x, xii, 2, 4, 25–9, 33, 35, 44, 47–9, 54, 57–61, 65–6, 81, 90, 97, 122–8, 136, 149, 169
    baby boomers, and 135
    counter-cultures, and 19, 29, 40–41, 69, 88, 91
    cultural ferment of xii, 4, 9, 11, 45, 49, 100, 134
    cultural revolution of 26
    early 27, 44
    generational schism and 31, 39, 120
    late 16, 75, 135, 139, 150
    long 26, 40, 47, 113, 119, 127, 150, 160–61
    mid- 60, 120
    post- xii
    radical politics, and 54
    sexual revolution, and 33, 46–9, 89, 101–2, 106–9, 111
    women's movement, and 40, 74
    youth sub-cultures, and 117, 160
1970s 9, 27, 44, 58, 73–5, 81, 97, 109, 120, 127, 134–6, 152, 162
    early 16, 26, 34–5, 40, 106
    late 40–41, 136, 141
    mid- 128, 161
1980s xi, 13, 25, 28, 41, 44, 60, 66, 76–9, 81, 91–2, 119–22, 135–41, 162, 165
    early 136, 141
    late 75, 92, 152
    mid- 127

A

abjection 78–9, 99–100, 139
actant ix

actinic keratosis 156
aesthetic surgery. *See under* cosmetic and/or plastic surgery
Africa 12, 39, 53
African American[s] 55–67
    ageing 53, 63
    beauty parlours 56
    community 55–7, 59–9, 65
    culture 12
    directors [film] 56
    discourses 56
    entrepreneurs 55–6
    families 60
    life expectancy 60
    longevity 61–2
    magazines 56
    middle-class 56
    mortality 61–2
    narratives 53, 57
    older 53, 60, 64, 66
    population 54, 65
    press 55
    society 54, 59
    studies 11–12, 52
    women 55–6, 65
    writers 55
    young 60
age 13, 17–27, 29–32, 35–6
    at marriage 36
    chronological vii, 22–4, 29–30, 48, 62, 83, 94, 97, 121, 127, 142, 155, 165
    clustering 24
    fourth vii, xii–xiii, 83, 139
    habitus of 29
    physical appearance of 23–4
    third vii, xii–xiii, 22, 46, 67, 69, 95–6, 99–100, 114, 138–9, 156, 161
agedness ix, xi, 17, 19, 22–4, 30–31, 41, 46–7, 53, 65, 81–2, 103, 115, 130, 151, 155

ageing
  and appearance 23, 36
  and disability 69–70, 81–2, 163
  and disability studies 19, 23, 80–81, 163
  and exercise 132–3
  and later life 26, 52
  and maximal performance 140
  and not becoming old 125, 165
  and old age vii–viii, 1, 21–2, 28, 52, 81, 136, 139
  and race 68, 81
  and sex 108
  and sexuality 107
  fears of 40
  healthy 102, 139
  the new vii, xii–xiii, 2–4, 17–18, 20, 25–6, 30–33, 43–49, 65, 69–70, 100–101, 114–15, 142–5, 160–61, 165–6
  successful 19, 29, 80, 96, 102, 109, 112–13, 122, 132, 138–9, 161
  studies 1, 42, 68, 83, 85, 93, 98, 159, 162–3
  the old 26
  without becoming old 51, 118
  See also anti-ageing
ageism 18, 68, 101, 108, 137, 155
agency xii, 2, 11, 16, 18, 42, 70, 74, 77–8, 94
  ageing with 44
  concepts of ix
  consumerist 117
  corporeal 7
  degrees of 48
  embodied 163
  identity and 2
  issues of 162
  human 19
  models of 11
  personal 6, 107
  positive 31
  potential 53
  sites of 82, 136
  social x, 17
  socially mediated 116
agonism 31, 45, 163, 166
America 11–12, 18, 27, 53–5, 58–60, 63, 67, 71, 75, 104, 106, 118–20, 149
American
  'blackness' 53
  consumer society 54
  culture 98
  identity 162
  military 119
  older 61
  social scientists 54
  society 12, 53–4, 56, 58–9, 62, 67, 162
  See also under African, Asian, Black, European, Hispanic and White
American Academy of Cosmetic Surgery 152–3
American Academy of Facial Plastic and Reconstructive Surgery 66
American Association for Aesthetic Plastic Surgeons 150
American Coalition of Citizens with a Disability 74
American Psychiatric Association 112
American Society of Plastic Surgeons 66, 152–3
American Society for Plastic and Reconstructive Surgery 149
anti-ageing 45–8, 63, 93, 146, 156
  cosmetics 42, 100, 117, 121–2, 165
  medicine 140
  messages 122
  practices 45–8
  procedures 42, 48, 124, 150–51, 153–4
  products 43, 48, 64–5, 121, 124, 151
  surgery 47, 150
appearance 22–3, 43–8, 65–66, 96, 104, 113, 116–19, 123, 125, 129–130, 145, 147–8
  bodily 16, 37, 44, 66, 129
  of fitness/health 153
  male/masculine 36, 123
  management 29, 43–6, 48, 116, 123, 150
  of ageing/agedness 23–4, 26, 28, 37–8, 41, 129
  physical 23–4, 42, 44, 46, 145
Asians 66, 144
  American 64
aspirational
  advertising 161
  medicine xii, 83, 145–147, 153–4, 156–7, 166
  science 121, 145

B

baby boom/ers 81, 120–21, 124, 128
  cohort 60, 66, 93
  generation 62, 135, 137

Bacon, Francis xii, 115–16, 131, 145, 161, 164
Bacon, Roger 147
Barnes, Colin 70, 74–5
Bauman, Zygmunt x–xi, 15, 22, 25, 137–8, 141
beauty xii, 25, 27, 38, 55–6, 64, 66, 78, 119, 130–32, 153–4, 156, 166
   culture 47–8, 55–6
   doctors 147–8
   health and 146
   ideology 43
   industry 40, 56, 65, 117–18, 120, 153, 165
   magazines 150
   makeover/s 150
   parlours/salons x, 56–7, 118, 122–4, 150
   products 26, 55, 118–19
   therapists 123
   work 120–22, 124–5, 165
Beck, Ulrich viii, x, 54, 84
Biggs, Simon 18
bio-power 6, 88–9, 154
black 17, 40, 51–4, 59–66, 98–9, 115, 166
   aged 52
   Americans 60
   Athena 12
   beauty products 55
   body/ies 11, 54, 56, 67
   community/ies 56–7, 59
   culture 58, 60
   fashion 58
   freedom 60
   householders 60
   identity 59, 67
   life/style 12, 59
   middle-class 57
   models 58, 120
   nationalism/ist 56–7, 59
   /non–black 12
   Panthers 54
   persons/people 2, 35, 55, 75
   politics 96
   post- 54, 58–9, 63
   power 11–12, 54–5, 57–9, 73–6, 162
   pride 58
   renaissance 55
   subject 12
   studies 2, 11, 52, 68
   white binary/differences 60–63, 87, 144, 160
   writers 56
blaxploitation (cinema) 58
blepharoplasty 64, 148, 154
Boston Women's Health Book Collective 34, 134
body
   aged 28
   ageing xi, xiii, 1, 4, 18, 21, 25, 27, 31, 36, 42, 66, 85, 99–100, 140, 162, 165
   bodysense 29
   in later life 31, 144
   materiality of the ix, 30,
   sociology of the x, xii, 2–4, 9, 11, 17, 21, 33, 76
   the turn toward xii, 49, 57, 99, 119
   thinking through 28, 33, 35, 69
   without organs (body) 13, 160
   See also corporeality; embodiment
body work x–xii, 25, 29, 47, 54, 56, 96, 116, 123, 131, 153
   as beauty work 165
   forms of xii, 102, 161
   practices 116–17, 153
body workers 123
body workout xi, 135
Botox 48, 64, 124, 147, 150, 152–4, 156
Brown-Séquard, Edouard 104–5
Butler, Judith 7, 10–12, 18, 22, 35, 77, 99

C

civil rights 11, 58, 65, 74
   legislation 60
   movement 2, 39, 57, 59–60, 73, 106, 162
class 12–13, 26, 40, 49, 57, 62, 98, 117–18, 126–8, 162, 164–6
   analysis 12
   based movements 2
   differentiation 126
   distinction 127
   leisure 119
   middle- 56–7, 62, 64, 73, 119, 120, 126–7
   position 2
   relations 34
   working- 24, 120, 126–7
clothing xii, 15, 47, 116–17, 120, 123, 128–131
   and dress 129
   and fashion 125, 131
   choices 47, 129
   industry 125, 165
   sizes 128

cohort[s] xi, 29–30, 46–9, 59–60, 69, 87, 91–4, 108, 115, 123, 127–8, 137, 160
  baby boom 60, 66, 93
  differences 97, 111, 124
  future 63, 123
  prewar 61–2
  recent 61, 63, 109, 113
  replacement 92
collagen 64, 121, 152
community 16, 38, 66, 73, 75, 90, 98
  African American 55–9, 65
  black 57, 59
  centres 147
  gay 44, 90, 92, 95
  heterosexual 93–4
  homosexual 92–3
  lesbian 95–6
  studies 28
consciousness
  dual/double 52, 124–5
  false 16
  fashion 128
  feminist 34, 90
  generational 31
  of gender 34
  raising 35
consumerism x, 15–16, 27, 43, 49, 58, 65, 95, 117, 139, 161
  anti-ageing 45, 93
  contemporary 67, 138
  corporeal 40
  mass 54, 137
  multicultural 67
consumers viii, 45, 53, 56, 95, 120, 129, 138, 156
  American 122
  citizen 142, 161
  individualised 53
  older people as 27, 46–7
  proxy 139
  society of xi, 138, 141
  young/younger 125
consumption 14–17, 42, 49, 95, 116, 121, 127, 138, 143, 146, 160–61
  compulsive 40
  culture x
  mass 48, 117
  maximal oxygen 140
  men's 122
  personal 31
  sites of xii, 27

cosmeceuticals 65, 121, 129, 153
cosmetics 28, 38, 43, 55, 100, 117–23, 125, 129
  anti-ageing 100, 165
  and clothing xii
  and fashion 16, 28, 131–2
  and self-care 116–17
  consumption of 48
  facial 118
  industries 119
  market for 118
  therapy 130
  traditional 121
  unnatural 55
cosmetic surgery 129, 148–150, 152, 154–5
  attitudes toward 155
corporeality ix, xi–xiii, 3, 12, 21, 34, 63, 80, 99, 116, 128–9, 159–60
  and human nature 3
  asocial 31
  chronology and xii, 21, 165
  elements 22
  embodiment and 4, 22, 30, 96, 159
  fleshy 30
  human 78, 83
  hegemony of 68
  meanings of 160
  of age/ing ix, 1, 23, 37, 65, 70, 99, 140, 147, 164
  of later life 1
  of old age 30, 51
  of physical impairment 74, 79
  of sexual difference 33
  substantive 35
  unmediated 9, 140
  women's viii
crip/cripple[d] 70–71, 74, 77, 79, 83
  crip theory 77
Crossley, Nick x, 7–8
cumulative advantage/disadvantage 162

D

de Beauvoir, Simone 10, 27, 36, 39, 109, 113, 119
Deleuze, Gilles 13–14, 22
democracy 16, 58
  consumerist 16
  of fashion 125
disability ix, xi–xii, 2–4, 14, 17, 32, 40, 42, 49, 69–88, 98–9, 108, 115, 143, 164–6
  activists 8, 19, 69–70, 74–5, 80, 130

aesthetic 130
age/ing and 69–70, 82–3
ageing with a 164
biomedical model of 85
chronic 62
cultures of 164
embodiment of 82
European vs. North American models 75
excess 73, 83
having vs. experiencing 73
health and 42, 61, 63
illness and 113
impairment and 14, 79
indices of 82
in later life 73, 82, 164
movement 6, 69, 72–6, 80–81, 84–5, 163
organisations 74, 78, 81
performing 77–8
politics 75
post-structural models of 76–7, 79, 84
prevalence of 62
pride 80
researchers 19
rights (*see under* movement)
sex and 78
social model of 19, 70, 75–6, 79, 163
sociology of 19, 76
sports 143–4
status 1, 61, 70, 82, 162
studies 2, 7, 14, 19, 75, 79–81, 83–5, 162
theory/ists 19, 32, 70
diversity xii, 2, 47, 59, 79, 84, 95, 137
   ethnic 65
   normativity of viii
   of difference 59
   of products 120
   of the ageing body 66–7, 128
Durkheim, Emile 3

E

Elias, Norbert 8–9, 13, 156
embodied identities xii, 2–4, 10, 16–17, 20, 29, 32, 36, 49, 115–16, 125, 159, 162, 164
   defined ix,
   embodied practices and ix, 87
   in later life 101
of gender/race xii, 52, 87, 143, 166
embodied practices ix–xii, 7, 12, 42, 45–49, 51, 91, 101–2, 116, 142–3, 157, 159
   and identities 87, 159, 164

lifestyles and 49
of exercise/fitness 123, 140
of self-care 67
sex and 101, 145
embodiment 7, 12–13, 15, 53, 77, 99, 114, 123, 126, 155, 159, 161–66
   ageing and/of 18, 32–3, 48–9, 53, 70, 87, 96, 125
   agency and/of 166
   alternative 30
   and/of identity ix, xi, 2, 28, 41, 87–8, 115, 160–62, 164
   and lifestyle 161
   and self-care 68
   and the 'new' ageing 30–32
   aspects of 116
   concept/ion of 13, 159
   contested 87
   corporeality and 4, 22, 30, 159
   enhanced 82, 96
   experience[s] of 7, 42
   forms of x, xii–xiii, 22, 32, 53, 67–8, 84, 159–60
   habits of 48
   idea of 14, 85
   in later life 32, 84
   issues of 4
   mode of 17
   narratives of 99
   of age/ageing 32–3, 48–9, 53, 87
   of blackness 54
   of desire 78
   of disability 17, 82
   of femininity 96
   of gender 4, 17, 45, 48–9
   of impairment 4, 69
   of race 4, 17
   of sexuality 17, 101, 115
   of youth 80
   post-modern 161
   practices of x, 42
   racialised 12
   sites for 31
   subjective 69
   vulnerable 162
entertainment x, 25, 28, 133
entertainment industries ix, 27, 58, 118
Erikson, Erik 29, 93–4
ethnic
   diversity 65
   group 90, 120
   ideals of beauty 154

multi- 59, 64
plastic surgery 66
skin 64
studies 11–12, 68, 162
sub-culture 75
Ethnic Skin and Hair Clinic 65
Ethnic Skin Research Institute 64
ethnicity 2, 12, 29, 51, 65–7, 116, 124–5, 128, 146
  quasi- 98
Europe viii, xi, 9, 13, 27, 53, 70–71, 75, 103–6, 118–20, 147
European
  Americans 54–5, 57, 62–3, 144
  aristocracy 9
  comparisons 141
  fashions 55
  models of beauty 64, 154
  society 36, 106
  standards of beauty 66
exercise 25, 42, 44, 116, 131–137, 142, 144, 146, 153
  aerobic 142
  ageing and 132–3
  and activity 141–2, 144
  and health 139
  collective 44, 134–5
  critique of 139
  fitness and xii, 46, 123, 135–6, 144, 164
  in later life 132–3, 139, 143
  individualisation of 135
  machines 142
  masculine/masculinity 44, 136, 142
  of virtue 141
  physical 131, 133–5, 139
  physiologists 139
  regimes of 135–6, 141, 143
  socialised 143
  women and 142

F

face 36, 63–4, 151,
  ageing 147, 153
  cream 48
  peel 148
  powder 121
facelift/ing 45, 147–50, 152, 154
face and forehead lifts 47
fashion x, 16, 27, 28, 38–40, 46, 55–56, 77, 107, 115–32,
  advisors 130

age ordering of 129
and the changing life course 127
and design 130
authentic 55
black 58
boutiques x
changes in 15
conscious 128–9
democratisation of 16, 25–6, 48
for all ages 117–18
house 84
industries 58, 117–18, 120, 125
magazines 57–8
models 120
sports 44
stores 128–9
styles 126
writers 126
youth and 126
Featherstone, Mike xi 15–17, 25, 29, 138, 156
feminism 2, 4, 11, 34, 42, 134, 155
  radical 32
  second-wave 33, 37, 39, 79, 135,
feminist
  activists 39
  concerns 18
  consciousness 90
  discourse 11
  gerontology/ists 41, 52, 162
  perspective 6
  project 6
  theorists 10
  theory 18, 79
  tradition 35
  views 129
  writers 10, 33–5, 39, 79
feminists 49, 90
  first-wave 148
  lesbian- 98
fillers 43, 45, 47–8, 64, 124, 147–8, 150–53, 156
Firestone, Shulamith 10, 33, 35
fitness 21, 29, 44, 46, 72, 119, 131–42, 166
  and beauty 25, 131, 146, 153
  and exercise xii, 123, 131, 135, 164
  and health 44, 147, 153
  and sexuality 29
  and sport 143
  centres x, 44
  culture of 135
  exercises 143

forms of 142–3
for work 133
idea of 131, 134, 137
ideals of 134, 138
men's 133, 136
practices of 44, 134, 140
pursuit of 131, 138, 143
regimes 30, 135
'forever feminine' 29, 43, 48, 108, 136
'forever functional' 29, 43, 136
Foucault, Michel xi, 4–14, 17, 22, 25, 31, 35, 46, 53, 88–9, 96, 98, 101, 103
fourth age. *See under* age
frailty xiii, 79, 83, 85, 103
Friedan, Betty 34, 40, 107

G

Galen, Claudius 131, 146, 164
gay 98–9, 114–15, 166
  activism 90
  ageing 93
  citizens 91
  community/ies 44, 90–92, 95–6, 101, 162
  consciousness 90
  culture 91–2, 95–7
  events 96
  identity 87, 91, 93, 101, 164
  liberation 44, 88–90
  lifestyles 92
  literature 92
  market 95
  men 17, 44, 90, 92–7, 100, 123
  movement[s] 76, 88, 91
  old age 92
  older 93–6
  partnerships 97
  pride 90–91
  relationships 39
  rights 74
  scene 93
  sex/sexuality 94–5, 100
  studies 162
  sub-cultures 93, 96, 101
gender viii–xii, 2–4, 10–13, 19–22, 29, 32–49, 110–11, 113, 160, 164
  agonisms of 45
  and age/ing 13, 36, 42, 53
  and ethnicity 124–5
  and its embodiment 10, 17, 47, 49
  and not becoming old 46
  and race viii, 4, 52, 55, 70, 87, 99, 124
  and sex/sexuality 34, 101–2
  and the body 3, 41
  and the cultural turn 42
  and generational schism 39
  bodily distinctions of 3
  differences 39, 42, 142
  identities of 3, 52, 87–8, 143
  in later life 41–2, 45
  issues of 3
  performance of 40, 45, 161
  performativity of 10, 41, 49
  performing 10–11, 17–18, 42, 45, 48, 51
  sex and 2
  studies 2, 162
  theorists of 10
geriatric medicine 71–2, 83, 85, 133
Gerontological Society of America (GSA) 41
Gilleard, Chris vii, xii, 1, 4, 23, 31, 44, 48, 83, 95, 97, 102, 142, 145, 161, 164–5
Goffman, Erving 7–8, 10, 18, 29
Greer, Germaine 34, 52
Guattari, Félix 13–14, 22
Gullette, Margaret M. xi, 18, 31, 87, 115

H

hair 38, 64
  care 65
  colour/colorant 118
  cream 27
  curlers 119
  dyes 42–3, 46–8, 117–20
  ethnic 64–5
  facial 48
  grey/greying 115, 123, 129, 147, 152
  loss of 23, 123, 156
  receding 65
  removal 42
  restoration 152
  salons x, 57, 124, 147
  shampoo 118
  sprays 120
  straightening 55, 155
  texture 65
  transplants 84, 146
  white/ning 22, 36
haircut 95
hairdo 58, 125
  pensioners' 125
hairdresser[s] 118, 123, 125
hairdressing salons 56, 153

hairstyle x, 27, 38, 55, 58, 96, 117–19, 126, 129, 154
   afro 58
   choice 58
   pensioner 130
   women's 40
Hahn, Harlan 73, 75, 77
Haraway, Donna ix
health 21, 23, 46, 133–4, 138, 141
   and beauty 166
   and disability 42, 61, 63
   and disease 5
   and fitness 131–2, 137
   and illness 63
   and longevity 162
   and sexuality 35
   and social care/welfare xi, 21, 69, 73, 75, 78, 109
   and social policy 76, 138
   and well-being 53, 62–3, 67, 112, 133, 145
   inequalities 63
   in later life 61, 138–9
   insurance 63
   men's 105
   positive 146
   promotion xiii, 112, 137, 145
   status 61, 139
   will to 138
healthcare viii, 23, 62–3, 72, 107
   system 63
hetero-normativity 75, 93
heterosexual 160
   community 93–4
   couples 100
   culture 88, 95
   difference 94
   discourses 98
   family 96
   family rights 91
   household 97
   identities 91, 115
   intercourse 88
   life course 100
   lifestyle 91
   marriage/married life 94, 97
   men 94, 100, 105, 111
   patterns 92
   relationship 94
   sex/sexuality 89, 95, 103
   white male vii, ix, 3, 115
   women 94, 100
   world 93
heterosexuals 90
heterosexuality 88, 93
Higgs, Paul vii, xii, 1, 4, 15, 23, 31–2, 43, 45, 47, 73, 83, 95, 97, 114, 137–8, 142, 144–5, 156, 161
hip replacement 146, 150
Hispanic/s 64, 66
homosexual 91, 160
   acts 89
   aged/ageing 87, 97
   community 91–3, 97
   desires 78
   identity 91–2, 96–7
   lifestyle 92
   men 90, 92, 94, 97, 100, 105, 111
   modern 88–9
   older 94, 97, 112
   partnership 94
   rights 89
   role 90
   scene 90
   sex 91
   women 90, 94, 97, 100
homosexuality 89– 94, 98
   decriminalisation of 90
   discourses of 89
   male 89
   modern ideas of 88–9, 98
   naming of 89
   performativity of 97
   politics of 98
   homosexuals 90, 107
hormone[s] 107–8
   female 106
   fluctuating 39
   levels 109
   male 106
   replacement 106, 108, 146
   systems 146
Hughes, Bill 7, 76, 79, 93, 95–6
Hurd-Clarke, Laura 42–3, 45, 47, 122, 124, 155

I

identity ix–xi, 1–21, 25, 34–5, 40, 57, 65, 70, 88–90, 107, 124, 129, 159
   age and 93
   aged/ness 51, 82
   ageing 18
   and lifestyle xi, 41, 55, 115–16, 161–2
   black 59
   bodily 33, 35, 51, 66, 163

corporeality and 21, 96
crisis 29
de-sexualised 101
development 93–4
disabled people, of 85
embodied xi, 17, 51–3, 69, 84, 87–8, 97–9, 101, 116–17, 163–4
embodiment and 28, 41, 49, 88, 102, 162
erotic 96
ethnic 66
formation 93
gay/lesbian 87, 91, 101
gendered 33, 45, 48, 51, 165
homosexual 91–4
ideals 49
labour 98
management 8
masculinity 136–7
men's 33
moral 26
movement 69
politics of xii, 19, 31, 49, 67, 76, 98, 101
queer 98
queering 164
racial[ised] 26, 51–3, 55, 58–9, 62–3, 67
self- 49
sexual 26, 89, 92–3, 98, 105, 130
sexualised 165
sociological 33
women's 33, 113
work 31
implants 111
   breast 149
   cochlear 83–4, 146
   dental 84, 146, 150
individualism 16, 95, 155
individuality 19, 21, 29, 88, 120
inequality/ies 34, 39–40, 52, 59, 65, 67, 162
   health 63
   racial 63
   ratio 60
   structural 66, 77
insurance 23, 63
Irigaray, Luce 35

J

jeopardy 67–8
   double 53, 61, 68, 162
   triple 61
Jones, Geoffrey 118–21
Jones, Ian R. 137–8

K

Kligman, Albert 43, 121–2, 130, 151, 153

L

laser correction 83
laser resurfacing 152
laser technology 150
lentigoes 156
lesbian 2, 94
   citizens 91
   community/ies 91, 95–6, 100–101, 162
   couples 97
   culture 97
   development 93
   events 96
   feminists 90, 98
   identity 87, 91, 101, 164
   life course 93
   lifestyles 92
   movement[s] 88, 91
   old[er] 94–5
   partnerships 97
   relationships 39
   sex/sexuality 95
   society 96
   studies 162
   sub-cultures 101
lesbians 91–3, 97, 100, 107, 114
   older 95–6, 100
liberation 39, 47, 52, 57, 98, 106–7, 120, 162
   black 57
   cripple 74
   gay 44, 88–90
   movements 74
   personal 111
   sexual 106, 109
   women's 106, 108
life course 19, 22–3, 46, 67, 81, 91, 93, 95, 97, 99, 108–9, 112, 164–6
   changing 127
   democratising the 83
   diversification in 62
   generationally defined xi
   heterosexual 101
   institutionalised vii–viii, 37
   lesbians' 93
   men's 37
   moral economy of 157
   moralised 30
   natural 103–4

queering the 93
transitions viii
'white'/white male 51, 67
women's vii–viii, 38
life stage 68
lifestyle viii–x, 56, 67, 74, 80, 83, 86–8, 101, 114–16, 122, 129, 137, 140–43, 159–65
    age-less 135
    ageing 31
    alternative viii, x, 101, 160
    authentic 35
    black 59
    consumerist 95
    embodied 47, 53, 59
    fashionable 57, 155
    flexible 49
    gay 92
    healthy 101–2
    heterosexual 91
    homosexual 90, 92
    identity and xi, 41, 55, 114–16, 160–62
    later xiii, 47, 97, 130, 143, 161
    magazines 129
    male 136
    marketing 87
    multiple 164
    personal 56
    post-war 119
    refashioned 142
    sybaritic 30
    viable 43
    women's 134
Lipovetsky, Giles x, 25, 29, 125–6
longevity 1, 36, 38, 48, 62, 115, 142, 153, 162–3
L'Oréal 64, 118, 121, 123
Luciano, Lynne 44, 91, 133–4

M

make-up 15, 117, 119
male climacteric 106, 108
Marshall, Barbara 3, 11, 29, 35, 43, 45, 47, 52, 100, 165
Marx, Karl 3, 13, 15
Marxist 34, 76
masculinity 37, 43–6, 113–14, 122, 133, 136
    ageing and 137
    crisis of 136
    hegemonic script of 43–5
    performance of 45
    postmodern 136
mass media ix, 16, 118–19
master athletes 44, 139–40, 143–4
'mattering' 30
McCruer, Robert 77–8, 99
menopause viii, 37–8, 52, 108
men's ageing 1, 36–8, 43, 45, 49, 105, 108, 113
men's studies 33
Merleau-Ponty, Maurice x, 7–8
micro-dermabrasion 124
Miller, Charles 147–9
Millett, Kate 33–5, 37–8
mini-facelifts 152
modernity 48, 54, 57, 102, 113, 118–19, 147, 160–62, 164–5
    classical 44, 52, 65–6
    early 146
    first 39, 46, 55, 59, 117, 141, 143, 160, 165
    late 41, 114, 145, 150
    'liquid' 137
    second 54, 65, 67, 87, 91, 113, 115, 143, 160, 165
moral economy 30, 157, 166
mortality 1, 92, 136
    black-white differences 61–3
    in later life 42
    risk of 21

N

new social movements x, 2, 4, 6, 13, 39–40, 69, 73–5, 80, 89–90, 101, 160–62
Noel, Suzanne 148–50
normativity viii, 47, 59, 66, 100, 137, 139
    diversity of viii

O

old age xi–xii, 17, 21–6, 28–31, 37–8, 87, 92, 95, 102, 116, 139, 156, 164–6
    abjection of xii
    ageing and vii–viii, 1, 21–2, 28, 52, 62, 71, 81, 136, 139
    and disability 81
    as a status vii
    Cicero's essay on 1
    corporeality of 30, 51
    'croning' of 99
    embodied 166
    embodiment of xii,
    fears about/of 29

gay 92
good 1, 139
healthcare in 72
healthy 102
infirmities of 73
lonely 93
men's vii
nature of 23
neutering of 43, 52, 87
'new' 161
old fashioned 128
pensions 24, 38
senile 105
social category, as vii
successful 1, 102
tyranny of 164
See also agedness; ageing
Oliver, Mike 8, 69–70, 75–7
Ongiri, Amy Abugo 58

P

panopticon 5–6
peak performance 140
Peiss, Kathy 27, 56, 118
pensions 24, 28
  occupational viii, 67
  old age 38
pensioners 28, 125, 135, 142,
performativity 10, 18–19, 41, 44, 47, 59, 67, 77, 87
  'ageless' 140
  of age 41
  of gender 10, 49
  of homosexuality 97
  in sex 100
plastic surgery 48, 66, 83, 146–9, 155
  See also cosmetic surgery
plastic surgeons 146, 148–150, 152
pop/popular culture 25–6, 28, 44, 56, 90, 103, 106–7, 126, 153
pop/popular music 107, 126
post-black 54
  See also black
postmodern 2, 16–17, 25, 65, 98, 100, 129, 134–8, 161
  writers 22
postmodernism 25
postmodernity 137
post-sixties 87
practices of freedom xi, 6, 95–6, 101, 136, 141, 153, 156, 161–6

pre-modernity 24–5
prolongevity 23, 30, 145
prostheses 78, 84, 130
prosthetic devices 72, 130
Pullin, Graham 78, 84, 130, 143

Q

queer
  ageing 93
  culture 95
  gerontology 162
  identity 98
  lens 99
  perspective 93
  theory 2, 32, 78–9, 88, 98–101
  theorists 99, 164
queerer way of ageing 97
queering 164
  age 99–101
  identity 164
  the life course 93

R

race viii, ix–xii, 2–4, 12, 18–22, 36, 40, 49, 51–9, 62–8, 82, 87–8, 98, 115–16, 124, 143, 160–62
  and ageing 51–3
  and class 98
  and ethnicity 51
  and identity 68
  legacy of 60
  prism of 52
  studies 18 (*see also* critical race)
  thinking 9
racialisation 51, 53–4, 59, 162
racialised
  body/ies 51, 62
  differently 53
  divisions 61
  embodiment 12
  identities 51–5, 59, 62–3, 65–68, 88, 143, 161
  oppression 62
  structuring of society 67, 162
radical sell 17, 40, 49, 58, 107
rehabilitation 71–4, 83
  medicine 71–3
Rehabilitation Act (US, 1973) 74
reflexivity 101–2, 112, 117
rejuvenation 29, 48–9, 64, 105–6, 147, 150–57

experiments 104
facial 151–2
of male sexuality 106, 108
medicine 147–8
practices 152
procedures 151–2
prolongevity and 23, 30
surgery 153
techniques of 152, 156
temporary 150
rejuvenation by grafting (Voronoff) 105
retinol 121
revolution 58–9
   Chinese Cultural 35
   consumerist 150
   cultural x, xii, 26, 29
   sexual 26, 33, 39–40, 46–7, 49, 89–90, 100–102, 106–8, 111, 113
   silent 127
   sixties' 120
rhytidectomy 148, 154
   See also face lift
Rooks, Noliwe M. 55–6
rosacea 156

S

sebaceous hyperplasia 156
Second World War x–xi, 25, 29, 35, 44, 49, 54, 57, 59, 71–2, 89, 106–7, 119, 127, 133, 146, 149
self-care xi–xii, 6, 17, 20, 29, 35, 43–4, 46–7, 67–8, 85, 115–16, 156–8, 164–6
   industries x, 27, 119–20
   male 91
   practices of ix, 20, 43, 67, 95, 125, 161
   products 26, 116, 120, 124
   routines xi
   technologies of 53, 101
senior citizen 142
senior citizenship viii
senior sports 46, 143
   See also master athletes
seniority 1, 36, 144
sex 2, 29, 33–8, 40–48, 53, 67, 90–91, 153–4, 165
   and age/ageing 101–114
   and disability 78
   and exercise 132
   and gender 2, 7, 33–5, 99, 103, 108, 165
   and sexual practices 165
   and sexuality 25
   and violence 13
   census of 89
   healthy 29, 78
   heterosexual 95
   homosexual 90, 94
   in later life 94
   manuals 47
   modern 89
   oral 111
   same-sex 95, 107
   therapist 78
sexual activity 47, 88, 94, 96, 100, 102, 106–12, 145
   in later life 96, 102, 109–11
sexual intercourse 94, 102, 109–10
sexual partners 88, 94, 101, 109
sexual practice xi–xii, 46, 87–8, 93–4, 102, 115, 164–5
sexual prowess 38
sexuality ix–xii, 2–4, 10, 17, 19, 21–2, 34–5, 40, 49, 77–9, 82, 87–101, 106–9, 112–16, 160–61, 166
   ageing and 107
   and age/ing 113
   and gender 33, 108
   celebrating 13
   declining 38
   gender and 101–2, 108
   gay 100
   history of 6, 88, 103
   ideas about 109
   in later life 108
   male 106
   sex and 25, 89, 98–9, 103, 108, 112, 114–15
   understanding of 38
   women's 39, 106
   youth and 130
sexual health and disability alliance 78
Shakespeare, Tom 74
sixties (age group) 30, 94, 97, 109
sixties (period) 26
skin 54, 147, 155
   ageing 64–5, 121, 123, 152
   black 64
   care 121–3
   colour 27, 51, 55, 65–6
   colorants 118
   creams 121
   ethnic 64
   fillers 148
   lifting 147
   lightening 55

moisturising 121
old 146
peels 45, 148, 156
pigmentation 156
products 43
punches 64
smoothing 152
structure 121
texture 121
tightening 147, 152, 156
types 64
white 64
wrinkling 65, 117
social gerontology 1, 21–2, 52, 65
society
    ageist 18
    civic 36
    consumer 14–16, 40, 55, 66, 119, 125–6, 137
    industrial 37
    mass consumer ix, 12, 15, 25, 31, 58–9, 73–4, 129, 165
    of consumers 138, 141
    of producers 15, 138, 141
    patriarchal 39
    post-industrial 26, 76
    somatic x, 25–6, 47, 57, 135, 160
sociology 4, 7, 22, 76
    embodied 11
    founding fathers of 3
    of ageing xiii, 1, 19, 21
    of disability 19, 76
    of not becoming old 20
    of the body x, xii, 2–4, 9, 11, 17, 21–2, 33, 76, 161
sociological canon 3–4
Steinach, Eugen 105–6
Stonewall 88, 90, 92–3, 97, 101
subjectivity 42, 77, 79, 85, 136, 163
    embodied 157
    fashioned 130
    human 6
    of disability 14
    modern 14, 31
surgery. *See under* cosmetic surgery; plastic surgery

T

theory 3
    crip 77
    critical race 2, 32, 78

disability 32, 70
Eriksonian 93
feminist 18
Marxist 34
of patriarchy 34
of power (Foucault) 35
queer 2, 32, 78–9, 88, 98–101
thinking through the body 28, 33, 35, 69
third age. *See under* age
tights 48, 126–8
toiletries 120, 123
    anti-ageing 123
    male market for 120, 123
Turner, Bryan 1, 3–4, 9, 25
Twigg, Julia 29, 42, 129
Twiggy 120

U

ugly laws 72
underwear 126–7
union suits 127

V

Viagra 45, 48, 100, 111–12, 165, 172

W

weathering 62, 162
well-being 80, 116, 119, 139
    and health 53, 62–3, 67, 112, 145
    financial 53
    global 155
    moral 133
    of older people 28
    personal 43, 113
    physical and mental 108
    psychological 109
    social 61
West, Cornel 99
white
    American 12, 53, 60, 62
    bodies 54, 66
    collar 38
    communities 54, 62, 64
    discourses 98
    European 154
    faces 63–4
    hair 22, 36
    male breadwinner viii
    male heterosexual ix
    male life course 67

men viii, 40, 98, 118
mortality 61–2
skin 64
society 2, 52, 58
women 64
worker viii
See also black-white differences
women/women's
  access to education 38, 120
  activists 107
  ageing 37–8, 51, 124
  bodies 10, 33, 37, 40–41, 147
  breasts 149
  cosmetic practices 123
  embodiment 43
  entry to later life viii, 37
  equality 39
  fashions 40
  fears of ageing 40, 47
  hairstyles 40
  identity/ies 33, 45, 113
  leisuretime 142
  liberation 35, 106, 108
  life course vii, 38
  lifestyle/s 134
  lives 100
  magazines 56, 107
  movement ix, 35, 37, 39–40, 42, 49, 73–4, 76, 91, 134
  oppression 34–5
  participation in sports 134
  position 35, 39, 49
  rethinking 45
  right to vote 37–8
  role 33–4
  sense of well-being 43
  sexuality 39, 106
  status 38–9,
  studies 41–2
  use of cosmetics 55
  work 124
wrinkles 64, 115, 123, 129, 147, 149, 151–3, 156

Y

youth 25–8, 30, 40–41, 48, 59, 71–3, 91–3, 117, 121, 124, 128, 131, 134, 164–5
  1960's 107, 127, 134
  affluent 27
  ageing of 69
  and age 20, 22, 49, 87, 116, 164
  and appearance 96
  and beauty 66, 119
  and fashion 126
  and sexuality 130
  and youthful[ness] 13
  celebration of 38, 119
  consumerism 137
  counter-culture 46, 58, 69
  culture of 4, 26, 57, 69, 80, 150
  decay of 23
  diseases of 146
  embodiment of xii, 80
  emphasis on 120
  experience of 45
  facial 64
  fears 37
  freedom of 136
  grafting 105
  market 126
  middle-class 73
  movements 39
  organisations 133
  oriented culture 92
  privileged 128
  qualities of 136
  restoration of 154
  styles of 126
  sub-culture x, 28, 117, 126, 160
  upper-class 126
  urban 58
  versus age 87, 153
  working-class 126

Z

Zerbi, Gabriele 24, 132, 147

ADVANCE PRAISE

'Chris Gilleard and Paul Higgs are two of our foremost theorists of age. Their work has helped transform how we understand later life. In this fascinating and insightful book, they address the key issue in ageing: embodiment, its meaning and significance. The text is set to become a classic.'

—*Julia Twigg, Professor of Social Policy and Sociology, University of Kent*

'The lively writing, exciting critical theories and wide-ranging explorations into fashion, fitness and consumerism in this work by Gilleard and Higgs transforms the cultural field of the "new ageing" into a new form of sociological inquiry. Finally we have a book that exposes how our deep ambivalence about growing older shapes generation, identity, lifestyle, corporeality and embodiment.'

—*Stephen Katz, Professor of Sociology, Trent University*

'Gilleard and Higgs break from the prevailing literature on the physicality of ageing and engage the reader in novel perspectives on the social aspects of the ageing body. This is an extraordinarily carefully written – and at times eloquent – narrative that is refreshingly original in its contribution.'

—*Scott A. Bass, Provost and Professor of Public Administration and Policy, American University*

'Gilleard and Higgs canvass a breathtaking range of work on embodiment and ageing, reviewing diverse theoretical trajectories and research contexts, and suggesting compelling questions that await investigation. This insightful book is agenda-setting, and will be an indispensable resource for both cultural gerontology and the sociology of the body.'

—*Barbara L. Marshall, Professor of Sociology, Trent University*

'Gilleard and Higgs bring their own brand of scholarship and critical reflexions to bear on Third Age corporeality and embodiment. This book confirms that sociology should take old age and ageing seriously, not treat it simply as the back end of the sociology of the body.'

—*Emmanuelle Tulle, Reader in Sociology, Glasgow Caledonian University*

'The stubborn, insistent fact of bodily ageing requires that we bring age into the sociology of the body and, likewise, bring the body into ageing studies. Arguing for this mutual enrichment, Gilleard and Higgs review historical and theoretical developments on both sides and analyse key practices of the "new ageing".'

—*David J. Ekerdt, Professor of Sociology and Director, Gerontology Center, University of Kansas*

CPSIA information can be obtained at www.ICGtesting.com
Printed in the USA
BVOW021501300613

324629BV00002B/7/P

9 780857 283290